AF572621

ANNUAL REVIEW OF GERONTOLOGY AND GERIATRICS

Volume 19, 1999

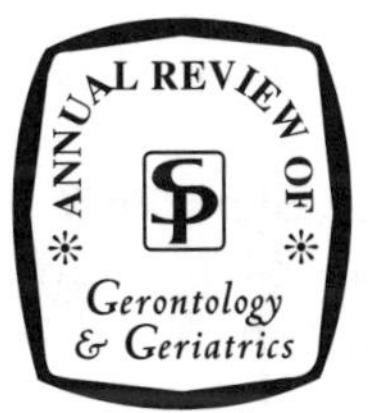

Editor-in-Chief

M. Powell Lawton, PhD
Philadelphia Geriatric Center
Philadelphia, Pennsylvania

Associate Editors

Risa Lavizzo-Mourey, MD, MBA
Director, Center on Aging
University of Pennsylvania
Philadelphia, Pennsylvania

Vincent Cristofalo, PhD
Wistar Institute
Philadelphia, Pennsylvania

John W. Rowe, MD
President and Chief
Executive Officer
Mount Sinai Medical Center
New York, New York

George L. Maddox, PhD
Duke University
Durham, North Carolina

K. Warner Schaie, PhD
The Pennsylvania State University
University Park, Pennsylvania

Managing Editor

Bernard D. Starr, PhD
Marymount Manhattan College
New York, New York

Founding Editor

Carl Eisdorfer, PhD, MD
University of Miami
School of Medicine
Miami, Florida

ANNUAL REVIEW of

Gerontology and Geriatrics

Volume 19, 1999

Focus on
Psychopharmacologic Interventions in Late Life

Ira Katz, MD, PhD
David Oslin, MD
Volume Editors

M. Powell Lawton, PhD
Series Editor

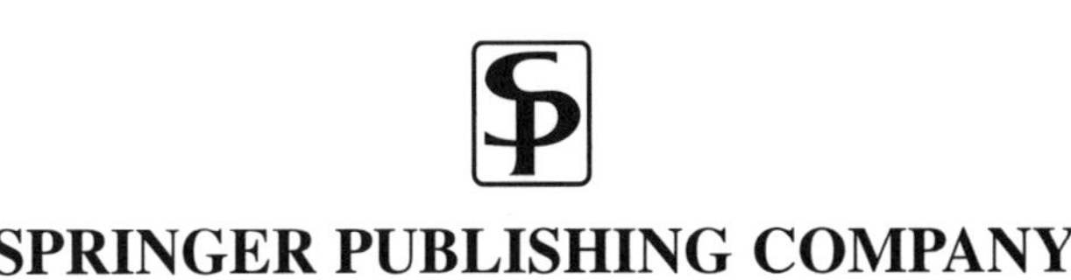

Copyright© 2000 by Springer Publishing Company, Inc.

All rights reserved

No part of this publication may be reproduced, stored in a retrieval system, or transmitted in any form or by any means, electronic, mechanical, photocopying, recording, or otherwise, without the prior permission of Springer Publishing Company, Inc.

Springer Publishing Company, Inc.
536 Broadway
New York, NY 10012-3955

Acquisitions Editor: Helvi Gold
Production Editor: J. Hurkin-Torres
Cover design by James Scotto-Lavino

99 00 01 02 03 / 5 4 3 2 1

ISBN 0-8261-6502-8
ISSN 0-198-8794

Contents

Contributors

George Alexopoulos, MD
Department of Psychiatry
Joan and Sanford I. Weill Medical College of Cornell University
White Plains, NY 10605

William Apfeldorf, MD, PhD
Department of Psychiatry
Joan and Sanford I. Weill Medical College of Cornell University
White Plains, NY 10605

Fred C. Blow, PhD
Department of Psychiatry
University of Michigan
Ann Arbor, MI 48113

Catherine J. Datto, MD
Geriatric Psychiatry
University of Pennsylvania
Philadelphia, PA 19104

David J. Greenblatt, MD
Department of Pharmacology and Experimental Therapeutics
Tufts University School of Medicine
Boston, MA 02111

Herbert W. Harris, MD, PhD
Adult/Geriatric Treatment & Prevention Research Branch
National Institute of Mental Health
Rockville, MD 20857

Bryan James, BS
Division of Geriatric Medicine
University of Pennsylvania
Philadelphia, PA 19104

Jason H. T. Karlawish, MD
Division of Geriatric Medicine
University of Pennsylvania
Philadelphia, PA 19104

Barry D. Lebowitz, PhD
Adult/Geriatric Treatment & Prevention Research Branch
National Institute of Mental Health
Rockville, MD 20857

Sarah H. Lisanby, MD
Columbia University
Columbia Presbyterian Medical Center
New York, NY 10032

Rebekah Loy, PhD
University of Rochester Medical Center
Departments of Psychiatry and Neurology
And Program in Neurobehavioral Therapeutics
Rochester, NY 14620

Sarah Meredith, MBBS, MSC
Department of Preventive Medicine
Vanderbilt University School of Medicine
Nashville, TN 37232

David W. Oslin, MD
University of Pennsylvania
Geriatric and Addiction Psychiatry
Philadelphia, PA 19104

Bruce G. Pollock, MD, PhD
Western Psychiatric Institute and Clinic
University of Pittsburgh Medical Center
Pittsburgh, PA 15213

Wayne A. Ray, PhD
Department of Preventive Medicine
Vanderbilt University School of Medicine
Nashville, TN 37232

Klara Rosenquist
University of Rochester Medical Center
Departments of Psychiatry and Neurology
And Program in Neurobehavioral Therapeutics
Rochester, NY 14620

Lon S. Schneider, MD
University of Southern California
Department of Psychiatry and the Behavioral Sciences
Los Angeles, CA 90033

Joel E. Streim, MD
Geriatric Psychiatry
University of Pennsylvania
Philadelphia, PA 19104

Robert A. Sweet, MD
Western Psychiatric Institute and Clinic
University of Pittsburgh Medical Center
Pittsburgh, PA 15213

Pierre N. Tariot, MD
University of Rochester Medical Center
Departments of Psychiatry and Neurology
And Program in Neurobehavioral Therapeutics
Rochester, NY 14620

Thomas R. Ten Have, PhD
Center for Epidemiology and Biostatistics
University of Pennsylvania
Philadelphia, PA 19104

Lisa L. von Moltke, MD
Department of Pharmacology and Experimental Therapeutics
Tufts University School of Medicine
Boston, MA 02111

Forthcoming

ANNUAL REVIEW OF GERONTOLOGY AND GERIATRICS

Volume 20: The End of Life: Scientific and Social Issues

Editor-in-Chief: M. Powell Lawton

Volume Editor: M. Powell Lawton

Contents

Preface

Increasingly over the next 20 years there will be a demand from clinicians for a better understanding of how to translate research from basic science and clinical trials into meaningful treatment recommendations for late life mental disorders. When deciding on the content and focus of this edition of the *Annual Review of Gerontology and Geriatrics,* this was our guiding principal. We have thus selected to focus both on the methodologies that will guide research over the next decade and on reviews of the current knowledge for the mental disorders that are the most common in late life.

We are indebted to the authors of each of the chapters for fulfilling our goals and raising critical issues for the field. Lebowitz and Harris have appropriately indicated the need for focusing on intervention research and the need to bring to the clinician the incredible advances that have been made in more purely clinical laboratory settings. This presents many challenges for mental health researchers, as highlighted in the chapter by Ten Have, in designing and implementing larger clinical studies and understanding interventions in populations of patients that are not highly selected for "pure disease states." In the same vein, the chapter by Streim points to the need for a better way of understanding the goals of treatment as not just symptom reduction but also as rehabilitation and improvement in functional capacity. We are also reminded by Karlawish and James about the responsibilities we have as clinicians and researchers to our patients and the ethical difficulties this raises in patients who may be cognitively impaired or vulnerable. Finally, the chapters by von Moltke and Greenblatt and Meredith and Ray remind us that there continues to be an important role for basic science research in understanding adverse effects of treatment, drugs, drug interactions, and pharmacodynamic changes that are specific to older adults.

The section on selected clinical diseases and syndromes is a timely and thorough review of the current state of knowledge of late life mental illness. The treatment of Alzheimer's disease continues to be an area that is poorly understood despite tremendous advances in the understanding of the pathophysiology of dementia. Noncognitive behavioral disturbances are common among most dementias and lead to enormous morbidity for patients and caregivers. Mental health professionals are a key resource for assisting in the care of patients with dementia both in the community and in specialized settings such as nursing homes and assisted care settings. Apfeldorf and Alexopoulous have demonstrated the public health problem of late life depressive disorders including minor and major depression. As reviewed, this is an area that we clearly have efficacious treatments that need to make their way to more patients. Oslin and Blow and Sweet and Pollock review disorders that are not typically thought of as diseases of the elderly. However, both chapters convincingly dispel this myth and show that both substance abuse and psychosis can be managed effectively in older adults. The final chapter by Datto and Lisanby provides a glimpse of the future and look to a past. ECT has been used in psychiatry for decades but only sparingly. The advent of Transcranial Magnetic Stimulation is an exciting advance for the field and one that hopefully sparks greater interest in understanding the intricacies of the brain.

We hope that reading this book will be useful to both clinicians and researchers for assimilating the current state of knowledge and ever more pressing ahead to advance the field of mental health. In closing we are grateful for the help of our staff in the Section of Geriatric Psychiatry at the University of Pennsylvania and to our families in supporting this effort.

Ira Katz
David Oslin

PART I

Methodologic Issues

CHAPTER 1

Efficacy and Effectiveness: From Regulatory to Public Health Models

BARRY D. LEBOWITZ & HERBERT W. HARRIS
ADULT/GERIATRIC TREATMENT & PREVENTION RESEARCH BRANCH
NATIONAL INSTITUTE OF MENTAL HEALTH

INTRODUCTION

Treatment works. A generation of research has led to this inescapable conclusion. A vast body of literature, including complete textbooks, chapters, and aggressive public and professional education campaigns, fully explicates this positive message (Geriatric Psychiatry Alliance, 1997; Niederehe & Schneider, 1998; Salzman, 1998). Yet, among ourselves, we are generally less positive about the impact of our treatments on our patients' lives. We will agree that most patients do pretty well most of the time on most treatments. But we will also agree that this is not nearly good enough and that much more needs to be learned about how treatments work.

What, in particular, don't we know as well as we would like? Why do treatments rarely work as well in practice as they do in clinical trials? Why are the approaches to treatment that are studied in research settings rarely the ones that are used in practice? Does treatment enhance functioning? Does early treatment predict a more favorable response? How can we keep people well once they have been made well? What approaches should be used for the treatment-resistant patient?

These are the sorts of questions that are raised within the context of what has been called a public health model of treatment (Lebowitz & Harris, 1998). These are questions we cannot yet answer as well as we would like, however, largely because the direction and culture of treatment research has been determined by a more narrowly defined regulatory model (Leber & Davis, 1998). This regulatory model has been the dominant force shaping treatment research in the past, and we will explore some of its limitations below.

TRADITIONAL (REGULATORY) CLINICAL TRIALS: STRENGTHS AND WEAKNESSES

Most treatment studies are done with a very specific purpose in mind: to gain approval or acceptance of a particular therapeutic modality. These studies are usually referred to as trials to establish efficacy. In a shorthand way, this type of consideration is appropriately referred to as a "regulatory" one.

Research following the regulatory model is specifically geared to the legal requirements of drug approval and registration. Although there is no equivalent to the Food and Drug Administration (FDA) for psychotherapy, the methodology of the regulatory model has been adopted in that field as well. In order to establish efficacy, it is essential that pure disease entities are isolated. This has led to the practice of eliminating from clinical trials all patients with comorbid illnesses, coexisting conditions, and even potentially compromising psychosocial or environmental characteristics. Dimensions of outcome are limited to the direct symptomatic measures of that disease. Observation periods are, typically, very short. In order to prevent administrative or delivery problems from masking the effect of the treatment, clinicians are carefully selected and trained. Intrusions such as the administrative requirements of a health care plan or third-party payer are minimized, and the treatment is provided in optimal form, often in an academic health center. Specific measures are taken to assure compliance of the clinician with the protocol and adherence of the patient to the procedures and treatments.

Formally speaking, efficacy studies define optimal treatment outcomes for narrowly selected patients treated under rigidly controlled and ideal conditions. With a primary focus on symptoms, the assessment of efficacy is based upon the degree to which the level of symptomatology is reduced or eliminated (Lohr, 1988; Scott, 1993). In an efficacy trial, treatment is provided by specially selected and trained clinicians who provide optimal treatment and who expend substantial resources to assure compliance and to minimize dropout.

Research supported for commercial purposes, particularly that supported by the drug companies themselves, has, of necessity, conformed to the regulatory model. This is the case regardless of whether the site of the study is an academic health center or a community treatment facility, and regardless of whether the coordination of the study is done directly by the sponsor or by an intermediary (contract research organization, or CRO). It is worth noting that those doing clinical psychotherapeutic or behavioral research have not (yet) adopted this CRO type of arrangement. The regulatory model has also been carried over into research that has no industrial sponsorship, even to research on mental disorders that has been directed to government agencies or foundations.

In a treatment study driven by a regulatory model of investigation, there is no minimum effect size or minimum proportion of responders necessary. In addition, there is no requirement that the subject population be representative of the kind of patient seen in actual practice. As such, a trial done in accordance with the regulatory model represents only the beginning of a process of clinical development. Efficacy studies define optimal treatment outcomes for narrowly selected patients treated under rigidly controlled and ideal conditions. The classic efficacy trial is used to define the gold standard of the best outcome under ideal circumstances. Because of the tight standard of control required in efficacy studies, the policy and practice relevance of these trials will always be limited (Wells, Sturm, Sherbourne, & Meredith, 1996).

The clinical trials of cognitive enhancers provide a useful example of the differences between regulatory and public health research. The trials of cognitive enhancers seek to show slowing or reversal of the progression of Alzheimer's disease or to demonstrate improved management of the symptoms of the disease. These trials typically attempt to show that the course of a progressive disease has been modified. The design of such trials involves great complexities even under optimal conditions (Leber, 1996). In an effort to demonstrate efficacy within the regulatory model, current clinical trials involving antidementia compounds typically exclude any patient with psychiatric or neurologic symptoms or substance abuse, and require the patient to be generally physically healthy and living with a caregiver. Schneider, Olin, Lyness, and Chui (1997) applied these criteria to a large, statewide database in California and excluded all but 10% of patients. The resulting sample was younger, less severely ill, more highly educated, more likely to be White, and with higher incomes than the population as a whole. These sorts of data provide little guidance to the patient, family, or clinician in the selection of treatment approaches.

In general, the rigid exclusions of most regulatory-oriented clinical trials have significantly distorted the conclusions of these studies. Age itself is the most common concern, with most studies being restricted, for all intents and purposes, to the "young-old" population of patients in their 60's. Few older patients have ever been studied (Salzman, Schneider, & Lebowitz, 1993) despite the clear impact of advanced age on pharmacokinetics, dynamics, and drug metabolism (von Moltke, Abernethy, & Greenblatt, 1998) and on treatment response (Reynolds, in press).

PUBLIC HEALTH MODEL INTERVENTION STUDIES

Studies that are informed by a public health model are often called "effectiveness" studies. We avoid use of that term, since it seems to convey multiple and conflicting meanings in different audiences. Public health studies bring us into the world of actual practice, with time-pressured clinicians taking care of large numbers of patients with uncertain clinical presentations, complex comorbidities, and varying degrees of interference with ideal levels of compliance. The exclusive focus on symptomatology is expanded to include outcomes related to issues of function, disability, morbidity, mortality, resource use, and quality of life. The classic public health trial is used to assess the expected outcome under usual circumstances of practice (DeFriese, 1990).

In contrast to the elegantly crafted efficacy trial, a public health trial must be bigger in size, simpler in design, broader in terms of inclusions and narrower in terms of exclusions, and more representative with respect to settings of care. These settings will not be limited to academic health centers or tertiary care institutions, but will include primary care, community settings, and long-term care institutions. Unlike efficacy trials, where specially trained clinicians carry out state-of-the-art assessment and treatment, public health trials are carried out in settings of usual practice, where there is a broad and variable range of clinician expertise and experience with the disorder under study. Outcome measures will necessarily extend beyond symptomatology to include function, disability, morbidity, mortality, health care and other resource use, family burden, institutionalization, and quality of life. Public health studies are not simply secondary analyses of administrative data collected in large and naturalistic databases, but are treatment trials that are broadly representative of clinical, family, and organizational factors (Dickey & Wagenaar, 1996).

TYPES OF INTERVENTION RESEARCH

We begin with the assumption that the mental disorders of late life are chronic, recurring conditions. Within this broad perspective, three types of studies would seem to be appropriate. First are treatment trials, including both short-term and long-term studies directed toward management of symptoms, optimization of function, and minimization of disability. Treatment trials of this kind are common and well-recognized in the field. The methodology of these trials is well-established and accepted by all those involved in clinical care. However, the conceptualization of the nature of treatment response is broader in public health trials than in regulatory trials. Rather than focusing exclusively on response as a dichotomous variable—responder or nonresponder—a public health approach requires in addition that attention be paid to speed of response, completeness of response, and durability of response.

An intervention directed at the speed of response fits within an overall conceptualization of treatment. The question is: "How can we accelerate the response to treatment?" and "how early in the treatment process can we know when an approach to treatment is likely to fail?" A related question concerns the management of treatment-resistant cases. Regardless of how treatment response is defined, we know that invariably a subset of patients show incomplete responses or nonresponse to any given treatment intervention. Under the regulatory model, the management of nonresponders and partial responders receives relatively little attention. Yet treatment resistant patients make up a significant portion of actual clinical practice, and they account for a major share of the mortality, morbidity, and cost of mental illness. Therefore, a public health orientation requires that the management of treatment resistance be a priority for investigation.

An intervention directed at the completeness of response is considered rehabilitative. The question is: "How well is well?" and can we improve the nature of response by targeting interventions to reduce residual symptomatology post-treatment? A rehabilitative strategy might entail augmentation with a new pharmacologic or psychotherapeutic agent/or some significant alteration in lifestyles and circumstance.

An intervention directed at durability of response is considered preventive. The question is: "Once well, how to stay well?" and can we reduce the risk of relapse (of the same episode) or recurrence (of a new episode) through some longer-term approaches to treatment? Interventions are also preventive if they target the excessive levels of disability that often characterize the mental disorders of older people. As we learn more about the risk factors, etiology, and pathophysiology of mental disorders in late life, it is conceivable that preventive interventions could be directed toward delaying the onset of disease or even preventing the onset entirely (Lebowitz & Pearson, in press).

INFRASTRUCTURE CONSIDERATIONS FOR PUBLIC HEALTH MODEL STUDIES

In order to carry out such studies, whether they are treatment studies, preventive interventions, or rehabilitative interventions, we need to identify the structural barriers in the ways in which research is organized and to innovate approaches to address these barriers.

Researchers and their laboratories are largely based in academic health centers. The role of the academic health center is being redefined in the context of health care system reorganization, and access to patients has become problematic. Patient-oriented research is seen as a particularly fragile enterprise at this point in time (Shine, 1997; Thompson & Moskowitz, 1997).

There are important opportunities emerging, however. Many academic health centers are part of clinical systems that include community hospitals, primary care and specialty care office practices, and capitated contracts. The nonacademic settings of these large networks are where the majority of patients are located. The new challenge for the field is how to turn these clinical and administrative networks into research networks for the development and management of intervention trials. At the same time, the parallel challenge is how to identify the critical elements of academically based protocols and paradigms and adapt them for use in the broader community.

Advancement for academic investigators is based on research productivity, usually measured by significant publications and success in developing extramural funding. Large-scale longitudinal public health oriented studies typically have a very long period of time before important publications are developed, and they usually involve the participation of a large number of investigators. Individual intellectual contributions can be difficult to assess in such projects. If there is a commitment to developing this type of research, the challenge for the field is how to adapt promotion and tenure policies to this situation so as to properly recognize individual contributions.

Similarly, much of the training of new investigators is based upon a model of individual scientific activity: the independent investigator directing a small group of junior colleagues, fellows, students, and technicians. Training typically does not prepare investigators for participation in large-scale endeavors, nor are there established training pathways into some of the newer roles in large-scale studies, database management, clinical coordination, site management etc.

ISSUES IN PRIORITY SETTING

Determination of priorities within this broad panorama of intervention research is always the result of the complex interaction of public health need and scientific opportunity. However, this is not so straightforward as it appears. We can estimate public health need in many ways. Death, disability, and societal and family burden have each been proposed as the sole criterion for policy determination. For example, in the influential

Global Burden of Disease (Murray & Lopez, 1996), major depression, bipolar disorder, schizophrenia, and obsessive compulsive disorder are all included on the list of the 10 leading causes of disability worldwide. In fact, major depression is identified as the leading cause of disability. On the other hand, in that same study, no mental disorder is included as a leading cause of death worldwide.

The identification of significant areas of scientific opportunity is equally problematic, with investigators from different fields advocating on behalf of substantial increases in the investment in their particular areas of interest. The National Advisory Mental Health Council, with the legislative mandate to guide policy development and program support, has become a valuable sounding board for the identification of promising scientific opportunities. This Council has produced recent reports on genetics research (1998), prevention research (1998b), and the interface of clinical trials and mental health services research (in press).

Priority-setting must be part of a continuing process of programmatic adjustment, readjustment, and redirection in the field. New treatments must be developed as our knowledge base of basic and clinical neuroscience and behavioral science expands. Established treatment approaches must be fine-tuned in accordance with the needs of patient populations and the settings in which they receive care. Research must catch up with practice, and evaluate the many common approaches to treatment that have developed without a firm base of research. Here we include such approaches as continuation and maintenance electroconvulsive therapy, reduction or taper strategies, treatment algorithms or decision trees for patients with treatment refractory illness, and unusual treatments, such as methylphenidate for minor depression. A wealth of potentially promising treatment approaches currently exists in the form of case reports, uncontrolled studies, letters to the editor, and internet postings. A major goal for the public health enterprise will be to organize and systematically study these interventions and identify those which are clinically valuable and those which are not.

As part of a public health mission, we must also attend to issues of safety and consumer protection. For example, the widespread use of over-the-counter, unregulated treatments needs to be carefully examined for possible benefit and for potential harm. Use of complementary and alternative approaches is very high (Astin, 1998; Eisenberg et al., 1993). Even in patients volunteering for participation in clinical drug trials, use of herbal medications is substantial; in a series of 150 such subjects, Emmanuel and Cosby (1998) report that 56% have used herbs in the last month. It is therefore incumbent upon us to evaluate these treatments including natural products such as St. John's Wort or kava, psychophysiologic approaches such as eye movement desensitization (EMDR), and somatic approaches, such as acupuncture, if for no other reason than that our patients are using these in large, uncontrolled, natural experiments.

A final priority must be dissemination. Our patients are not helped by treatments that are available in only in scientific journals. A recent example highlights the problem. Lehman and Steinwachs (1998) report that fewer than half the patients with schizophrenia in the United States received a level of care that was consistent with the current state of the art. This is an important finding that cannot be ignored. As a field, we must take on the challenge of translating our research into practice and placing the most powerful clinical tools in the hands of patients, their families, and the clinicians that take care of them. The Geriatric Psychiatry Alliance initiatives on depression (1997) and Alzheimer's disease represent important and potentially valuable approaches to this problem.

CONCLUSION

The mental health field in general, with geriatrics in the lead, is significantly altering the culture of treatment research by moving from a narrowly defined regulatory model to a more inclusive public health model. This new approach to intervention promises to improve patient care by addressing the types of practical questions and functional outcomes that are typically brought to the attention of clinicians. This new generation of research is directed toward defining standards of appropriate and cost-effective treatment for the diverse population of patients seen in all health care settings. This should not be taken to indicate that there is no place for the highly controlled efficacy research needed to establish that a treatment has merit. Rather, we believe that efficacy is the beginning of a process of inquiry and not the end. The interdependence of challenge and opportunity, often used as a cliché, should be considered real and entirely appropriate in this instance. The challenge to all of us: patients, clinicians, scientists, and educators is great. We are having to learn to do new things. At the same time, there is a wonderful opportunity to have a significant impact on improving patient care. This opportunity is too good to miss.

REFERENCES

Astin, J. A. (1998). Why patients use alternative medicine: Results of a national study. *Journal of the American Medical Association, 279,* 1548–1553.

DeFriese, G. H. (1990). Measuring the effectiveness of medical interventions: New expectations of health services research. *Health Services Research, 25,* 691–695.

Dickey, B., & Wagenaar, H. (1996). Evaluating health status. In L. I. Sederer & B. Dickey, (Eds.), *Outcomes assessment in clinical practice,* (pp. 55–60). Baltimore, MD: Williams and Wilkins.

Eisenberg, D. M., Kessler, R. C., Foster, C., Norlock, F. E., Calkins, D. R., & Delbanco, T. L. (1993). Unconventional medicine in the United States: prevalence, costs, and patterns of use. *New England Journal of Medicine, 384,* 246–252.

Emmanuel, N. P., Cosby C. (1998 November), *Prevalence of herbal products use by subjects evaluated for pharmacological clinical trials.* Poster presentation, 38th Annual New Clinical Drug Evaluation Unit (NCDEU) meeting, Boca Raton, FL.

Geriatric Psychiatry Alliance. (1997). *Depression in late life: Not a natural part of aging. Bethesda, MD: American Association for Geriatric Psychiatry.*

Leber, P. D. (1996). Observations and suggestions on antidementia drug development. *Alzheimer Disease and Associated Disorders,* 10, 31–35.

Leber, P. D., & Davis, C. S. (1998). Threats to the validity of clinical trials employing enrichment strategies for sample selection. *Controlled Clinical Trials, 19,* 178–187.

Lebowitz, B. D. & Harris, H. W. (1998). Treatment research in geriatric psychiatry: From regulatory to public health considerations. *American Journal of Geriatric Psychiatry, 6,* 101–103.

Lebowitz, B. D., & Pearson, J. L. (in press). Prevention in mental disorders of late life: elements of a model. *Psychiatric Services.*

Lehman, A. F., Steinwachs, D. M., (1998). Patterns of usual care for schizophrenia: Initial results from the Schizophrenia Patient Outcomes Research Team (PORT) client survey. *Schizophrenia Bulletin, 24,* 11–20.

Lohr, K. (1988). Outcome measurement: Concepts and questions. *Inquiry, 8,* 25, 37–50.

Murray, C. J. L., & Lopez, A. D. (Eds.) (1996), *The global burden of disease.* Cambridge: Harvard University Press.

National Advisory Mental Health Council. (1998a). *Genetics and mental disorders.* (NIH Publication 98-4268).

National Advisory Mental Health Council, (1998b). *Priorities for prevention research at* NIMH, (NIH Publication 98-4321).

National Advisory Mental Health Council (in press). *Clinical Trials and mental health services research.*

Niederehe, G., & Schneider, L. S. (1998). Treatments for anxiety and depression in the aged. In P. E. Nathan, & J. M. Gorman, (Eds.) *A guide to treatments that work,* (pp. 270–287). New York: Oxford University Press.

Reynolds, C. F., Frank, E., Dew, M. A., Hoock, P. R., Miller, M., Mazumbar, S., Perel J. M., & Kupfer, D. J. Treatment of 70(+) year olds with recurrent major depression. *American Journal of Geriatric Psychiatry, 7,* 64–69.

Salzman, C. (Ed.) (1998). *Clinical geriatric psychopharmacology,* (3rd ed.) Baltimore, MD: Williams and Wilkins.

Salzman, C., Schneider, L. S., & Lebowitz, B. D. (1993) Antidepressant treatment of very old patients. *American Journal of Geriatric Psychiatry, 1,* 21–29.

Schneider, L. S., Olin, J. T., Lyness, S. A., & Chui, H. C. (1997). Eligibility of Alzheimer's disease clinic patients for clinical trials. *Journal of the American Geriatrics Society, 45,* 1–6.

Scott, J. D. (1993). Hypothesis generating research: The role of medical treatment effectiveness research in hypothesis generation. In N. K. Wenger, (Ed.), Inclusion of elderly individuals in clinical trials (pp. 119–125). Kansas City, MO: Marion Merrill Dow.

Shine, K. 'I. (1997). Some imperatives for clinical research. *Journal of the American Medical Association, 278,* 245–246.

Thompson, J. N., & Moskowitz, J. (1997). Preventing the extinction of the clinical research ecosystem. *Journal of the American Medical Association, 278,* 241–245.

Von Moltke, L. L., Abernethy, D. R., & Greenblatt, D. J. (1998). Kinetics and dynamics of psychotropic drugs in the elderly. In C. Salzman, (Ed.), Clinical geriatric psychopharmacology (3rd ed.) Baltimore, MD: Williams and Wilkins.

Wells, K. B., Sturm, R., Sherbourne, C. D., & Meredith, L. S. (1996). *Caring for Depression.* Cambridge, MA: Harvard University Press.

CHAPTER 2

Assessing Outcomes of Psychopharmacological Treatments in the Elderly: Evolving Considerations for Research and Clinical Practice

JOEL E. STREIM
GERIATRIC PSYCHIATRY
UNIVERSITY OF PENNSYLVANIA

INTRODUCTION

Over the past few years, the research literature has reflected a broader range of concerns about assessing outcomes of drug treatment in geriatric patients. Dilemmas in measuring the outcomes of psychopharmacologic interventions in older adults have been addressed most intensively by investigators who study degenerative dementia and late-life depression. This chapter explores key issues in outcome assessment, including the determinants of clinical relevance, the expanding range of domains to be measured, indicators and parameters of positive response, safety and tolerability considerations, and confounding effects. Recent progress in this area is summarized and discussed.

DETERMINANTS OF CLINICAL RELEVANCE

One of the greatest challenges to investigators is the need to ascertain which outcomes of treatment are clinically relevant (Prien & Robinson, 1994). It cannot be assumed that what a scientist considers relevant is the same as what the patient, the family caregiver, the clinical practitioner, the third-party payer, the public health official, the government regulatory agency, or the pharmaceutical company consider relevant. For example, in a study of the efficacy of a drug to treat Alzheimer's disease, an investigator may choose to examine the frequency of behavioral disturbances, but the patient may care most about the ability of the treatment to help him maintain functional independence, and the family caregiver may believe that delay in nursing home placement is the most clinically important outcome. In contrast, the managed care company, which is not responsible for the cost of either home health aides or nursing home care, may not view these variables as clinically meaningful; instead, it may value the treatment if it reduces the frequency of office visits and hospital admissions. The pharmaceutical company may be most interested in research designed to measure a reduced rate of cognitive decline, which would be recognized by the U.S. Food and Drug Administration (FDA) as evidence of efficacy for the treatment of Alzheimer's disease. Thus, clinical relevance is not merely what is interesting or important to the investigator; it is multiply determined, and must be understood from the perspectives of several different individual and group stakeholders. Although there may be some coincidence of values assigned to outcomes by these groups, there is often a substantial divergence of opinion about what domains and dimensions of outcomes are most important to measure. Recognizing that these differences in the valuation of clinical outcomes are important in defining clinical relevance, ethicists have urged the inclusion of consumer values in specifying outcome measures for research.

Choice of outcome measures is an integral and necessary component of research design. By contrast, standardized outcome measures are seldom used by clinical practitioners. However, there is a growing trend for regulatory agencies, payers, and health care systems to require that practicing clinicians employ standardized measures to assess treatment response and tolerance. This has resulted, in part, from an increasing emphasis on establishing standards of quality care by developing practice guidelines and implementing clinical pathways that require more objective evaluations of treatment response. Objective outcome measures are needed in clinical practice to determine whether an individual has responded to treatment, to assess the degree of response (i.e., full or partial remission or improvement), to evaluate tolerability and monitor for adverse effects of treatment, and to assess ongoing treatment benefits. Such information is crucial for the provision of high quality care, as well as for ensuring that care is cost-efficient. Thus, there is a need for the development and application of valid, reliable, and clinically relevant treatment outcome measures in clinical practice, as well as in research. The tools and methods for measuring outcomes in clinical settings must be user-friendly and acceptable to both the provider and the consumer of clinical care. Acceptability to patients and their families will be determined, in part, by their perception of clinical relevance, that is, whether the outcome being measured is important to them.

OUTCOME DOMAINS

Clinically relevant outcomes of psychopharmacologic treatment in older adults can include a wide range of measurable phenomena. Psychopharmacologic treatment studies traditionally are designed to demonstrate efficacy of a drug for the treatment of a specific disease or disorder, with a focus on symptom reduction. As discussed by Lebowitz, the relevance of symptom reduction as a measure of drug efficacy derives in part from regulatory requirements for approval of drugs for specific indications by the FDA (Lebowitz & Harris, 1998). However, the amelioration of the symptoms or signs of an illness represents only one of the important aspects of treatment outcome. Other important patient-focused domains include comorbidity, disability, patient functional capacity and performance of activities of daily living (ADLs), role functioning, patient satisfaction, quality of life, and mortality. In addition, there are several related systems-focused domains such as caregiver burden, health care resource utilization, and institutionalization. Although the field of geriatrics has led the way in turning our attention to these domains, outcomes in these domains are not often measured in psychopharmacologic research and clinical care settings (Meyers & Bruce, 1997).

Nowhere has the scrutiny of outcome measures for psychopharmacologic interventions in late life been more intense than in research on treatment of Alzheimer's disease. The prime example of this is the effort by the Alzheimer's Disease Cooperative Study (ADCS), a National Institute on Aging (NIA)-sponsored, multisite clinical trials consortium. The ADCS has undertaken systematic evaluation of new measures of efficacy for their utility in assessing treatment outcomes in Alzheimer's research (Ferris et al., 1997). The Instrument Development Project evaluated the sensitivity, reliability and validity of new or improved measures in each of five assessment domains: (a) cognition, (b) clinical global change, (c) activities of daily living, (d) behavioral symptoms, and (e) cognition in severely impaired patients. This project also addressed the need to develop sensitive and reliable measures of longitudinal change, which is important for efficacy assessment in Alzheimer's disease, in which the natural course of the illness is progressive. In addition, Spanish versions of these instruments were developed, acknowledging the need to measure outcomes in different ethnic populations. Evidence that existing measurement instruments may not be reliable across cultural groups should inspire caution in their use and in the interpretation of outcomes (Jacobs, et al., 1997).

Prototypical clinical trials to demonstrate the efficacy of drugs that are indicated for the treatment of Alzheimer's disease have focused on the measurement of change in cognitive symptoms over time. Recent studies have generally used the mean change from baseline scores on cognitive assessment instruments such as the Alzheimer's Disease Assessment Scale-Cognitive Subscale (ADAS-cog) among their primary outcome measures (Knapp et al., 1994; Rogers et al., 1998, Rosen, Mohs, & Davis). Randomized controlled trials of several cholinesterase inhibitors have demonstrated drug-placebo differences in the range of approximately 2 to 4 points (mean change from baseline) on the 70-point ADAS-cog, indicating a statistically significant treatment effect in the direction of clinical improvement. However, it is generally appreciated by researchers and clinicians that statistically significant changes in scores on cognitive assessment instruments alone may not reflect treatment benefits that are readily apparent or clinically valuable to the patient or caregiver. There is a need to determine whether modest but statistically significant differences in performance on cognitive measures translate into "real-life" treatment benefit for patients and their caregivers. For this reason, the FDA now requires that a drug approved for Alzheimer's disease have not only a cognitive effect, but a clinically meaningful effect as well. Consequently, most studies of pharmacologic interventions for Alzheimer's disease also use instruments that measure clinical global impression of change (CGIC) to demonstrate the clinical utility of the treatment.

Schneider and Olin (1996) have reviewed the history of the development of CGIC instruments. Although these instruments have been used for several decades across a wide range of antidepressant, antipsychotic and anxiolytic medication trials, they have undergone various modifications for the study of drugs for Alzheimer's disease. An international working group reached a consensus that "clinician's global ratings are intended to assess clinically meaningful change based on multidimensional clinical assessment and take into account the clinical heterogeneity of dementia by assessing at least cognition, behavior, and functioning" (Reisberg et al., 1997, p. 8). The ADCS has developed its own CGIC, responding to concerns that instruments that rely on anchor points tend to measure severity rather than change; and instruments with too much structure tend to be overly sensitive, measuring small changes that may not be clinically meaningful (Schneider et al., 1997). The ADCS-CGIC assesses the domains of cognitive, behavioral, social, and daily functioning without excessive reliance on anchor points, and it utilizes semistructured interviews with an informant as well as with the patient.

While cognitive measures and clinical global impressions have served as primary outcome measures in Alzheimer drug trials, behavioral symptoms, daily functioning, caregiver burden, and quality of life have been examined as secondary outcome measures that are thought to reflect clinically meaningful treatment effects. Instruments have been developed that specifically assess activities of daily living in Alzheimer clinical trials (Galasko et al., 1997; Gauthier, Gelinas, & Gauthier, 1997), and strategies are being developed to measure quality of life (Albert et al., 1996; Lawton, 1994), although the latter poses special challenges in patients with dementia. Various instruments have been used to measure psychiatric and behavioral symptoms in Alzheimer patients, and some investigators have recently employed these as primary outcome measures (Cummings, 1997). Some investigators have explored the use of Goal Attainment Scaling (GAS) to measure treatment effects (Rockwood, Stolee, Howard, & Mallery, 1996). This employs an individualized approach to setting goals in areas of self-care, behavior, cognition, and leisure activities; and then measuring attainment of individual goals to determine treatment benefit. Effect sizes were greater with the GAS than with the ADAS-cog, the CGIC, or the Mini-Mental State Examination.

Similar issues arise in studying the drug treatment of depression in late life. A widely accepted research criterion for determining whether an individual has responded to an antidepressant drug is a 50% reduction in the score on the Hamilton Depression Rating Scale (HAM-D). As discussed by Lebowitz, such an end point is a useful measure for demonstrating the efficacy of a drug, i.e., determining whether the drug can work to treat depression; but it does not tell us whether the drug is effective in clinical practice, i.e., whether it really produces a clinically meaningful treatment benefit for the individual patient (Baldwin, 1995). In the clinical practice setting, it is also important to measure latency of treatment response, completeness of remission, and maintenance of remission, as discussed in the next section on indicators of positive response. The delay in onset of treatment effects is a characteristic of virtually all available antidepressant drugs. This is a serious shortcoming for geriatric patients whose depression is associated with severe nutritional compromise (leading to medical comorbidity and increased mortality, and sometimes introducing the need for feeding tubes), severe psychomotor retardation and akinetic states (leading to prolonged bedrest and its many complications), inability to participate in and benefit from rehabilitation during a hospital stay (resulting in increased risk of long-term institutionalization), intractable somatic symptoms (often leading to unnecessary invasive procedures and treatments, and causing excess disability), and high risk of suicide. For this population, as well as patients with less severe symptoms but with significant distress and disability, accelerating responses to antidepressant treatment is an important objective. Recent trials of pindolol to hasten the response to selective serotonin reuptake were designed to measure rates of partial remission (Berman, Darnell,

Miller, Arnand, & Charney, 1997) and to detect changes very early in the course of treatment inhibitors (Tome, Isaac, Hartz, & Holland, 1997). Rate of change of symptoms is another outcome measure that can reflect the "recovery trajectory" in patients who are treated for depression.

An extensive literature on late-life depression has revealed the importance of measuring outcomes in the other domains discussed above, such as comorbidity, disability, role functioning, caregiver burden, health care resource utilization, institutionalization, patient satisfaction, quality of life, and mortality (Meyers & Bruce 1997). A classic study by Borson and colleagues (1992) demonstrated improvement in physical symptoms and function as primary outcome measures in a study of nortriptyline for the treatment of depression in patients with chronic obstructive pulmonary disease. Treatment with nortriptyline was associated with increased tolerance of mild exertion and decreased breathing-related symptoms in the absence of an effect on physiological measures of pulmonary function. Other health-related benefits of antidepressant treatment have been demonstrated by studies that measured outcomes such as glycemic control in diabetics (Lustman et al., 1997), as well as weight loss (Connolly, Gallagher, & Kesson, 1995), and electroencephalographic sleep (Reynolds et al., 1997).

Social adaptation and role functioning are novel outcomes for depression treatment trials. Work on this frontier has already yielded interesting results. A study comparing the selective noradrenaline reuptake inhibitor reboxetine to the elective serotonin reuptake inhibitor fluoxetine employed a self-evaluation scale to rate social adaptation (Dubini, Bosc, & Polin, 1997). On this outcome measure, both noradrenergic and serontonergic antidepressants improved social motivation and behavior; but reboxetine was found superior to fluoxetine in improving negative self-perception and motivation towards action. This furnishes evidence for differential effects of treatment among classes of antidepressant drugs that may become apparent only as we begin to measure outcomes in a wider range of ecologically significant domains (Montgomery, 1997).

Another novel approach to measuring functional outcomes used an experience sampling method (ESM) (Barge-Schaapveld, Nicolson, van der Hoop, & DeVries, 1995). This assessed involvement in household chores, leisure and social activities by sampling 10 times a day for 6 days pre- and post-treatment, yielding a quantitative measure of real-life time use. Antidepressant responders showed greater increases in time spent in chores, and greater decreases in passive leisure time. This outcome measure may be a reflection of productive activity, not just functional capacity.

Quality of life (QOL) measures that have been developed and validated in recent years may be better adapted for assessing outcomes of psychopharmacologic interventions. Quality of life has been conceived by some investigators as a multidimensional construct, though others have used unidimensional approaches to measuring QOL (Kerner, Patterson, Grant, & Kaplan, 1998; Lawton, 1994; Stewart, Hays, & Ware, 1988). Kerner, Kaplan and colleagues have conceptualized outcomes in terms of Quality-Adjusted Life Years (QALYs). QALYs integrate mortality and morbidity to express health status in terms of equivalents of well years of life. These investigators have validated the Quality of Well-Being (QWB) Scale for evaluating patients with Alzheimer's disease and late-life psychosis (Patterson, et al., 1996). Their goal in QWB assessment is to generate a single number that expresses disease impact as a function of the number of QALYs lost to the disease. Ultimately, such instruments may be used to measure treatment benefits in terms of QALYs spared by treatment interventions. Recent antidepressant trials have used more traditional QOL scales that measure multiple dimensions such as role functioning, social functioning, disability, and self-perceived well-being (Meyers & Bruce, 1997). For example, a placebo-controlled trial of fluoxetine employed the Medical Outcomes Study 36-Item Short-Form Health Status Survey (SF-36), and demonstrated that the fluoxetine-treated group improved more on measures of mental health, role limitations due to emotional problems, physical functioning, and bodily pain (Heiligenstein et al., 1995).

Treatment outcomes related to occupational disability, caregiver burden and the need for institutional care may be measured in terms of the reduction in associated economic costs. Pharmacoeconomic studies attempt to compare the value of treatment to no treatment based on measures of cost and benefit (Hylan, Buesching, & Tollefson, 1998). For geriatric patients with depression or dementia, it is possible to assign costs to lost productivity and to caregiver services (Clipp & Moore, 1995); but it is more difficult to assign an economic value to functional independence or quality of life for patients with these disorders. Other outcomes related to cost of care include treatment failures necessitating alternative therapy, additional physician visits and/or hospitalization (Lapeirre, Bentkover, Schainbaum, & Manners, 1995). These are outcomes of treatment that are of interest to policymakers and payors.

INDICATORS AND PARAMETERS OF POSITIVE RESPONSE

Psychopharmacologic treatment research in geriatric populations must also identify appropriate indicators of positive response within each outcome domain—whether an investigator chooses to measure symptoms, disability, quality of life, mortality or other dependent variables. Indicators of positive response to a pharmacologic intervention should reflect clinically meaningful treatment goals. These can include prevention, delayed onset, arrested or delayed progression, palliation, improvement, maintenance of gains, prevention of relapse or recurrence, and cure (Holmes, Hurley, & Lawton, 1997). For example, an investigator might choose to study whether an antidepressant drug treatment has an effect on disability in patients with late-life depression. A measurable indicator of positive response in the domain of "disability" might be improvement in ability to perform instrumental activities of daily living; or it might be the maintenance of functioning; or perhaps the prevention of decline in the patient's functional status.

Parameters of positive response must also be specified. In the example just cited, measuring the maintenance of the patient's functional status requires that the investigator specify the level of functioning to be maintained, and the time interval over which it must be maintained. These parameters define what will be interpreted as clinically meaningful treatment benefit, i.e., a positive response to treatment.

The literature on pharmacologic treatment of Alzheimer's disease illustrates the evolution of this approach to measuring clinically meaningful indicators of positive response. A panel of experts convened by the FDA previously suggested that for drug treatment of dementia, an improvement of 4 points or more on the ADAS-cog should be considered a clinically significant effect (FDA Advisory Committee, 1989). However this parameter by itself is not a meaningful way to judge the benefits of treatment, because it fails to consider the rate of decline in the corresponding placebo cohort or the degree of decline expected in untreated patients, and because it does not specify the time interval for detecting treatment benefits.

Since then, it has generally been recognized that arrested or delayed progression is an important indicator of positive response in the pharmacologic treatment of a progressive degenerative illness. In the cholinesterase inhibitor trials mentioned above, cognitive performance usually improved modestly, if at all, when scores at 24 or 26 weeks were compared to baseline measures. If this were the only indicator of treatment response, the cognitive performance parameters defining a positive response would need to be set at a level high enough so that individual patients and caregivers could readily appreciate the difference from the pretreatment baseline. However, Alzheimer's is a degenerative disease, and an inexorable progressive decline in cognitive function is expected during the natural course of the untreated illness (Brooks, Kraemer, Tonke, & Yesavage, 1993). Therefore, a pharmacologic treatment that did not result in higher levels of cognitive performance could still be considered beneficial if it maintained cognitive performance without decline, or with a rate of decline that was slower than would be expected from the natural course of the illness.

In this scenario, arrested or delayed progression of cognitive decline is a meaningful indicator of positive response to treatment. With this indicator, parameters of positive response should include not only the slope of the cognitive performance curve, but the duration of the delay in symptom progression as well. Outcome measures can then describe continuous change over time. A modest treatment effect that is detected when outcomes are measured over a 26-week follow-up period may be substantially magnified if the effects are shown to be durable over several years, during which time untreated patients continue to deteriorate.

Investigators have begun to employ response-interval analyses of cognitive change to assess treatment benefits for individual patients. This type of outcome assessment could be adapted for use in clinical practice. It defines meaningful treatment benefit, and would enable the practicing clinician to make decisions about how long to continue treatment, and when to discontinue treatment, based on objective measures of treatment outcome. This approach to assessing treatment outcomes should include measurement of functional as well as cognitive domains. Stern and colleagues (1996) have pioneered the application of growth curve models to characterize functional change in Alzheimer patients over time. Using repeated measures of cognitive function and measures of basic and instrumental activities of daily living, they demonstrated that the expected progression of Alzheimer's disease is nonlinear, and that the pattern of decline differs across the three domains that were measured. It follows from this that the measurement of outcomes in treatment studies must take into account these expected changes across cognitive and functional domains.

Under the auspices of the ADCS, Sano et al. (1996) designed a multicenter study of selegiline and alpha-tocopherol in the treatment of Alzheimer's disease that employed novel clinical outcomes, using survival analysis techniques to measure the time it takes to reach particular end points. Subjects were randomized to receive selegiline, alpha-tocopherol, the combination of selegiline and alpha-tocopherol, or placebo for a period of 2 years (Sano et al., 1997). The primary outcome was the time it took to reach any one of the following four end points: death, institutionalization, loss of the ability to perform two of three basic activities of daily living, or progression from stage 2 to stage 3 on the Clinical Dementia Rating instrument. These outcomes were chosen in part because they represent significant indicators of disability, loss of quality of life, and economic impact that are considered clinically meaningful. The end points are readily observable, and outcome measurement is highly reliable. Furthermore, the investigators identified end points, intuitively and empirically, that appear to represent true progression of the underlying neurodegenerative disease, rather than acute fluctuation in the symptoms of the illness. By measuring the delay in the time it takes patients to reach these end points, especially the nonreversible end points, they focused on a primary outcome that they believe is more indicative of a "neuroprotective effect," and not limited to interpretation as merely an indicator of "symptomatic benefit." It is hoped that this approach will eventually help discriminate pharmacologic interventions that only modify the clinical manifestations and course of the illness (e.g., by producing symptomatic effects on cognitive performance) from those treatments that actually alter the course of the underlying disease process.

This trial highlights another dilemma in specifying indicators and parameters of positive response to a treatment that is designed to slow the progression of a degenerative illness with a long, chronic course. In the example of Alzheimer's disease, currently available treatments might be considered most beneficial if they prolonged the period of highest functioning and quality of life, i.e. the earlier rather than the later stages of the illness. However, Sano and colleagues chose, as an indicator of positive response, delay in reaching end points that are usually observed in the later stages of the illness. Design of this study therefore called for recruitment of patients with Alzheimer's disease of moderate severity, in part so that the end points could be observed over a shorter follow-up period. In order to observe the end points in this study among patients with early Alzheimer's disease, a much longer follow-up interval would have been required. Although it might seem desirable to design a study with indicators of positive response that can be more easily measured early in the course of the illness, indicators of progression of functional impairment and loss of quality of life are not well developed for the study of patients in the earliest stages of Alzheimer's disease. Thus, for the patients who are probably the most likely to benefit from the treatments currently available, the measurement of clinically meaningful outcomes may be more difficult.

Another crucial outcome parameter is the proportion of patients who have a favorable response to treatment. Even if a drug is capable of producing a positive response in some patients, it may not achieve the desired effects in many. This is illustrated by the experience with antidementia and antidepressant drugs. Approximately 40% of patients completing a 30-week trial of tacrine had ADAS-cog improvements of 4 points or greater (Knapp et al., 1994). Although this meets FDA criteria for a positive treatment response, 73% of subjects dropped out of this study, and only 12% of patients originally randomized to the highest-dose group achieved this level of improvement. Similarly, antidepressant drugs have been shown to produce a treatment response, defined as a 50% reduction in HAM-D scores, in approximately 60% of geriatric patients treated (Schneider & Olin, 1995). More than a third of geriatric patients fail to respond to initial treatment with antidepressant drugs. Thus, parameters that are currently used to define a positive outcome are designed to yield a categorical measure of treatment response. Patients are categorized as either responders or nonresponders. This, in turn, is used to establish the capacity of the drug to produce a positive response. These parameters do not specify the minimum proportion of patients who must have a positive outcome in order for the treatment to be considered effective.

Outcome parameters must also establish the degree of improvement or the completeness and durability of remission required for a treatment response to be considered positive. Among patients classified as antidepressant responders in most clinical trials, a substantial proportion achieve only partial remission of symptoms, and are still left with residual distress and disability, as well as increased risk of relapse (Frank, 1994; Kupfer, 1991). There is a dire need for pharmacologic studies to employ outcome measures that do a better job of describing the extent and adequacy of treatment response. In fact, most clinical trials currently use assessment instruments that yield dimensional measures of treatment outcome, and can be adapted to achieve these research goals, as discussed in chapter 3. Relevant, measurable outcomes include not only the degree to which individuals experience improvement, but also the proportion of patients who improve to a sufficient degree, and the proportion who have sustained remission over specified follow-up periods. Reynolds, Frank, and Perel (1995) have studied outcomes of maintenance therapy for late-life depression, reporting this as the percent of patients who remain well at long-term follow-up. Other investigators have measured relapse rates to determine effectiveness of continuation therapy for relapse prevention (Lauritzen et al., 1996).

SAFETY AND TOLERABILITY AS OUTCOME MEASURES

Safety is routinely assessed as an important outcome in drug treatment trials, with emphasis on adverse events that occur while the patient is taking the drug. Recognizing that older adults experience a disproportionately large number of adverse drug reactions, investigators have called for the increased attention to dose-toxicity relationships (O'Neill, 1995). Although the risk of adverse drug reactions may not increase with advancing age by itself (Gurwitz & Avorn, 1991), the tolerability of a psychopharmacologic intervention must also be addressed, and is especially critical as an outcome in geriatric patient populations. The concept of tolerability relates to the patient's ability and willingness to initiate and continue treatment, given the characteristics of the treatment with respect to the occurrence of unwanted side effects or inconveniences in the delivery of the treatment. Older adult populations often differ from younger patients in their ability to tolerate a drug treatment. Conversely, a drug can be expected to have a different profile of tolerability when administered to geriatric patients. Tolerability is therefore an outcome that must be assessed across age groups, and especially in the context of the illnesses and disabilities of late life. Tolerability also affects other outcome measures. For example, low tolerability can confound efficacy studies by leading to high dropout rates.

Drug side effects that might be regarded as merely "nuisance symptoms" by some adults may be considered "intolerable" by others. For example, drugs with anticholinergic effects can cause constipation. Some patients tolerate or "put up with" mild constipation, and others follow a bowel regimen that helps them accommodate the treatment. However, some still find even mild symptoms intolerable, and choose not to continue treatment. In a study comparing the efficacy and safety of paroxetine and imipramine, overall rates of adverse events were 51.5% and 50.5% respectively; but when specific categories of adverse experiences were analyzed, imipramine was associated with a higher rate of anticholinergic adverse experiences that could affect its tolerability in patients with specific health problems (Katona, Hunter, & Bray, 1998). This illustrates the need to assess specific tolerability outcomes that are relevant to geriatric patients with medical comorbidity.

Geriatric patients are more likely than younger patients to be taking multiple medications and to have concurrent medical illnesses that render drug side effects or administration regimens less tolerable. In some cases, safety is diminished as well as tolerability. A symptom that is annoying but tolerable for a younger adult can become a serious threat to health and can introduce excess disability in an older adults. In the example of the anticholinergic drug that can cause constipation, older adults are at greater risk for developing an ileus or a fecal impaction that in some cases may require hospitalization. Similarly, drugs with alpha-1 adrenergic antagonist effects may cause orthostatic blood pressure changes that cause dizziness on arising. When the dizziness is mild and transient, some patients dismiss it and tolerate the treatment; others find it unacceptable and choose to discontinue treatment. Older adults who have preexisting dizziness or unsteady gait may have lower tolerability for this treatment. However, older adults with conditions such as diabetic autonomic neuropathy, Shy-Drager syndrome, or intravascular volume depletion, or those who are taking diuretics or afterload reducers are even more susceptible to severe orthostatic hypotension that can lead to falls and serious injuries. For these patients, safety, not just tolerability, is the outcome that limits treatment.

Roose and colleagues (1998) have employed specific objective measures of cardiovascular safety in antidepressant trials in depressed patients with ischemic heart disease. These include heart rate and rhythm, supine and standing systolic and diastolic blood pressures, electrocardiogram conduction intervals, indices of heart rate variability, and rate of adverse events. Of note, these investigators found a reduction in heart rate variability in patients treated with nortriptyline, although the clinical significance of this outcome unclear.

Unfortunately, most safety data from clinical trials usually comes from adverse event reporting, whether by patient self-report or observer rating. Unfortunately, observer ratings may not be sufficiently sensitive to significant subclinical changes, and are subject to examiner bias. Self-report may be influenced by education and other personal characteristics. To address these problems, Lebowitz, Pollock, Caligiuri, Luger, Laghrissi-Thode, (1995) have made a case for increased use of instrumental measures in psychopharmacologic research in geriatric populations. These are mechanical measures of performance or function that are adapted from the fields of psychophysiology or rehabilitation. They point out that instrumental measures can identify subtle or subclinical effects of drug treatment that are clinically important, such as motor and cognitive effects, and are often overlooked by other outcome measures. An application of this strategy can be found in a study of the effects of nefazodone and imipramine on highway driving performance, psychomotor function, and sleep latency in healthy adult and elderly subjects (van Laar, van Willigenburg, & Volkerts, 1995).

Another major shortcoming of patient- and observer-based ratings of adverse drug effects is the common difficulty in distinguishing symptoms due to illness from symptoms due to the pharmacologic effects of the drug. This is exemplified by elderly patients with depression, with or without medical comorbidity. A symptom such as fatigue might be attributable to the drug effect, to medical comorbidity (e.g. from anemia or congestive heart failure), or to the depression itself. In the absence of a "gold standard" for discriminating among these causes of fatigue, the attribution is left to the clinical impression of the rater. Assessment of side effects or other adverse events must be adapted to avoid this confounding effect of the illness on the measurement of drug toxicity or tolerability.

OTHER OUTCOME MEASUREMENT DILEMMAS IN OLDER ADULTS

Uncertainty in assigning the correct attribution for the symptom is especially problematic when measuring depression in medically ill older adults (Kurlowicz & Streim, 1998). Most of the commonly used measures of depression include somatic symptoms that, according to standard diagnostic criteria, are among the constellation of signs and symptoms that can be counted toward establishing the diagnosis of a major depressive episode. These symptoms include fatigue, anorexia, weight loss, sleep disturbance, and psychomotor slowing, all of which can be variously caused by medical illness or its treatment, as well as by depression (Koenig, Cohen, Blazer, Rama-Krishnan, & Sibert, 1993). Considered by themselves, these symptoms are not specific for any one illness. Aside from the challenge this presents for establishing clear entry criteria for depressed elderly subjects in antidepressant drug studies, it can be equally problematic when measuring improvement in depressive symptoms as an outcome of drug treatment. To illustrate, a frail nursing home resident with lung carcinoma may show improvement in mood and diminished guilt when treated with antidepressant medication, but may have residual fatigue, anergy, anorexia and weight loss. This subject may therefore experience clinically significant relief of psychological symptoms, but not appear to have improved sufficiently with respect to somatic symptoms to be counted as a case in remission.

Over the past 15 years, investigators have deliberated about the relative merits of using an "inclusive" approach to measuring depression—in which the somatic items on assessment instruments are taken as indicators of depression, regardless of their actual cause—versus an "etiologic" approach, in which somatic symptoms are counted as "depressive" symptoms only if they are determined not to be due to a medical illness—versus an "exclusive" approach, in which somatic items are eliminated from assessment instruments to avoid potential confounding. The Geriatric Depression Scale (GDS) is a well-validated self-report assessment tool that was designed to exclude somatic items (Yesavage et al., 1983). However, the GDS is not widely used for measuring improvement in depression in clinical trials, and the HAM-D, which includes somatic symptoms, still remains an FDA and industry standard. Some investigators have described a divergence of scores on the GDS and HAM-D when used to assess the response of medically ill geriatric patients treated with antidepressant drugs, but the reasons for this may have more to do with the differences between self-report and observer ratings.

Self-reporting of outcomes is fraught with limitations. Although the validity of self-reported health status has been established in community samples, self-reporting of depression and ADL function may be affected by depression and cognitive impairment in treatment study samples. For example, in Borson and coworkers' study (1992) of nortriptyline treatment of depression in patients with chronic obstructive pulmonary disease, pretreatment self-ratings of functioning, made while the subjects were still depressed, might reflect the tendency of the depressive illness to result in a more negative perception of functional status. That is, self-reports may be tainted by the subjects' depression, which tends to result in a subjective appraisal of functional status that may be bleak compared to more objective ratings of an independent observer. Conversely, one might also expect that self-reports of functioning would be positively affected by improvement in outlook as depressive symptoms respond to treatment. Thus, treatment could be associated with improvement in self-rated function because of improvement in negativism (which is a cognitive symptom of the depressive illness itself), rather than actual improvement in functional capacity or performance as treatment outcome.

Self-report instruments that have been well-validated for measuring depression appear to lose their utility in subjects with severe cognitive impairment, but may still be useful in those with mild dementia. In a recent review, Katz (1998) discussed the controversy about the reliability and validity of self-report instruments for rating the severity of depressive symptoms in patients with dementia. McGivney, Mulvihill, & Taylor 1994) found that the GDS remained valid and reliable in nursing home residents with Mini-Mental State Examination scores of 15 or greater. However, Gilley and Wilson (1997) examined the agreement between the self-report GDS and the clinical diagnosis of major depression and HAM-D total scores, the latter two derived from structured interviews with a collateral informant to circumvent the effect of cognitive impairment. They administered the GDS to 715 community-dwelling subjects with Alzheimer's disease and 93 controls with normal cognitive function, and found a decrement in GDS validity coefficients across a broad range of cognitive impairment. Other investigators have suggested that self-report instruments such as the Beck Depression Inventory, the Zung Self-Rating Scale for Depression, and the Centers for Epidemiological Studies-Depression Scale remain valid in populations with mild to moderate dementia (Gottlieb, Gur, & Gur, 1988; Lewisohn, Seeley, Roberts, & Alan, 1997; Miller, 1980).

Although the HAM-D is not a self-report instrument, it relies on information gathered in a semistructured interview, and the rating of many items depends on the patients' memories regarding recent depressive symptoms. Despite the fact that it has been used to demonstrate treatment response in clinical trials of treatment for depression in patients with dementia, and high levels of interrater reliability have been established with the use of the HAM-D in patients with dementia, there must be questions about the reliability of ratings on those items that depend on patients' recall of symptoms. One remedy is to obtain information from collateral informants. To address this concern in populations with moderate and severe cognitive impairment, Alexopoulos and colleagues (Alexopoulos, Abrams, Young, & Shamoian, 1988) developed the Cornell Scale for Depression in Dementia (CS), in which the scoring of items relies not only on input from the patient, but also on the caregiver interview and direct observations of the examiner. This instrument has been shown to have high internal and interrater reliabilities in cogntively intact and demented patients, and a high level of concurrent validity relative to other measures of depression used in subjects with dementia (Maixner et al., 1995; Teri & Wagner, 1991).

In more severely demented patients, where self-reports of mood are obviously unreliable or even unobtainable, measurement of depression must rely on objective signs rather than subjective symptoms. Lawton, Van Haitsma, & Klapper (1996) have explored the use of direct observation of affective expression and of the signs of depression in patients with dementia on multiple occasions by trained observers. This is the type of approach that needs to be developed to permit measurement of affective outcomes in treatment trials involving patients with advanced dementia.

Limitations of self-report measures are found in virtually all outcome domains in clinical trials that include patients with dementia. Cognitive impairment interferes with self-reporting of activities of daily living. A study in old-old hospitalized and community-dwelling subjects (≥75 years old) used the Barthel Index to assess functional status, and found a substantial lack of agreement between the subject's self-report and an independent rater's observation of performance (Sinoff & Ore, 1997), with Kappa scores in the range of 0.103 and 0.398. The discrepancy in ratings was explained in part by the presence of cognitive impairment. This suggests that for treatment studies in demented patients, performance-based measures should be used to assess functional outcomes.

Similarly, studies of drugs used to treat agitation and psychosis in patients with dementia must rely on observer ratings. Subjects in these clinical trials generally have severe dementia, and are not reliable reporters. Several instruments have been used for this purpose, including measures of frequency and severity of psychiatric symptoms. These generally use caregivers and examiners as raters.

One outcome domain that necessarily relies on the response of the demented patient is cognitive function. As patients progress to the moderate and severe stages of dementing illnesses, such as Alzheimer's disease, many neuropsychological and mental status assessment tools become limited in their ability to measure cognitive function (Schmitt et al., 1997). Floor effects on cognitive tests are often encountered due to severely impaired language function, and when test scores are at or near floor levels, further changes in cognitive function cannot be measured. Patients at this stage may still be ambulatory, and even able to perform a few basic activities of daily living, but their language and communication deficits make it impossible to detect changes in cognitive function using instruments like the Mini-Mental State Examination, the ADAS-cog, or other structured cognitive tests that work well for measuring change early in the course of Alzheimer's disease (Schmitt & Sano, 1994). Furthermore, clinical trials that enroll patients in the early or middle stages of Alzheimer's disease may be designed to study the outcomes of treatment after a period of years, during which time patients deteriorate beyond the test range of standard measures of treatment outcome. In response to this problem, measures have been developed that minimize the need for expressive language skills, and instead rely on gestures, pointing, and limited verbalization for patient responses. The best studied of these instruments is the Severe Impairment Battery (Panisset, Roudier, Saxton, & Boller, 1994), which has been shown to be a reliable and valid measure of cognitive change in patients with moderate to severe Alzheimer's disease (Schmitt et al., 1997).

Although this chapter has focussed on clinical outcome measures, it is worth noting that progress is being made in the use of biological markers to demonstrate efficacy of psychopharmacologic treatments for Alzheimer's disease. Enhancement of cerebral metabolic response with propentofylline has suggested that it may be useful for slowing the progression of Alzheimer's disease (Mielke et al., 1998). Regional cerebral glucose metabolism was increased in Alzheimer patients treated with transdermal nicotine, suggesting a role for positron emission tomography in clinical trials (Parks et al., 1996). Quantitative electroencephalography has also been explored as an outcome measure in treatment trials for Alzheimer's disease (Mohr et al., 1995; Schellenberg, Todorova, Dimpfel, & Schober, 1995). Meaurement of brain function may ultimately help demonstrate the effects of pharmacologic treatment on the disease process.

SUMMARY

Measuring outcomes of psychopharmacologic interventions in late life has been a challenging frontier for investigators. Practical and ethical considerations demand that we recognize the key stakeholders, and choose to study outcomes that are relevant to them. Clinical realities in this area require that we pay attention to an array of outcome domains that define treatment benefit beyond improvement of symptoms. Research design must include appropriately defined parameters of positive response. Tolerability, as well as safety, should be more fully explored as an outcome measure. Confounding effects of medical illness and medication effects;

limitations of self-reporting and floor effects; and the natural course of chronic and progressive illnesses must all be taken into account when measuring outcomes. Great progress has been made in our evolving approaches to measuring outcomes in research on psychopharmacologic interventions in late life.

REFERENCES

Albert, S. M., Del Castillo-Castaneda, C. Sano, M., Jacobs. D. M., Marder, K., Bell, K., Bylsma, F., Lafleche, G., Brandt, J., Albert, M., & Stern, Y. (1996). Quality of life in patients with Alzheimer's disease as reported by patient proxies. *Journal of the American Geriatrics Society, 44,* 1342–1347.

Alexopoulos, G. S., Abrams, R. C., Young, R. C., & Shamoian, C. A.; (1988). Cornell scale for depression in dementia. *Biological Psychiatry, 23,* 271–284.

Baldwin, R. C. (1995). Antidepressants in geriatric depression: What difference have they made? *International Psychogeriatrics, 7,* 55–68.

Barge-Schaapveld, D. Q., Nicolson, N. A., van der Hoop, R. G., & De Vries, M. W. (1995). Changes in daily life experience associated with clinical improvement in depression. *Journal of Affective Disorders, 34,* 139–154.

Berman, R. M., Darnell, A. M., Miller, H. L., Anand, A., & Charney, D. S. (1997). Effect of pindolol in hastening response to fluoxetine in the treatment of major depression: A double-blind, placebo-controlled trial. *American Journal of Psychiatry, 154,* 37–43.

Borson, S., McDonald, G. J., Gayle, T., Deffeback, M., Lakshminarayan, S., & Van Tuinen, C. (1992). Improvement in mood, physical symptoms, and function with nortriptyline for depression in patients with chronic obstructive pulmonary disease. *Psychosomatics, 33,* 190–201.

Brooks, J., Kraemer, H. C., Tanke, E. D., & Yesavage, J. A. (1993). The methodology of studying decline in Alzheimer's disease. *Journal of the American Geriatrics Society, 41,* 623–628.

Clipp, E., & Moore M. J. (1995). Caregiver time use: An outcome measure in clinical trial research with Alzheimer's disease. *Clinical Pharmacology and Therapeutics, 58,* 228–236.

Connolly, V. M., Gallagher, A., & Kesson, C. M. (1995). A study of fluoxetine in obese elderly patients with type 2 diabetes. *Diabetic Medicine, 12,* 416–418.

Cummings, J. L. (1997). The neuropsychiatric inventory: Assessing psychopathology in dementia patients. *Neurology, 48* (supplement 6), S10–S16.

Dubini, A., Bosc, M., & Polin, V. (1997). Noradrenaline-selective versus serotonin-selective antidepressant therapy: Differential effects on social functioning. *Journal of Psychopharmacology, 11,* (supplement 4), S17–23.

FDA Advisory Committee (1989). *Peripheral and central nervous system drugs Advisory Committee Meeting, July 7, 1989.* Rockville MD: Dept of Health and Human Services, Public Health Service, Food and Drug Administration, Publication #227.

Ferris, S. H., Mackell, J. A., Mohs, R., Schneider, L. S., Galasko, D., Whitehouse, P. J., Schmitt, F. A., Sano, M., Thomas, R. G., Ernesto, C., Grundmanm M., Schafer, K., Thal, L. J., and the Alzheimer's Disease Cooperative Study. (1997). A multicenter evaluation of new treatment efficacy instruments for Alzheimer's disease clinical trials: Overview and general results. *Alzheimer's Disease and Associated Disorders, 11* (supplement 2), S1–S12.

Frank, E. (1994). Long-term prevention of recurrences in elderly patients. In L. S. Schneider, C. F. Reynolds, B. D. Lebowitz (Eds.), *Diagnosis and treatment of depression in late-life* (pp. 31`7–329). Washington, DC: American Psychiatric Press.

Galasko, D., Bennett, D., Sano, M., Ernesto, C., Thomas, R., Grundman, M., Ferris, S., and the Alzheimer's Disease Cooperative Study. (1997). An inventory to assess activities of daily living for clinical trials in Alzheimer's disease. *Alzheimer Disease and Associated Disorders, 11* (supplement 2), S33–S39.

Gauthier, S., Gelinas, I., & Gauthier, L. (1997). Functional disability in Alzheimer's disease. *International Psychogeriatrics, 9* (supplement 1), 163–165.

Gilley, D. W., & Wilson, R. S. (1997). Criterion-related validity of the Geriatric Depression Scale in Alzheimer's disease. *Journal of Clinical and Experimental Neuropsychology, 19,* 489–499.

Gottlieb, G. L., Gur, R. E., & Gur, R. C. (1988). Reliability of psychiatric scales in patients with dementia of the Alzheimer type. *American Journal of Psychiatry, 145,* 857–860.

Gurwitz, J. H, & Avorn, J. (1991). The ambiguous relation between aging and adverse drug reactions. *Annals of Internal Medicine, 114,* 956–966.

Heiligenstein, J. H., Ware, J. E. Jr., Beusterien, K. M., Roback, P. J., Andrejasich, C., & Tollefson, G. (1995). Acute effects of fluoxetine versus placebo on functional health and well-being in late-life depression. *International Psychogeriatrics, 7* (supplement), 125–137.

Holmes D., Hurley A., & Lawton M. P. (1997). Outcome measures for Alzheimer disease research: The continuum of domains to be measured. *Alzheimer Disease and Associated Disorders 11* (supplement 6), 175–178.

Hylan, T. R., Buesching D. P., & Tollefson, G. D. (1998). Health economic evaluations of antidepressants: A review. *Depression and Anxiety, 7,* 53–64.

Jacobs, D. M., Sano M., Albert S., Schofield P., Dooneief G., & Stern Y. (1997). Cross-cultural neuropsychological assessment: A comparison of randomly selected, demographically matched cohorts of English- and Spanish-speaking older adults. *Journal of Clinical and Experimental Neuropsychology, 19,* 331–339.

Katona, C. L., Hunter, B. N., & Bray J. (1998). A double-blind comparison of the efficacy and safety of paroxetine and imipramine in the treatment of depression with dementia. *International Journal of Geriatric Psychiatry, 13,* 100–108.

Katz, I. R. (1998). Diagnosis and treatment of depression in patients with Alzheimer's disease and other dementias. *Journal of Clinical Psychiatry, 59,* 38–44.

Kerner, D. N., Patterson T. L., Grant I., & Kaplan, R. M. (1998). Validity of the quality of well-being scale for patients with Alzheimer's disease. *Journal of Aging and Health, 10,* 44–61.

Knapp, M. J., Knopman, D. S., Solomon, P. R., Pendlebury, W. W., Davis, C. S., & Gracon, S. I., for the Tacrine Study Group. (1994). A 30-week randomized controlled trial of high-dose tacrine in patients with Alzheimer's disease. *Journal of the American Medical Association, 271,* 985–991.

Koenig, H. G., Cohen, H. J., Blazer, D. G., Rama-Krishnan K., & Sibert, T. E. (1993). Profile of depressive symptoms in younger and older medical inpatients with major depression. *Journal of the American Geriatrics Society, 41,* 1169–1176.

Kupfer, D. J. (1991). Long-term treatment of depression. *Journal of Clinical Psychiatry, 52* (supplement 5), 28–34.

Kurlowicz, L. H., & Streim, J. E. (1998). Measuring depression in hospitalized, medically ill, older adults. *Archives of Psychiatric Nursing, 12,* 209–218.

Lapeirre, Y., Bentkover, J., Schainbaum, S., & Manners, S. (1995). Direct cost of depression: Analysis of treatment costs of paroxetine versus imipramine in Canada. *Canadian Journal of Psychiatry, 40,* 370–377.

Lauritzen, L., Odgaard, K., Clemmesen, L., Lunde, M., Ohrstrom, J., Black, C., & Bech, P. (1996). Relapse prevention by means of paroxetine in ECT-treated patients with major depression: A comparison with imipramine and placebo in medium-term continuation therapy. *Acta Psychiatrica Scandinavica, 94,* 241–251.

Lawton, M. P. (1994). Quality of life in Alzheimer's disease. *Alzheimer Disease and Associated Disorders, 8* (supplement), S138–150.

Lawton, M. P., Van Haitsma, K., & Klapper, J. (1996). Observed affect in nursing home residents with Alzheimer's disease. *Journal of Gerontology, B, Psychological Sciences and Social Sciences, 51,* P3–P14.

Lebowitz, B. D., Pollock, B. G., Caligiuri, M. P., Kluger, A., & Laghrissi-Thode, F. (1995). Instrumental measure in geriatric psychopharmacology. *Psychopharmacology Bulletin, 31,* 641–649.

Lebowitz, B. D., & Harris, H. W. (1998). Treatment research in geriatric psychiatry: From regulatory to public health considerations. *American Journal of Geriatric Psychiatry, 6,* 101–103.

Lewisohn, P. M., Seeley, J. R., Roberts, R. E., & Alan, N. R. (1997). Center for Epidemiologic Studies Depression Scale (CES-D) as a screening instrument for depression among community-residing older adults. *Psychology and Aging, 12,* 277–287.

Lustman, P. J., Griffith, L. S., Clouse, R. E., Freedland, K. E., Eisen, S. A., Rubin, E. H., Carney, R. M., & McGill, J. B. (1997). Effects of nortriptyline on depression and glycemic control in diabetes: Results of a double-blind, placebo-controlled trial. *Psychosomatic Medicine, 59,* 241–250.

Maixner, S. M., Burke, W. J., Roccaforte, W. H., & Wengel, S. P. (1995). A comparison of two depression scales in a geriatric assessment clinic. *American Journal of Geriatric Psychiatry, 3,* 60–67.

McGivney, S. A., Mulvihill, M., & Taylor, B. (1994). Validating the GDS depression screen in the nursing home. *Journal of the American Geriatrics Society, 42,* 490–492.

Mielke, R., Ghaemi, M., Kessler, J., Kittner, B., Szelies, B., Herholz K., & Heiss, W. D. (1998). Propentofylline enhances cerebral metabolic response to auditory memory stimulation in Alzheimer's disease. *Journal of the Neurological Sciences, 154,* 76–82.

Meyers, B. S., & Bruce, M. L. (1997). Outcomes for antidepressant trials in late-life depression. *Psychopharmacology Bulletin, 33,* 701–705.

Miller, N. E. (1980). The measurement of mood in senile brain disease: Examiner ratings and self-reports. In J. O. Cole, J. E. Barrett (Eds.) *Psychopathology in the aged.* (pp. 97–122) New York: Raven Press.

Mohr, E., Knott, V., Sampson, M., Wesnes, K., Herting, R., & Mendis, T. (1995). Cognitive and quantified electroencephalographic correlates of cycloserine treatment in Alzheimer's disease. *Clinical Neuropharmacology, 18,* 28–38.

Montgomery, S. A. (1997). Reboxetine: Additional benefits to the depressed patient. *Journal of Psychopharmacology, 11* (supplement 4), S9–15.

O'Neill, R. T. (1995). Statistical concepts in the planning and evaluation of drug safety from clinical trials in drug development: Issues of international harmonization. *Statistics in Medicine, 14,* 1117–1127.

Panisset, M., Roudier, M., Saxton, J., & Boller, F. (1994). Severe Impairment Battery: A neuropsychological test for severely demented patients. *Archives of Neurology, 51,* 41–45.

Parks, R. W., Becker, R. E., Rippey, R. F., Gilbert, D. G., Matthews, J. R., Kabatay, E., Young, C. S., Vohs, C., Danz, V., Keim, P., Collins, G. T., Zigler, S. S., & Urycki, P. G. (1996). Increased regional cerebral glucose metabolism and semantic memory performance in Alzheimer's disease: A pilot double blind transdermal nicotine positron emission tomography study. *Neuropsychology Review, 6,* 61–79.

Patterson, T. L., Kaplan, R. M., Grant, I., Semple, S. J., Moscona, S., Koch, W. L., Harris, M. J., Jeste, J. V. (1996). Quality of well being in late life psychosis. *Psychiatry Research, 63,* 169–181.

Prien, R. F., & Robinson, D. S. (Eds.) (1994). *Clinical Evaluation of Psychotropic Drugs: Principles and Guidelines.* New York: Raven.

Reisberg, B., Schneider, L., Doody, R., Anand, R., Feldman, H., Haraguchi, H., Kumar, R., Lucca, U., Mangone, C. A., Mohr, E., Morris, J. C., Roigers, S., & Sawada, T. (1997). Clinical global measures of dementia: Position paper from the International working group on Harmonization of Dementia Drug Guidelines. *Alzheimer Disease and Associated Disorders, 11* (supplement 3), 8–18.

Reynolds, C. F., Frank, E., Perel, J. M. (1995). Maintenance therapies for late-life recurrent major depression: research and review circa 1995. *International Psychogeriatrics, 7* (supplement), 27–29.

Reynolds, C. F., Buysse, D. J., Brunner, D. P., Begley, A. E., Dew, M. A., Hoch, C. C., Hall, M., Houck, P. R., Mazumdar, S., Perel, J. M., & Kupfer, D. J. (1997). Maintenance nortriptyline effects on electroencephalographic sleep in elderly patients with recurrent major depression: double-blind, placebo- and plasma-level-controlled evaluation. *Biological Psychiatry, 42,* 560–567.

Rockwood, K., Stolee, P., Howard, K., & Mallery, L. (1996). Use of Goal Attainment Scaling to measure treatment effects in an anti-dementia drug trial. *Neuroepidemiology, 15,* 330–338.

Rogers, S. L., Farlow, M. R., Doody, R. S., Mohs, R., Friedhoff, L. T., and the Donepezil Study Group. (1998). A 24-week, double-blind, placebo-controlled trial of donepezil in patients with Alzheimer's disease. *American Academy of Neurology, 50,* 136–145.

Roose, S. P., Laghrissi-Thode, F., Kennedy, J. S., Nelson, J. C., Bigger, J. T Jr., Pollock, B. G., Gaffney, A., Narayan, M., Finkel, M. S., McCafferty, J., & Gergel, I. (1998). Comparison of paroxetine and nortriptyline in depressed patients with ischemic heart disease. *Journal of the American Medical Association, 279,* 287–291.

Rosen, W. G., Mohs, R. C., & Davis, K. L. (1984). A new rating scale for Alzheimer's disease. *American Journal of Psychiatry, 141,* 1356–1364.

Sano, M., Ernesto, C., Klauber, M. R., Schafer, K., Woodbury, P., Thomas, R., Grundman, M., Growdon, J., Thal, L. J., and members of the Alzheimer's Disease Cooperative Study. (1996). Rationale and design of a multicenter study of selegiline and a-tocopherol in the treatment of Alzheimer disease using novel clinical outcomes. *Alzheimer Disease and Associated Disorders, 10,* 132–140.

Sano, M., Ernesto, C., Thomas, R. G., Klauber, M. R., Schafer, K., Grundman, M., Woodbury, P., Growdon, J., Cotman, C. W., Pfeiffer, E., Schneider, L. S., & Thal, L. J., for the members of the Alzheimer's Disease Cooperative Study. (1997). A controlled trial of selegiline, alpha-tocopherol, or both as treatment for Alzheimer's disease. *The New England Journal of Medicine, 336,* 1216–1222.

Schellenberg, R., Todorova, A., Dimpfel, W., & Schober, F. (1995). Pathophysiology and psychopharmacology of dementia—a new study design. I. Diagnosis comprising subjective and objective criteria. *Neuropsychobiology, 32,* 81–97.

Schmitt, F., & Sano M. (1994) Neuropsychological approaches to the study of dementia. In Morris JC (ed)., *Handbook of dementing illnesses.* (pp.89–124) New York: Marcel Dekker.

Schmitt, F. A., Wesson, A., Ernesto, C., Saxton, J., Schneider, L. S., Clark, C. M., Ferris, S. H., Mackell, J. A., Schafer, K., Thal, L. J., and the Alzheimer's Disease Cooperative Study. (1997). The severe impairment battery: concurrent validity and the assessment of longitudinal change in Alzheimer's disease. *Alzheimer Disease and Associated Disorders, 11* (supplement 2), S51–S56.

Schneider, L. S., & Olin, J. T. (1995). Efficacy of acute treatment for geriatric depression. *International Psychogeriatrics, 7* (supplement), 7–25.

Schneider, L. S., & Olin, J. T. (1996). Clinical global impression of change: clinical global impressions in Alzheimer's clinical trials. *International Psychogeriatrics, 8,* 277–290.

Schneider, L. S., Olin, J. T, Doody, R. S., Clark, C. M., Morris, J. C., Reisberg, B., Schmitt, F. A., Grundman, M., Thomas, R. G., Ferris, S. H., and the Alzheimer's Disease Cooperative Study. (1997). Validity and reliability of the Alzheimer's Disease Cooperative Study-Clinical Global Impression of Change. *Alzheimer Disease and Associated Disorders, 11* (supplement 2), S22–S32.

Sinoff, G., & Ore L. (1997). The Barthel activities of daily living index: self-report versus actual performance in the old-old. *Journal of the American Geriatrics Society, 45,* 832–836.

Stern, Y., Liu, X., Albert, M., Brandt, J., Jacobs, D. M., Del Castillo-Castaneda, C., Marder, K., Bell, K., Sano, M., Bylsma, F., Lafleche, G., & Tsai, W–Y. (1996). Application of a growth curve approach to modeling the progression of Alzheimer's disease. *Journal of Gerontology: Medical Sciences, 51A,* M179–M184.

Stewart, A. L., Hays, R. D., & Ware, J. E. (1988). The MOS Short-Form General Health Survey. *Medical Care, 26,* 724–745.

Teri, L., & Wagner, A. W. (1991). Assessment of depression in patients with Alzheimer's disease: concordance among informants. *Psychology and Aging, 6,* 280–285.

Tome, M. B., Isaac, M. T., Harte, R., & Holland, C. (1997). Paroxetine and pindolol: A randomized trial of serotonergic autoreceptor blockade in the reduction of antidepressant latency. *International Clinical Psychopharmacology, 12,* 81–89.

Van Laar, M. W., van Willigenburg, A. P., & Volkerts, E. R. (1995). Acute and chronic effects of nefazodone and imipramine on highway driving, cognitive functions, and daytime sleepiness in healthy adult and elderly subjects. *Journal of Clinical Psychopharmacology, 15,* 30–40.

Yesavage, J. A., Brink, T. L., Rose, T. L., Lum, O., Huang, V., Adey, M.,. & Leier, V. O. (1983). Development and validation of a geriatric depression scale: A preliminary report. *Journal of Psychiatric Research, 17,* 37–49.

CHAPTER 3

Statistical and Design Issues in Geriatric Psychiatric Research

THOMAS R. TEN HAVE
CENTER FOR EPIDEMIOLOGY AND BIOSTATISTICS
UNIVERSITY OF PENNSYLVANIA

> Far better an approximate answer to the right question, which is often vague, than an exact answer to the wrong question, which can always be made more precise.
>
> —John Tukey (1962)

Statisticians, as well as the investigators with whom they collaborate need to heed such wisdom during the multiple phases of any study. This advice is especially pertinent for researchers in geriatric psychiatry, where confounding factors such as competing risks for drop-out (e.g., dementia and death) and multiple comorbidities and medications play havoc with analyses both elaborate and simple unless these factors are accounted for in the study design.

This chapter covers both study design and analysis issues of clinical trials that prospectively assign treatments to groups of psychiatric patients with longitudinal follow-up. Study design is first considered not only because it precedes data analysis in the progression of a study, but also because of its importance in ensuring valid inference. The choice of design impacts not only validity or bias but also precision or power.

STUDY DESIGN

Comparison Group

Clinical trials designs may be first classified according to the specification of the comparison group for contrast with the treatment of interests. Assigning depressed geriatric patients to a placebo as the comparison treatment may not be ethical. In such a case, low or high doses of a treatment (e.g., nortriptyline) may be administered with the expectation that the resulting dose response curve will allow extrapolation of the response to a zero-dose level. Through regression models, the predicted response at this level may serve as the placebo mean response for comparison with the mean response of the nortriptyline treatments. This approach was implemented in comparing mean fractional decreases in Hamilton Depression Scores from a randomized dose-response study of nortriptyline to an estimated average fractional decrease in the Hamilton Depression Score from an open-label sertraline trial (Katz, Streim, Oslin, Bilker, & Cooper, 1997). Such an approach should be used with caution, because of the unverifiable assumptions underlying the extrapolation to zero dose.

Another form of a comparison group may be an alternative treatment. For interventions involving changes of provider behavior, the comparison group may be usual care, in which case the approach to analysis is the same as if the alternative treatment is a placebo. Equivalence studies provide similar examples of comparison groups (e.g., standard treatment). Instead of trying to reject an equality in favor of an alternative hypothesis involving an inequality, equivalence studies typically entail tests to reject a null hypothesis of a difference in favor of an alternative hypothesis of equality. This reversal of the hypothesis-testing process may be undertaken with confidence intervals, and their comparison with pre-specified endpoints within which the confidence interval must lie to help support equivalence. For example, in a study of severely depressed patients, confidence intervals were compared to pre-specified intervals to show that while St. John's Wort extract LI 160 reduced on average the Hamilton Depression Scale, the reduction was not equivalent to the larger average reduction with imipramine (Vorbach, Arnoldt, & Hubner, 1997). An equivalence study also may be useful in showing that the well-understood medication, nortriptyline, does as well as newer but more costly and less well-understood pharmacological treatments of depression in the elderly.

Related to choice of comparison groups is the issue of deciding between parallel and cross-over designs. Under the parallel treatment design, each participant is assigned (e.g., randomized) to one treatment group. Examples of randomized parallel studies pervade the geriatric psychiatric literature (e.g., Geretsegger, Bohmar, & Ludwig, 1995; Geretsegger et al. 1994; Katona 1998; Roose et al., 1998), including comparisons of such pharmacological treatments as imipramine, paroxetine, nortriptyline, amitriptyline, and fluoxetine in comorbid subgroups such as those with cognitive deficits. As an example of a cross-over trial in geriatric psychiatry, 25 frail nursing home subjects were randomized to the two reverse sequences of carbamazepine and placebo, to investigate the former's toxicity (Tariot et al., 1995). As another example, the cognitive effects of two antispasmodic agents and a placebo were compared in a three-treatment, three-period cross-over study of normal elderly volunteers (Katz et al., 1998).

Parallel Versus Cross-Over Designs

Although both parallel and cross-over designs rely on within-subject changes to estimate treatment effects, the cross-over trial is more efficient in a statistical sense. Under a cross-over design, the treatment contrasts are compared to within-subject residual variation, which tends to be less than between-subject residual error used in parallel studies. Consequently, smaller sample sizes are typically needed for cross-over studies than for parallel studies, all other things (i.e., probabilities of type I and II errors, effect size) being equal. Of course, the main disadvantage of the cross-over trial is the potential for carry-over effects, which often require a long wash-out period between treatment administrations to the same subject. Wash-out of the effects of treatment must consider both the plasma levels of the drugs (determined by pharmokinetics) and tissue-level effects (determined by pharmacodynamics). Ensuring the absence of carry-over effects on psychiatric effects is, in general, difficult. There do exist cross-over designs involving more time points than treatments to allow the unconfounding of carry-over and other factors, although it is often unfeasible or unethical to change the drug treatment of geriatric psychiatric patients multiple times, let alone just once.

Randomization

Regardless of the design, randomization is one of the most effective ways of ensuring that Tukey's correct question will be addressed. However, because the decision to randomize may sacrifice ethics in the face of the individual physician's desire to administer the best treatments to individual patients, adaptive randomization strategies have been developed. With such strategies, the probability of being randomized to one of the treatments under study depends on the results of previously randomized patients. The likelihood of being randomized to more effective treatments increases, whereas the likelihood for less effective treatments decreases. Such strategies require quick responses so that information from previous and current patients can be incorporated into randomization for future patients. Moreover, the logistics of these strategies mandate small sample sizes and thus large treatment effects. Studies comparing quick-acting treatments (e.g., ECMO; Bartlett et al., 1985) for acute outcomes in premature newborns provide an appropriate context for these adaptive randomization strategies. In most geriatric psychiatric studies, the time to response of study participants is not sufficient to allow for adaptation of randomization schemes. Moreover, the sample sizes of many geriatric studies are too large for these strategies to be practically feasible. In cases where nonrandomized allocation is performed, it is imperative that all baseline differences between treatment groups be adjusted for in the analysis of treatment effects. Even then, there may be unknown confounders biasing the results.

The unit of randomization is a critical factor, especially with trials using multiple clusters of subjects, e.g., patients within distinct clinical practices. For certain types of interventions that require involvement on the part of providers, such as increased screening for depression in primary care practices, randomization of practices may be more feasible than randomizing patients. The latter strategy may lead to contamination between intervention and usual care patients within a practice. On the other hand, randomization of practices likely will lead to less power than randomization of patients for a given sample size. Consequently, any gain in precision or reduction of bias through prevention of contamination by randomizing practices may be lost through a decrease in power to detect clinically significant differences (Murray, 1997). Furthermore, it is more difficult to ensure relatively equal distributions of confounders among treatment groups with randomization of practices than of patients, because the numbers of practices available for randomization is typically smaller than the numbers of patients randomized.

To prevent bias resulting from unequal distributions of confounders among treatment groups regardless of the unit of randomization, one may randomize within the strata of a confounder or combinations of confounders. A refined special case of stratification is matching, where the matching or stratification criteria are so stringent that each matched set contains a small number of randomized units (e.g., matched pairs). In the case of randomizing clusters of subjects such as practices, matching may lead to more problems than benefits, in which case crude stratification may be more useful (Klar & Donner, 1997). An important advantage of crude stratification over matching is that stratification ensures the balance necessary to investigate interactions involving treatment (e.g., outcomes of treating depression in patients with and without dementia), whereas paired matching precludes the assessments of interactions (Klar & Donner, 1997; Meinert, 1986).

Because sample sizes within the levels of a potential confounder may not be sufficient to achieve a pre-specified randomized allocation ratio (e.g., 1:1), blocked randomization is sometimes employed within the strata of the confounder (Meinert, 1986). Under block randomization, patients to be randomized are grouped into blocks of a certain size according to the order of entry into a study, and then randomized assignments are constrained such that the prespecified allocation ratio is maintained within each block. For example, if in a randomized clinical trial, under 1:1 randomization, patients were grouped into blocks of size 4, one would have randomly assigned the first two subjects of each block. If both of these first two subjects within a block were to be assigned to the same treatment, then the remaining two subjects in the block would be assigned to the other treatment. Otherwise, the third subject is then randomized, and the fourth is given the assignment that will result in two subjects in the block being assigned to each treatment. In blinded studies where investigators and/or patients are blinded to the randomization assignment, one may randomly vary the length of blocks across time, to reduce the possibility of unblinding by determining the blocking schedule. Finally, block randomization may also be applied to the randomization of practices, because they will be of a fewer number than the typical patient pool from which random subjects are selected.

Confounding

Whereas the randomization and comparison group selection strategies represent attempts to preclude selection biases that would confound any treatment differences, there exist other potential confounding biases in clinical trials. These include center effects in multicenter trials, drop-out, compliance, and regression to the mean. Differences among centers in multicenter randomized trials will only have the potential to cause confounding if the treatment allocation varies across centers. In this case, treatment will be associated with center, thus allowing any association between center and the outcome of interest to lead to confounding due to center. Of course, such confounding can be prevented by randomization within center. This type of confounding is more likely in observational trials, where nonrandomized allocation of treatments depends on factors like quality of health care providers which vary across center (Berlin, Kimmel, Ten Have, & Sammel). Similar confounding due to subject differences has also been controlled for in the context of longitudinal studies (Kleban, 1992).

Regression to the mean is another type of confounding that may be resolved somewhat by randomized assignments to groups including a placebo. In this context, selecting on the basis of scores at one end of a population distribution (e.g., GDS for severe depression; Reynolds 1997) likely will lead to a decrease in the average score due to regression to the mean, regardless of treatment. If the different groups under comparison vary in terms of their pretreatment average outcome score, then tests and estimates of treatment differences in post-treatment responses may be analyzed by including pretreatment responses as a covariate or independent variable. Under such adjustments, the interpretation of treatment differences assumes that the baseline value is held fixed for all groups under comparison. Furthermore, when estimating differences in treatment effects, it may be assumed that the regression to the mean effect is the same in each group, in which case this effect cancels out. However, the absolute treatment effects within each group are still affected by regression to the mean. The inclusion of a placebo in a randomized study should help facilitate adjustments for regression to the mean. Of course, other effects may be included in the overall placebo effect, such as that due to receiving any type of attention. If including a placebo group is unfeasible from an ethical point of view, multiple baseline run-in observations may facilitate some adjustment for regression to the mean (Lin & Hughes, 1995).

The negative impact of noncompliance may not be precluded by randomization, although in many cases the biases resulting from noncompliance can be resolved to some extent with the help of randomization. The changing nature of treatments across time in some studies may be due to noncompliance on the part of study subjects resulting from side effects or poor treatment outcomes in geriatric psychiatric studies (Rao et al., 1996; Reynolds 1997; Salzman, 1995). Moreover, provider noncompliance may occur, especially when treatment modalities involve changes in behavior on the part of the provider (e.g., intensified screening and referral efforts). The intent-to-treat approach (i.e., analyze all patients according to the group to which they were randomized disregarding their compliance status) has been the traditional strategy for addressing this issue, under the pretense that the analysis of differences between groups determined at baseline (e.g., randomized assignments) has the highest priority. While intent-to-treat hypothesis tests of treatment differences are in general unbiased under noncompliance, it has been shown that treatment effect estimates based upon intent-to-treat analyses may severely underestimate the true causal relationships between treatments and outcomes, and reliance on intent-to-treat analyses may lead to loss of power under strong noncompliance (Mark & Robbins, 1993). We consider some alternative analysis strategies for accommodating non-compliance in the analysis half of this chapter.

Drop-outs may cause problems for analyses of longitudinal data from clinical trials, if the propensity of drop-out is related to the dependent variable in a longitudinal analysis. For instance, dropping out may be related to insufficient decreasing of depression as reflected in smaller changes in GDS scores. Differing degrees of such a relation have been defined in the statistical literature to accommodate the variety of ways statistical methodologies account for missing data (Little & Rubin, 1987).

Even if there is no relation between the dependent variable and missingness, naive analyses of longitudinal data in the presence of missing data may still lead to biased results in the case of time-varying covariates, such as treatment in a cross-over design or change in depression scores in a parallel trial (Neuhaus & Kalbfleisch, 1997; Ten Have, Landis, & Weaver, 1995). In particular, the pooling of within- and between-subject effects of time-varying covariates may confound overall estimates of time-varying. Hence, it is imperative that longitudinal clinical trials make every effort to retain participants so that the chances of drop-out are minimized.

Sample Size Calculations

Even with randomization, good compliance, and minimal drop-out, a study may not be worthwhile or possibly even ethical if the sample size is not sufficient to show that a clinically significant treatment effect is statistically significant. Sample size calculations serve to maximize the precision of study results given a sample size constrained by resource limits and an effect size. A number of different approaches are available for computing sample sizes for randomized clinical trials involving repeated measures data. One approach entails calculations based upon theoretical formulae that take into account the correlated nature of the repeated measures data (Hedeker, Gibbons, & Waternaux, in press). Such formulae are more common and implemented in software for continuous responses than for categorical responses.

A second approach entails adjusting well-known sample size formulae for cross-sectional data to accommodate correlated data. Such a procedure was employed in planning for a placebo-controlled randomized assessment of subacute challenges of several medications in terms of cognitive and affective toxicities (Ira Katz, personal communication, July 1998). In general, this sample size approach consists of first computing the sample size (number of subjects × number of observations per subject) under a cross-sectional assumption that the observations within each subject are independent. The resulting sample size is then multiplied by a factor (design effect) accounting for the correlation among repeated observations on an individual subject (Diggle, Liang, & Zeger, 1994). For a comparison of different treatment groups in a parallel study, this design effect is DE1=(1+(m-1)*rho), where rho is the within-subject correlation for the dependent variable and m is the number of observations for each subject. In contrast, for treatment comparisons within each subject, such as in a cross-over trial, the design effect is DE2=(1-rho), which is not a function of the number of observations per subject. A comparison of the two design effects, DE1 and DE2, indicates that DE1 inflates the sample size (again number of subjects × number of observations per subject) as calculated under the independence assumption, while DE2 deflates it. The increase in sample size due to DE1 also occurs for studies in which practices are randomized. If m, the average practice size, is large, the design effect is large even for small within-practice correlations.

A third, less common approach to computing power relies on simulations. At each iteration of the simulation, data are generated under the alternative hypothesis model and the hypothesis test is performed on the simulated data. The percentage of times the hypothesis test rejects the null hypothesis is the power of the test. This power analysis may be performed for different sample sizes.

ANALYSIS

As a corollary to John Tukey's maxim, a well thought-out study design should yield approximately the same answer with either crude or more exact analyses. However, as was discussed above, even the best designs may be hamstrung by poor compliance and/or drop-out, which may be especially true for geriatric psychiatric studies. Moreover, with small sample sizes, randomization may not lead to balanced distributions with respect to potentially confounding factors. Hence, even for the best study designs, the data analyses may need to account for these factors. In the subsequent discussion, we begin with more basic issues of data analysis before proceeding to the issues of accounting for noncompliance and drop-out in the analysis. The basis for these more fundamental issues hinges on the feasibility of testing the study hypotheses, which depends heavily on the type of response variable (continuous versus categorical).

Clustering and Correlation

As is well-known, methods for continuous responses are much more widely available and sophisticated than methods for categorical responses. However, there have been recent statistical developments for longitudinal categorical data that are now implemented in some major statistical packages (e.g., SAS). Many of the recent developments in the biostatistical literature have recently focused on accommodating different types of clustering of data that result in correlations among individual responses (Gibbons & Hedeker, 1997; Hedeker & Gibbons, 1994; Ten Have et al., 1995; Zeger & Liang 1986). In longitudinal trials, the major contributor to such clustering and correlation is the repeated observations on study subjects. With the emphasis on multicenter trials to obtain sufficient sample sizes and generalizability, the collection of data from multiple subjects within each center also leads to clustering and correlation that need to be accounted for in the analysis.

The correlations arising from such designs have a number of consequences. First, as was discussed previously with respect to power, the most well-known ramification is that the variances of treatment effect estimates accounting for such correlation differ from the variances assuming independent observations within each subject. The direction of this change in variance due to correlated observations within individuals depends on whether the treatment effect is a between- or within-subject comparison (as noted in the discussion of power). A second ramification is that different approaches to analyzing correlated data lead to different interpretations. The types of models that are commonly used to account for different types of clustering and correlated data fall into two categories: 1) subject-specific models; and 2) population-averaged models. The term "subject-specific" should be replaced with "cluster-specific" for the general case that also includes higher-level clustering such as that due to clinical centers.

Subject-Specific vs. Population-Averaged Models

Subject-specific models typically include random subject effects that are assumed to derive from a normal distribution (i.e., mixed effects or hierarchical linear models). In these models, treatment effect parameters correspond to differences between observations from the same subject but under different treatments. Frequently, not only are intercepts assumed to be random, but so are slopes characterizing change across time. Population-averaged models do not include subject effects, so that treatment effect parameters represent differences between the averages of groups of observations under different treatments, regardless of which subject they correspond to. Linear regression and logistic regression as performed in most statistical packages yield results for population-averaged models. Although regression parameter estimates from these packages are typically valid for correlated data, the corresponding standard errors are usually not, unless they are adjusted to accommodate correlated data (Zeger & Liang, 1986).

For correlated normally distributed continuous data, population-averaged and mixed effects linear models in general yield the same treatment effect parameters. The implication of this equivalence is that ordinary linear regression programs in such packages as SAS and SPSS theoretically provide valid estimates of the same fixed effects parameters as do sophisticated programs such as HLM, MLN, and Proc Mixed in SAS. However, the standard errors produced by the ordinary linear regression programs in general are not valid (Zeger & Liang, 1986).

The equivalence between multilevel and population-averaged parameters in linear models does not hold for logistic or probit models fitted to binary or ordinal data. Population-averaged effects are typically of smaller magnitude than subject-specific effects under these models (Ten Have, Landis, & Hartzel, 1996; Zeger, Liang, & Albert, 1988). Even when adjusted to be valid, standard errors under the population-averaged models are smaller than multilevel or mixed effects standard errors. Hence, for binary or ordinal responses, the distinction between population-averaged and subject-specific models is critical, whereas it is not as critical for continuous data. It has been shown, however, that because both population-averaged estimates and standard errors are smaller than their multilevel counterparts (by the same proportionality factor), tests of significance are approximately the same between the two types of models (Zeger et al., 1988). The choice of which type of model to use in the case of binary or ordinal data depends on the scientific question of interest and the study design. In general, multilevel models are more suitable for studies in which treatment or biological conditions change over time (e.g., cross-over trials), as the effects of such changes under population-averaged models are difficult to interpret. In contrast, population-averaged models may be more suitable for cases where covariates are constant across time (e.g., treatment in a parallel study design).

With multilevel models, there are many packages available for fitting linear-normal error versions of these models, e.g., HLM, BMDP5V, SAS Proc Mixed, and MLN. All of these packages allow random intercepts, slopes, and higher-order regression terms. There is less commercial software for analyzing binary, ordinal, and count data with mixed effects or hierarchical models. Hedeker and Gibbons offer a suite of free menu-driven programs for these types of models (Gibbons & Hedeker, 1997; Hedeker & Gibbons, 1994).

Generalized Estimating Equations (GEE) is an alternative approach for fitting mixed effects (hierarchical) and population-averaged models (continuous, binary, ordinal, and count data) entails. This procedure allows the user the latitude in specifying the correlation structure of repeated measures data, as long as the mean and variance are specified correctly. There are few commercial software packages that employ GEE to fit mixed effects models. However, there is a growing number of packages that offer GEE for estimating population-averaged models (without random effects). Currently, the major packages that offer GEE for this type of model are SAS (Proc Genmod), STATA, and SUDAAN.

Missing Data

In consonance with Tukey's maxim, the above approaches with their elaborate model specifications and estimation techniques succumb to the more naive approaches to the pitfalls of certain types of missing data and noncompliance, which are commonplace in geriatric psychiatric studies. The hierarchical models are indeed more robust with respect to missing data than to other procedures such as GEE or weighted least squares regression. However, there are two cases where most of these approaches are vulnerable to the consequences of missing data. First, estimates and tests of within-subject effects may be confounded by between-subject information under missing data, regardless of the cause of the missing data (Neuhaus & Kalbfleisch, 1997; Ten Have, Landis, & Weaver, 1996). A similar type of bias is more likely with multi-center observational trials, where the treatment allocation ratio varies across centers (Berlin et al., in press). Such bias is easily prevented by decomposing arithmetically the within-subject covariate (treatment dummy variable in a cross-over trial) into within- and between-subject components. In the context of cross-over trials, the parameter for the within-subject component is then the true within-subject treatment effect, whereas the parameter for the between-subject effect represents differences among subjects with different treatment patterns (e.g., those who only received one treatment would be compared to those who received both). For multi-center trials with varying treatment allocation ratios, similar decompositions of treatment effects into between- and within-center effects may to be performed (Berlin et al., in press).

It is not as easy to prevent the second type of bias resulting from certain types of missing data, which plagues most types of modeling approaches available in software packages (e.g., Proc Mixed in SAS, MLN, HLM, and BMDP5V). When missing data are informative, i.e., dependent on the outcomes that would have been observed had they not been missing (e.g., missed visit due to bout of depression), hierarchical or mixed effects models are thought to produce biased estimates (Little, 1995). However, there is some evidence that between treatment-group (e.g., two different antidepressants) comparisons may not be biased when hierarchical models are used. Comparisons across time within a treatment group (e.g., temporal effects within subject, such as treatment effects in a cross-over study) do appear to be biased by informative missing data (Ten Have, Pulkstenis, Kunselman, & Landis, 1998).

For such investigations of temporal effects in the presence of informative missing data, two classes of modeling approaches prevail in the statistical literature: selection and pattern mixture models. The selection model approach consists of two components: (Vorbach et al., 1997) the missing data or "selection" process (e.g., missed clinic visits), which is a function of the outcome variables (e.g., functional status or depression) and covariates (e.g., treatment); and the outcome process, which depends upon covariates such as treatment (Katz et al., 1998). This approach provides reasonable interpretations in the presence of missing data, although the results may be very sensitive to the specification of the missing data model depending upon the amount of missing data. The other class of missing data procedures, the pattern mixture approach, entails estimating separate model parameters for each pattern of missing data and then averaging the parameters across the missing data patterns (Hedeker & Rose, in press; Little, 1995). This approach is easier to implement than selection models, but is harder to interpret in light of informative missing data. Furthermore, there is evidence that the pattern mixture approach does not perform very well for between-treatment comparisons (Ten Have et al., 1998).

Other simpler approaches to handling missing data have been proposed in the medical literature. These include imputing missing data after drop-out with the last observed data point (last-observation-carried forward) or the respective group mean, or analyzing only those subjects with complete data. Because these approaches have been shown to produce biased inference under certain conditions, multiple imputation, which accounts for the variability of estimated missing values, is recommended if imputation is desired (Lavori, Dawson, & Shera, 1995; Little & Rubin, 1987). Finally, one may want to analyze the sensitivity of inference to a conservative form of imputation, which entails replacing the comparison group missing data with the treatment group mean; and vice versa. The resulting estimated group differences likely will be narrower than they would be otherwise.

Noncompliance

Noncompliance represents a form of missing data in that the noncomplier fails to provide information for the treatment to which they are assigned. As discussed previously, the traditional intent-to-treat approach underestimates treatment differences if they do exist. As an alternative, "as treated" analyses, which incorporate compliance information as time-dependent covariates in traditional regression approaches (e.g., hierarchical models), also may be problematic. They require additional assumptions about the comparability of treatment groups beyond those assumptions guaranteed by randomization (Kelsey, Thompson, & Evans, 1986). Hence, there is a need for alternative approaches when outcomes, noncompliance, and treatment influence each other across time. At least two approaches have been proposed in the statistical literature for accounting for noncompliance in the framework of potential outcomes: 1) estimating the treatment effect for different levels of compliance (Goetghebeur, Molenberghs, & Katz, 1998); and 2) estimating the treatment effect for the combined populations of compliers and noncompliers (Mark & Robbins 1993).

CONCLUSIONS

A critical premise to Tukey's maxim is that one can assess the "approximateness" of the answer to the right question. Methods of performing this assessment for simple linear models for normal-error independent data are well-developed and incorporated into statistical packages. The stable of procedures for investigating lack-of-fit in this more traditional context include testing or gauging the significance of lack-of-fit statistics (e.g., R-square as the percentage of the total variance explained), and analyzing residuals for departures from normality, constant variance, and outliers in terms of the dependent and independent variables. Validation of logistic models using the following is also important: the shrinkage coefficient to test for overfitting, the area under the receiver operating characteristic (ROC) curve statistic and related rank-order statistics, which assess how well the model discriminates between positive and negative test results, and the Hosmer-Lemeshow goodness-of-fit statistic. To account for additional variability under models fitted to longitudinal data and to penalize for overfitting, these statistics may be computed in terms of predicted values obtained with the bootstrap approach (Harrell, Lee, & Mark, 1996).

With models for longitudinal data, such as mixed effects models, additional issues arise in relation to assessing lack-of-fit. These include performing sensitivity analyses of the random effects assumptions by comparing results under different sets of assumptions (e.g., random intercept only versus random intercept and random slope). With these approaches, one likely can gauge the "approximateness" of the answer to what is hopefully the right question.

REFERENCES

Bartlett, R. H., Roloff, D. W. Cornell, R. G., Andrews, A. F., Dillon, P. W., & Zwischenberger J. B. (1985) Extracorporeal circulation in neonatal respiratory failure: A prospective randomized study. *Pediatrics, 76,* 479–87.

Berlin, J. A., Kimmel, S. E., Ten Have, T. R., & Sammel, M. D. (in press). An empirical comparison of several clustered data approaches under confounding due to cluster effects in the analysis of complications of coronary angioplasty. *Biometrics.*

Diggle, P. J., Liang, K. –Y., and Zeger, S. L. (1994) *Analysis of Longitudinal Data.* New York: Oxford University Press.

Geretsegger, C., Bohmer, F., & Ludwig, M. (1994) Paroxetine in the elderly depressed patient: Randomized comparison with fluoxetine of efficacy, cognitive and behavioural effects. *International Clinical Psychopharmacology, 9,* 25–29.

Geretsegger, C., Stuppaeck, C. H., Mair, M., Platz, T., Fartacek, R., & Heim, M. (1995) Multicenter double blind study of paroxetine and amitriptyline in elderly depressed inpatients. *Psychopharmacology, 119,* 277–281.

Gibbons, R. D. & Hedeker, D. (1997) Random-effects probit and logistic regression models for three-level data. *Biometrics, 53,* 1527–1537.

Goetghebeur, E., Molenberghs, G., & Katz, J. (1998) Estimating the causal effect of compliance on binary outcome in randomized controlled trials. *Statistics in Medicine, 17,* 341–355.

Harrell, F. E., Lee, K. L., & Mark, D. B. (1996). Multivariate prognostic models: Issues in developing models, evaluating assumptions, and adequacy, and measuring and reducing errors. *Statistics in Medicine, 15,* 361–387.

Hedeker, D., & Gibbons, R. D. (1994) A random-effects ordinal regression model for multilevel analysis. *Biometrics, 50,* 933–944.

Hedeker, D., Gibbons, R. D., & Waternaux, C. (in press). Sample size estimation for longitudinal designs with attrition: Comparing time-related contrasts between two groups. *Journal of Educational and Behavioral Statistics.*

Hedeker, D. & Rose, J. S. (in press). The natural history of smoking: A pattern-mixture random-effects regression model. In J. S. Rose, L. Chassin, C. C. Presson, & S. J. Sherman (Eds.) *Multivariate applications in substance use research.* Erlbaum: Mahwah, NJ.

Katona, C. L., Hunter, B. N., & Bray, J. (1998). A double–blind comparison of the efficacy and safely of paroxetine and imipramine in the treatment of depression with dementia. *International Journal of Geriatric Psychiatry, 13,* 100–108.

Katz, I. R., Sands L. P., Bilker W., DiFilippo S., Boyce A., & D'Angelo K. (1998). Identification of medications that cause cognitive impairment in older people: The case of oxybutynin chloride. *Journal of the American Geriatrics Society, 46,* 8–13.

Katz, I. R., Streim, J. E., Oslin, D. W., Bilker, W., & Cooper T. (1997). An alternative comparator for antidepressant trials. *Gerontologist, 37,* 17.

Kelsey, J. L., Thompson, W. E., & Evans. A. S. (1986). *Methods in observational epidemiology,* New York: Oxford University Press.

Klar, N., & Donner, A. (1997) The merits of matching in community intervention trials: A cautionary tale. *Statistics in Medicine, 16,* 1753–1764.

Kleban, M. H., Lawton, M. P., Nesselroade, J. R., & Parmelee, P. (1992). The structure of variation in affect among depressed and nondepressed elders. *Journal of Gerontology, 473,* P190–198.

Lavori, P. W., Dawson, R., & Shera, D. (1995). A multiple imputation strategy for clinical trials with truncation of patient data. *Statistics in Medicine, 14,* 1913–1925.

Lin, H. M. & Hughes, M. D. (1995). Use of historical marker data for assessing treatment effects in phase I/II trials when subject selection is determined by baseline marker level. *Biometrics, 51,* 1053–1063.

Little, R. J. A. (1995). Modeling the drop-out mechanism in repeated-measures studies. *Journal of the American Statistical Association, 90,* 1112–1121.

Little, R. J. A, & Rubin, D. B. (1987). *Statistical Analysis with Missing Data.* New York: Wiley.

Mark, S. D., & Robbins, J. M. (1993). A method for the analysis of randomized trials with compliance information: An application to a multiple risk factor intervention trial. *Controlled Clinical Trials, 14,* 79–97.

Meinert, C. L. (1986). *Clinical Trials: Design, Conduct, and Analysis.* New York: Oxford University Press.

Murray, D. M. (1997). *Design and Analysis of Group Randomized Trials.* New York: Oxford University Press.

Neuhaus, J., & Kalbfleisch, J. D. (1997) Between- and within-cluster covariate effects in the analysis of clustered data. *Biometrics, 54,* 638–645.

Rao, M. L., Deister, A., Laux, G., Staberock, U., Hoflich, G., & Moller, H. J. (1996). Low serum levels of tricyclic antidepressants in amitriptyline- and doxepin-treated inpatients with depressive syndromes are associated with nonresponse. *Pharmacopsychiatry, 29,* 97–102.

Reynolds, C. F., 3rd. (1997). Treatment of major depression in later life: A life cycle perspective. *Psychiatric Quarterly, 68,* 221–246.

Roose, S. P., Laghrissi-Thode, F., Kennedy, J. S., Nelson, J. C., Bigger, J. T., Pollock, B. G., Gaffnet, A., Narayan, M., Finkel, M. S., McCafferty, J., & Gergel, I. (1998). Comparison of paroxetine and nortriptyline in depressed patients with ischemic heart disease. *JAMA, 279,* 287–291.

Salzman, C. (1995). Medication compliance in the elderly. *Journal of Clinical Psychiatry, 56,* 18–23.

Tariot, P. N., Frederiksen, K., Erb, R., Leibovici, A., Podgorski, C. A., Asnis, J., & Cox, C. (1995). Lack of carbamazepine toxicity in frail nursing home patients: A controlled study. *Journal of the American Geriatrics Society, 43,* 1026–1029.

Ten Have, T. R., Landis, J. R., & Hartzel, J. (1996). Population-averaged and cluster-specific models for clustered ordinal response data. *Statistics in Medicine, 15,* 2573–2588.

Ten Have, T. R., Landis, J. R., & Weaver, S. L. (1996). Association models for periodontal disease progression: A comparison of methods for clustered binary data [letter]. *Statistics in Medicine, 15,* 1227–1229.

Ten Have, T. R., Landis, J. R., & Weaver, S. L. (1995). Association models for periodontal disease progression: A comparison of methods for clustered binary data. *Statistics in Medicine, 14,* 413–429.

Ten Have, T. R., Pulkstenis, E., Kunselman, A., & Landis, J. R. (1998). Mixed effects logistic regression models for longitudinal binary response data with informative drop-out. *Biometrics, 54,* 367–383.

Tukey, J. W. (1962). The future of data analysis. *Annals of Mathematical Statistics, 33,* 13.

Vorbach, E. U., Arnoldt, K. H., & Hubner, W. D. (1997) Efficacy and tolerability of St. John's wort extract LI 160 versus imipramine in patients with severe depressive episodes according to ICD–10. *Pharmacopsychiatry, 30* Suppl 2, 81–85.

Zeger, S. L., Liang, K.-Y., & Albert, P. A. (1988). Models for longitudinal data: A generalized estimating equation approach. *Biometrics, 44,* 1049–1060.

Zeger, S. L., & Liang, K.-Y. (1986). Longitudinal data analysis for discrete and continuous outcomes. *Biometrics, 64,* 121–130.

CHAPTER 4

Pharmacokinetics of Psychotropic Drugs in the Elderly*

LISA L. VON MOLTKE & DAVID J. GREENBLATT
DEPARTMENT OF PHARMACOLOGY AND EXPERIMENTAL THERAPEUTICS, TUFTS UNIVERSITY SCHOOL OF MEDICINE, AND THE DIVISION OF CLINICAL PHARMACOLOGY, NEW ENGLAND MEDICAL CENTER

Prescription and nonprescription drug use increases with age, and psychotropics rank high among the therapeutic classes that are most utilized. The elderly, usually defined as those over 65 years of age, are a highly heterogenous group, with large variability in their overall health status (Avorn, 1998; Chrischilles et al., 1992; Lebowitz, et al., 1997; Lebowitz, Pearson, & Cohen, 1998). In the aggregate, they are more vulnerable to the hazards of pharmacotherapy (Campbell, 1991; Cumming, 1998). Both pharmacokinetic and pharmacodynamic differences have been described after psychotropic drugs are administered to aging individuals (Bertz et al., 1997; Greenblatt, Harmatz, & Shader, 1991; 1991b; Nikaido, Ellinwood, Heatherly, & Gupta, 1990; von Moltke, Greenblatt, & Shader, 1993; von Moltke, Greenblatt, Harmatz, & Shader, 1995). Concern centers overwhelmingly on those differences and circumstances that lead to increased toxicity or exaggerated (and unwanted) therapeutic effects. Examination of the more frail subpopulations within the large "elderly" group reveals an increased risk of medication-related problems and more serious sequelae resulting from them. The use of multiple medications, which also increases with age, is intimately connected with the number of adverse drug events reported in older patients. Adverse events can also be tied to kinetic changes, where decreases in drug elimination because of physiologic changes or because of drug-drug interactions lead to increased drug levels in plasma and target organ

*Supported by Grants MH-01237, MH-34223, DA-05258, MH-19924, and RR-00054 from the Department of Health and Human Services.

tissue. It is these kinetic changes and interactions that we will focus on below. Any discussion of kinetic drug interactions must include a description of the cytochrome P450 system, which is responsible for the metabolism (and therefore clearance) of the majority of psychotropic drugs used.

KINETICS IN THE ELDERLY

The kinetic changes of greatest concern in psychopharmacology are those leading to increased drug amounts in the body with the potential for a corresponding increase in effect and an increase in accumulation (under situations of chronic dosing). The most important changes involve differences in volume of distribution and clearance, both renal and hepatic. Half-life, which may be the most widely discussed kinetic variable, is not an independent kinetic variable but simply reflects changes in either clearance and/or volume of distribution (Figure 4.1) (Greenblatt, von Moltke, & Shader, 1998; von Moltke, Greenblatt, Harmatz, & Shader, 1995; von Molke, Abernethy, & Greenblatt, 1998).

Absorption

In the absence of overt gastrointestinal (GI) tract pathology, there is no evidence that aging alone changes the ability of the GI tract to absorb medications. Accompanying medications may interfere with GI motility and absorption (e.g., anticholinergics) or may act as chelators and impair absorption (e.g., antacids), just as they could in an individual of any age. However, there may be a higher likelihood of encountering such a situa-

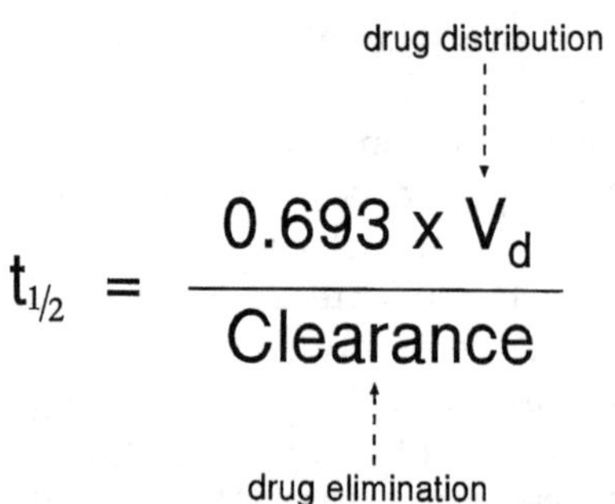

FIGURE 4.1 Mathematical relationship between elimination half-life (t1/2), volume of distribution (Vd) and clearance. Elimination half-life is the dependent variable, varying in direct proportion to the physiochemical property of drug distribution(Vd), and inversely with clearance, which reflects the capacity for drug elimination.

tion under circumstances involving polypharmacy, which are more common in the elderly. The medications for which no age related differences in absorption have been found include chlordiazepoxide, diazepam, lorazepam, midazolam, trazodone, and flumazenil (von Moltke et al., 1998).

Distribution and Protein Binding

Following absorption, a drug is distributed. How extensively, and to what tissues, is determined in large part by solubility, protein binding and blood flow to various tissues. Drugs in the systemic circulation may bind to albumin, alpha-1-acid glycoprotein (AAG), or red blood cells. This distribution process is described by "volume of distribution," Vd, a hypothetical quantity with units of volume (i.e. liters). Drugs which are more water-soluble and whose distribution is restricted to the vascular system and lean tissues (the central compartment) usually have smaller volumes of distribution than those drugs which are lipid-soluble and can distribute into adipose tissue. Nearly all psychotropic drugs are overwhelmingly lipid soluble entities (the most notable exception being lithium) which distribute extensively into peripheral tissues, including adipose tissue. Psychotropics, except lithium, are all moderately to extensively protein-bound.

Body composition changes with aging are well documented. In general, lean muscle mass and total body water decrease, while percentage of total body fat increases. Women generally have a greater percentage of body fat than men at any age. Consequently, lipid-soluble psychotropic drugs are more extensively distributed in peripheral tissues of elderly individuals than those of younger patients. Lithium, however, has a smaller volume into which it is distributed and is therefore more concentrated in the central compartment. In the case of plasma proteins, albumin levels tend to decrease with age, while AAG levels tend to increase.

The implications of changes in Vd under conditions of continuous drug therapy (chronic dosing) involve the amount of time it takes to reach any given steady-state concentration or the amount of time it takes for all of the drug to be eliminated if therapy is stopped. This relationship can be understood mathematically by examining the equation in Figure 4.1 and remembering that attainment of steady state during chronic fixed dosing (or attainment of a "zero level" after therapy cessation) is more than 90% complete in approximately 4 half-lives (Figure 4.2). Hence, the larger the Vd (assuming no other physiologic changes such as changes in clearance), the longer the half-life. The longer the half-life, the longer it takes to achieve any given steady-state concentration or to wash out drug after stopping therapy. Note that the amount of drug accumulated, that is, the

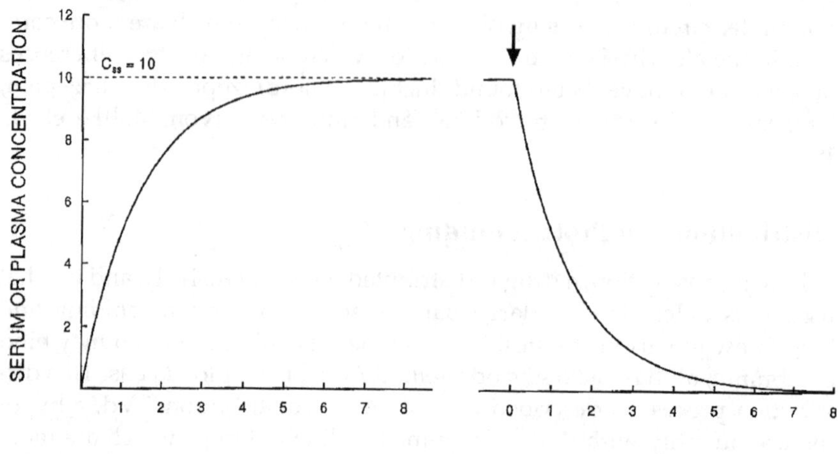

FIGURE 4.2 After initiation of drug administration of a constant dosing rate (without a loading dose) at time zero, the mean serum or plasma drug concentration approaches the steady-state value (C_{ss} = 10 units) exponentially. The steady-state condition is more than 90% attained after an interval of 4 times the elimination half-life has elapsed. Drug administration is stopped at the arrow, after which the serum or plasma concentration falls to zero exponentially. The concentration has fallen to less than 10% of its initial value after four times the elimination half-life elapses after drug discontinuation.

actual concentration at steady state, is not affected by Vd or by half-life, but is strictly a function of dosing (rate of drug administration) and clearance, which is discussed below. The potential for changes in volume of distribution underlie part of the well-known adage to "start low and go slow" with regard to initial dosing and escalation in the elderly, since steady-state concentrations may take longer to reach.

For psychotropic drugs, the tissue into which distribution is obviously of greatest interest is the brain. For many drugs that are avidly bound to albumin, it is not clear that differences secondary to aging in the amounts of albumin available for binding meaningfully change distribution into target tissue. Significantly lower albumin levels are, however, associated with other situations that may influence drug activity, such as the changes in AAG levels or changes in clearance that might be associated with cirrhosis, renal insufficiency, or debilitating disease.

In general, any bound drug, free drug, and distributed drug reaches a state of equilibrium under steady-state conditions. The extent to which protein binding limits distribution of various drugs to a spectrum of sites of biologic activity may vary, and is incompletely understood. For example, binding to albumin does not always seem to restrict the access of drugs to the active intrahepatocytic sites of enzymes responsible for metabolic clearance. Simply substituting the free plasma concentration of some drugs into in vitro to in vivo scaling models fails to accurately predict changes in clearance secondary to enzyme inhibition observed in vivo. While there are a number of possible explanations for why these models sometimes fail to predict clinical reality, one is that a full picture of how drugs dissociate and distribute vis-a-vis protein binding has yet to fully emerge. It may also be useful to remember that triazolam (~90% protein-bound) and midazolam (~97% protein-bound) have iv clearance values substantially higher (~2.6 and 9.0 ml/min*kg, respectively) than the less protein bound alprazolam (70% bound, 0.7 ml/min*kg) (Greenblatt et al., 1984; Greenblatt & Wright, 1993; Kroboth et al., 1995). Clearly, protein binding alone is not a predictor of the ability of the drug to become engaged with the enzyme of metabolic clearance. Testosterone is another example of a substance where bioactivity is not restricted by albumin. The free and albumin-bound portions of the total serum concentration are considered available for bioactivity, while that bound to sex hormone binding globulin is not (Manni et al., 1985; Nahoul & Roger, 1990).

In the case of AAG, there is now in vitro and animal data to suggest that changes in the level of this protein may significantly affect distribution of drugs that bind to this protein (Billelo et al., 1996). Work done in transgenic mice which have AAG levels greater than 8 times control has shown that brain distribution of imipramine, desipramine, and fluoxetine was markedly lower in those animals with elevated AAG, in spite of higher serum levels (Holladay, Dewey, & Yao, 1996, 1998a). The fluoxetine-treated mice were reported to show a corresponding decrease in antidepressant activity (Holladay, Dewey, & Yao, 1998b). This is of potential significance since AAG, an acute phase reactant, has been shown to increase (in general) with age, and specifically increase with many disease processes, including depression (Maes et al., 1997). How the animal data may relate to the more modest AAG levels seen in human aging and/or psychiatric states needs further clarification. Previous work looking at changes in AAG and alterations in imipramine binding with age in humans shows modest and widely varying changes in AAG in the absence of any other overt medical illnesses, and suggests that there will not be clinically significant changes in the percentage of unbound drug (Abernethy & Kerzner, 1984).

Additional issues involving protein binding include whether the changes in protein concentrations affect how plasma measurements of total drug concentrations should be interpreted and whether the elderly are at risk (equally or more) for drug interactions that might occur if one drug displaces another drug from its site of protein binding. Most reported drug levels are total plasma concentrations, which include the sum of bound and unbound portions. In settings where a specific plasma level has been targeted and achieved, an increase in binding protein and therefore bound drug will result in a higher total plasma level determination even if the free amount, the presumably active and available constituent, remains the same. This could lead to the erroneous assumption that a deviation from the desired therapeutic range has occurred and that a therapeutic maneuver to compensate should occur (lower the dose), though the free concentration has stayed the same. One often-cited situation where this is felt to be important is in the case of lidocaine levels in the setting of acute myocardial infarction, where drug levels are stabilized but as AAG levels rise the total amounts of lidocaine measured rise also, though free lidocaine concentrations remain unchanged (Shand, 1984). The concern is that reacting to the high total lidocaine level by lowering the infusion rate will subsequently drop the free portion into the subtherapeutic range with resultant loss of antiarrhythmic activity. The resulting caveat is that when using a highly AAG bound drug in the setting of changing AAG levels, total plasma concentrations should be interpreted with caution and the determination of free drug levels should be considered under certain clinical situations.

The question of protein displacement interactions has been reviewed by many authors (Rolan, 1994; Sansom & Evans, 1995), and the evidence seems clear that in the absence of perturbations in clearance, displacement of drugs from their site of protein binding will usually have a transient and usually clinically insignificant effect. Drugs which meet such criteria as having a very narrow therapeutic indices and small volumes of distribution have more potential to cause any meaningful effect. But as long as clearance mechanisms have not been simultaneously impaired, equilibrium states are quickly restored or a new equilibrium state is rapidly established. It is worth noting that many of the early reports documenting protein displacement interactions were simultaneous episodes of clearance impairment, i.e., the displacing drug also and more importantly impaired clearance of the displaced drug, often by what we can now identify as inhibition of the cytochrome P450 enzyme responsible for metabolism.

A non-circulating protein that can affect drug bioavailability and distribution is p-glycoprotein (p-gp), a plasma membrane glycoprotein that functions as a drug efflux pump for a wide variety of substances. P-gp is encoded by MDR1 in humans, and although long recognized as an important factor in multidrug resistance in cancer cells, it is present in normal tissues as well. In brain endothelial cells, it is felt to function as part of the blood brain barrier (bbb), limiting the access of many drugs to the brain. No currently used psychotropic drugs have yet been found to be important p-gp substrates. However, CNS distribution and toxicity of many other drugs in a wide variety of therapeutic classes can be drastically altered in mice which are p-gp deficient. Whether p-gp amount and/or function in the bbb changes with age is currently under investigation. We have seen decreased CNS permeability to known p-gp substrates (suggesting increased amount and/or function) with animal maturation. Similar findings have been described in human lymphocytes (Gupta, 1995). P-gp also shares a significant number of substrates with the cytochrome P450-3A subfamily (see below), and their coexistence in the GI tract may affect drug bioavailability and extent of "first pass metabolism" (Wacher, Wu, & Benet, 1995). The role of aging in GI p-gp amount and function is also under investigation.

Clearance

"Clearance" is the term describing the volume of blood, plasma or serum from which a substance is completely removed during a given unit of time. Typical units are ml/min or liters/hour. It is the most useful parameter in assessing an individual's capacity to remove any given drug. Renal excretion, hepatic biotransformation, or a combination of both are the most clinically relevant mechanisms of clearance. Decrements in clearance lead to prolonged half-life and to drug accumulation under situations of chronic dosing. For any given dosing regimen, this results in a "final" steady-state level that takes longer to achieve and is higher than in an individual with higher clearance.

Renal clearance declines predictably with age. Creatinine clearance (Clcr), used to estimate glomerular filtration rate, is often used as an indicator of renal function. The empiric formula for estimation, Clcr (ml/min) = (140 –age) × weight (kg)/72 × serum Cr (mg/dl) (× 0.85 for women), incorporates age. Lithium is the psychotropic medication most affected by this decrement, although a number of hepatically generated active metabolites of other psychotropics, such as antidepressants, are also renally cleared (Rudorfer & Potter, 1997). An increased risk of lithium toxicity in aging individuals can be expected.

Changes in hepatic metabolism and clearance in elderly individuals are not as predictable. Both phase I (e.g., cytochrome P450) and phase II (e.g., glucuronidation) mediated reactions can be involved in clearance. In addition, hepatic blood flow regulates the upper limit of clearance, since clearance cannot exceed delivery to the organ of clearance. There are no routinely available tests for quantitation of hepatic blood flow. Individual variability is considerable but values usually fall between 1500 and 1800 ml/min. Consistent changes in blood flow secondary to aging are not fully established. Using clearance of low-dose intravenous lidocaine as an index of hepatic blood flow, we previously demonstrated age-dependent decrements in men, but not in women (Figure 4.3).

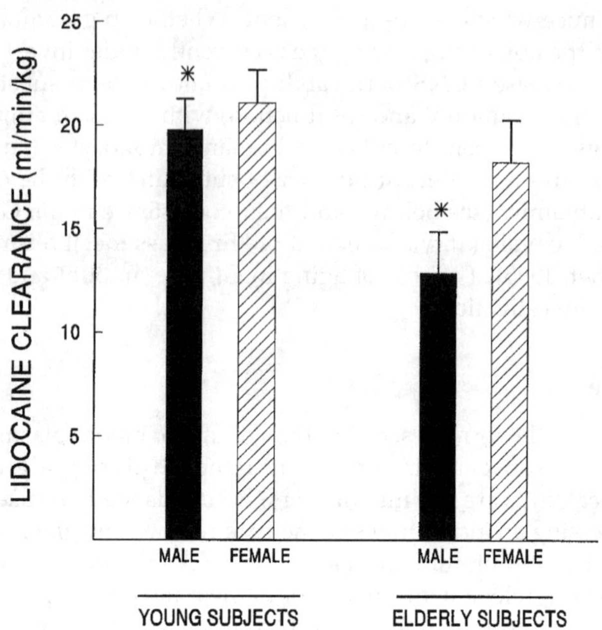

FIGURE 4.3 Mean (±SE) values of lidocaine clearance in groups in young male, young female, elderly male, and elderly female volunteers. Young subjects were aged 20–39 years, while elderly subjects were aged 60–79 years. Differences between young and elderly men were significant (*Ip.01). See Abernethy and Greenblatt (1983) for details.

While the bulk of research points to preservation of conjugation (phase II) metabolic capacity, some oxidative metabolic steps become impaired in aging individuals. Specifically, a number of studies indicate that metabolic transformations mediated by CYP3A enzymes (of great importance because of their participation in large numbers of the metabolic biotransformations of xenobiotics in humans) and some other cytochrome P450 enzymes are compromised, resulting in reduced clearance of the substrates in the elderly.

The cytochrome P450 system is a superfamily of heme containing enzymes responsible for the bulk of drug metabolism in humans. Although present in many locations in the body, those in the liver and intestine are the most important with regard to drug availability and clearance. The nomenclature of the enzymes is based on amino acid and/or nucleotide sequence, with the first number denoting family, the second letter identifying subfamily, and the last number specifying the unique and specific enzyme. Generally, CYP450 enzymes with less than

TABLE 4.1 Psychotropic Drugs that Are Substrates for Cytochrome P450-3a (CYP3A) in Humans

Complete or Nearly Complete CYP3A Substrates	Partial CYP3A Substrates
Triazolam	Diazepam
Alprazolam	Desmethyldiazepam
Midazolam	Zolpidem
Nefazodone	Sertraline
Trazodone	Citalopram
Buspirone	Imipramine
	Amitriptyline

Note: Evidence is available indicating reduced clearance of all of these drugs in the elderly (buspirone is the exception).

40% actual or deduced amino acid similarity are classified in different gene families. Enzymes that are at least 55% identical are classified in the same subfamily. In the case of CYP3A, the subfamily designation reflects primarily the activity of CYP3A4 when the discussion centers around enzyme activity in the intestine and liver (Maurel, 1996; Thummel & Wilkinson, 1998). CYP3A3, which is reported to have ~98% homology with CYP3A4, cannot be distinguished immunochemically and may be a laboratory artifact. Given the substrate similarities of these and other CYP3A members, the collective designation of CYP3A is generally used.

It is important to remember that individual enzymes can exhibit distinct behavior with regard to substrate specificity (which drugs they metabolize) and susceptibility to inhibition or induction. Some, like CYP2D6, CYP2C9 and CYP2C19, are subject to genetic polymorphisms, while others, like CYP3A, show large interindividual variability, but no true polymorphism. As noted above, the intestinal component of "first pass" metabolism that contributes to overall clearance may be a net result of CYP3A and p-gp activity for many CYP3A substrates, but so far no psychotropics have been identified for which this is true.

The CYP response to aging also seems variable, with CYP3A and CYP1A2 showing the most significant changes in vivo. Some 2C9 decrement has been established as well. Studies of CYP2D6 have shown varying results. Some estimate that about 50% of the drugs used in humans require CYP3A for all or a meaningful part of their clearance. In psychopharmacology, the list of CYP3A substrates is long and includes drugs like triazolam, alprazolam, diazepam, amitriptyline, nefazodone and haloperidol (Table 4.1). Many of these have shown age-related decrements in clearance, some of which are disproportionately present in older men. The reason for this is not clear, but proposed explanations have included the idea that the testosterone status of young men may set them apart from older men as well as women. Considering that young men have historically formed the major cohort in pharmacokinetic studies, their potential difference in CYP3A activity could have large implications for extrapolating pharmacokinetic data to older patients or women.

Drug interactions involving psychotropics and the CYP450 system can take a number of forms. The metabolism, and thus clearance, of these drugs can be inhibited, leading to potential toxicity (though if a given drug is a prodrug requiring metabolism for activation, inhibition results in loss of efficacy). For a clinically meaningful interaction to occur, the amount of inhibition has to be substantial enough to drive levels into a range corresponding to toxic effects. Very potent inhibitors of metabolism such as ketoconazole (inhibition of CYP3A), quinidine (CYP2D6) and the others listed in Table 4.2 are often involved in these interactions as are substrates with narrow therapeutic indices.

Interactions involving induction usually result in loss of efficacy because of the accelerated metabolism and clearance, though induction can cause toxic effects if a normally minor toxic metabolite is produced in an increasing amount. A number of potent inducers are also listed in Table 4.2. Analogous to the situation with inhibition, potent inducers and/or drugs with narrow therapeutic windows are most often involved in clinically relevant induction interactions. Though less often recognized and discussed, induction can cause important and unrecognized therapeutic failures that could be corrected by simple dosage adjustment.

In examining Table 4.2, it is evident that a number of the newer antidepressants are potent inhibitors of the cytochrome system (Greenblatt,

TABLE 4.2 Partial Listing of Potent Inhibitors and Inducers of the Cytochrome P450 System in Humans

Inhibitors	Inducers
Quinidine (2D6)	Phenobarbital (multiple, including 3A4)
Ketoconazole (3A4)	Rifampin (multiple, including 3A4)
Itraconazole (3A4)	Ritonavir (multiple, including 3A4)
Fluoxetine (2D6)	Dexamethasone (3A4)
Fluvoxamine (multiple, including 3A4)	Carbamazepine (3A4)
Paroxetine (2D6)	Phenytoin (3A4)
Nefazodone (3A4)	Ethanol (2E1)
Ritonavir (multiple, including 3A4)	
Delavirdine (3A4)	
Clarithromycin (3A4)	
Erythromycin (3A4)	
Ciprofloxacin (1A2)	

von Moltke, Harmatz, et al., 1998a; Richelson, 1997). Clinicians prescribing these entities must therefore be vigilant not only for perturbations in the activity profiles of the drugs they prescribe, but in those of other coprescribed drugs as well. As an example, the fluoxetine package insert cautions that therapy with medications as diverse as flecainide, vinblastine, and tricyclic antidepressants (all at least partial CYP2D6 substrates) should be initiated at the low end of the dosage range during fluoxetine therapy or within 5 weeks of cessation (because of the continued presence of the inhibiting metabolite norfluoxetine) due to the anticipated impairment of CYP2D6 mediated clearance. In addition, patients on stabilized phenytoin therapy have developed increased phenytoin levels and toxicity when fluoxetine was added, and patients receiving alprazolam had increased benzodiazepine levels and increased impairment when fluoxetine was coadministered.

It is not known whether the elderly have any physiologic differences in sensitivity to metabolic inhibition, and the data on induction are inconclusive as well (Crowley et al., 1988; Salem, Rajjayabun, Shepherd, & Stevenson, 1978). But the larger the number of medications administered to any given patient, the greater the odds of an interacting combination (Bergendal, Friberg, & Schaffrath, 1995). Consequently, the elderly as a group are at greater risk for the kinds of drug-drug interactions discussed above.

IN VITRO MODELS

Because the population is aging and drug therapy is a frequent component of elderly life, the realization that oxidative metabolism may be impaired is important, yet full elucidation of the mechanism behind this observation remains incomplete. As noted above, and by many other authors, changes in cytochrome mediated clearance with aging are not explained by hepatic blood flow, hepatic mass or protein binding. In vitro investigations utilizing hepatic microsomes, cDNA expressed enzymes, and other tools have yielded large bodies of fundamental information in many areas of drug metabolism, and such systems have been useful in attempting to predict in vivo metabolic behavior (Houston, 1994; Ito, Iwatsubo, Kanamitsu, Nakajima, & Sugiyama, 1998; Iwatsubo, Hirota, Ooie, Suzuki, & Sugiyama, 1996; Obach et al., 1997). Crucial to these studies are the sources of viable hepatic tissue, which has been a limiting factors for investigators in past years. Still of great concern is the variation in premortem drug exposure and clinical circumstances that occur before hepatic tissue in vivo becomes tissue available for in vitro studies. Much of the usable available tissue comes for patients who have died and have made their organs available for transplant. Some tissue donors have undergone some resuscitation efforts of various intensities and duration, while others have received drug therapy for head injury in attempts to treat increased intracranial pressure. Additional drugs are often added to treat or prevent secondary problems such as gastritis or infection. Such circumstances could lead to situations as diverse as decreased enzyme activity because of anoxic insult or increased activity secondary to drug stimulated enzyme induction. This variability makes it extremely difficult to assign any differences in donor enzyme amount or activity to a particular donor characteristic, such as age or gender. In fact, in vitro attempts to quantify enzyme amount or enzyme activity and correlate the results with age have yielded conflicting results (George, Byth, & Farrel, 1995; Hunt, Westerkam, & Stave, 1992; Transon, Lecoeur, Leeman, Beaune, & Dayer, 1996) One study done using liver biopsies in volunteers who also agreed to take a P450 metabolic probe, antipyrine, showed a decrease in total P450 content and activity with age (Sotaniemi, Arranto, Pelkonen, & Pasanen, 1997). No individual P450s were investigated.

Animal models which allow control of the in vivo-in vitro tissue transition may prove helpful in investigating metabolic changes. Initial data in our lab show a clear decrement in activity secondary to a unequivocal decrease in amount of CYP3A in aging mice. Studies to examine the mechanism behind the decrease in enzyme amount are ongoing in our laboratory. Another interesting avenue of research regards the possibility of changes in hepatic oxygen diffusion with aging which has an impact on oxygen requiring metabolic reactions, such as those mediated by P450 (Le Couteur & McLean, 1998).

CLINICAL IMPLICATIONS

The studies of age-related decrements in clearance of psychotropic drugs have shown consistent changes for substrates of CYP3A (Table 4.1). Drugs affected include commonly used treatments for anxiety as well as depression (Greenblatt et al., 1991, 1998; von Moltke et al., 1993, 1995, 1998). Of the newer antidepressants, venlafaxine clearance seems to show little change with aging while nefazodone, citalopram, paroxetine and fluvoxamine all show sizable decrements (Barbhaiya, Buch, & Greene, et al., 1996; Brennan et al., 1998; Kaye et al., 1989; Klamerus, Parker, Rudolph, Derivan, & Chiang, 1996; Overo, Toft, Christophersen, Gylding-Sabroe, 1985). Sertraline data do show a decrease in clearance in men only when men and women are considered separately (Figure 4.4) (Ronfeld, Tremaine, & Wilner, 1997). Given that many drugs have been shown to show gender- and age-dependent reductions in clearance, it would seem essential to examine each gender separately, thereby examining the vari-

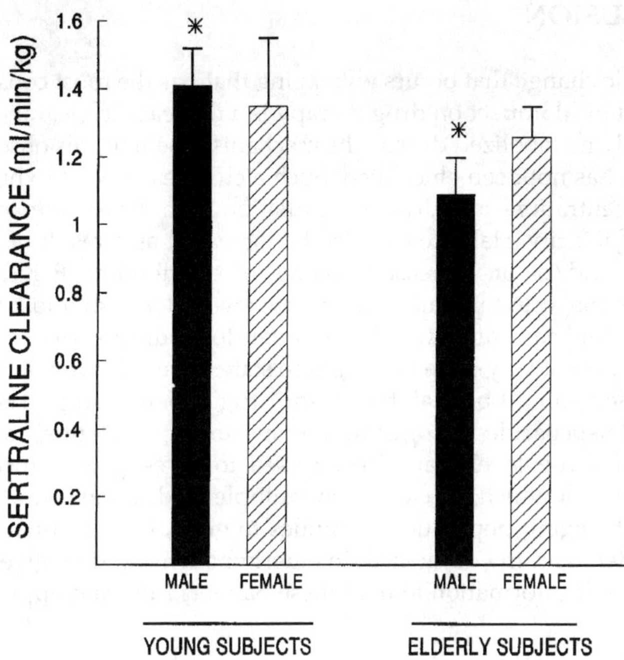

FIGURE 4.4 Mean (±SE) values of sertraline clearance in groups of young male, young female, elderly male, and elderly female volunteers. Differences between young and elderly men are significant (p*<.06) when male and female groups are considered separately (original data presented in Ronfeld et al., 1997).**

able of interest, age, against a background of minimized secondary variation. Data on fluoxetine kinetics in the elderly have been primarily limited to extrapolations from data on file with the manufacturer which showed no changes in half-life (Lemberger et al., 1985), and an abstract reportedly showing a significant increase in half-life (Preskorn, Shad, Alderman, & Lane, 1998). Data on steady-state levels suggest decreased clearance in the elderly (Preskorn, 1993). It is imperative that data needed for clinical decisions be in the public domain and subject to peer review. Clinicians should be wary of review articles, especially in nonpeer-reviewed supplements, which cite no peer-reviewed data as a basis for their conclusions. Unfortunately, as in the case of fluoxetine, the initial unreviewed data in one source was repeatedly cited as a basis for the conclusion that there was no evidence of impaired clearance in the elderly. When a potential change in kinetics can be anticipated and controlled for, as in the case of sertraline in elderly men, the chance for therapeutic success can be higher since the level of vigilance for toxicity is higher. Anticipated kinetic changes alone need not be a contraindication.

CONCLUSION

The kinetic change that occurs with aging that has the most consistent significant clinical impact on drug therapy is a decrease in clearance of some oxidatively metabolized drugs. The mechanism behind this observed phenomenon has not been elucidated. Such a change can lead to higher peak drug concentrations and drug accumulation with the accompanying possibility of toxicity. Half-life can also be increased as a result of decreased clearance and/or an increased volume of distribution. For drugs with known or suspected impaired clearance, lower doses should be used initially and clinicians must wait longer after dose adjustment or drug cessation for a new steady-state or drug-free state to be achieved. A high index of suspicion should be maintained for drug toxicity. Drug plasma levels can be indispensable in adjusting therapy to keep potential toxicity to a minimum. Drug levels can also be used to investigate suspected drug interactions for which the elderly on multiple medications are at increased risk. As the aging population continues to grow, it is essential that clinicians understand the differences in elderly patients and be given the necessary kinetic information to treat these patients fully and appropriately.

REFERENCES

Abernethy, D. R., & Kerzner, L. (1984.) Age effects on alpha-1-acid glycoprotein concentration and imipramine plasma protein binding. *Journal of the American Geriatrics Society, 32,* 705–708.

Abernethy, D. R., & Greenblatt D. J. (1983) Impairment of lidocaine clearance in elderly male subjects. *Journal of Cardiovascular Pharmacology, 5,* 1093–1096.

Avorn, J. (1998). Drug prescribing, drug taking, adverse reactions, and compliance in elderly patients. In C. Salzman (Ed.), *Clinical Geriatric Psychopharmacology.* (pp. 21–47). Baltimore: Williams and Wilkins

Barbhaiya, R. H, Buch, A. B., & Greene, D. S. (1996). A study of the effect of age and gender on the pharmacokinetics of nefazodone after single and multiple doses. *Journal of Clinical Psychopharmacology, 16,* 915–923.

Bergendal, L., Friberg, A., & Schaffrath, A. (1995). Potential drug-drug interactions in 5,125 mostly elderly out-patients in Gothenburg, Sweden. Pharmacy World and Science, 17, 152–157.

Bertz, R. J., Kroboth, P. D., Kroboth, F. J., Reynolds, I. J., Salek F., Wright, C. E, & Smith, R. B. (1997). Alprazolam in young and elderly men: Sensitivity and tolerance to psychomotor, sedative and memory effects. *Journal of Pharmacology and Experimental Therapeutics, 281,* 1317–1329.

Bilello, J. A., Bilello, P. A., Stellrecht, K., Leonard J., Norbeck, D. W., Kempf, D. J., Robins, T., & Drusano, G. L. (1996) Human serum 1 acid glycoprotein reduces uptake, intracellular concentration, and antiviral activity of A-80987, an inhibitor of the human immunodeficiency virus type 1 protease. *Antimicrobial Agents and Chemotherapy, 40,* 1491–1497.

Brennan, J., Hui, J., Pullen ,R., Yang, H. M., Baars, M., & Tolbert D. (1998). Steady state pharmacokinetics of fluvoxamine in young and elderly volunteers (abstract). *Clinical Pharmacology and Therapeutics, 63,* 164.

Campbell, A. J. (1991). Drug treatment as a cause of falls in old age: A review of the offending agents. *Drugs & Aging, 1,* 289–302.

Chrischilles, E. A., Foley, D. J., Wallace, R. B., Lemke, J. H., Semla, T. P., Hanlon, J. T., Glynn, R. J., Ostfeld, A. M., & Guralnik, J. M. (1992) Use of medications by persons 65 and over: Data from the established populations for epidemiologic studies of the elderly. *Journal of Gerontology, 47,* M137–M144.

Crowley, J. J., Cusack, B. J., Jue, S. G., Koup, J. R., Park, B. K, & Vestal, R. E. (1988). Aging and drug interactions. II. Effect of phenytoin and smoking on the oxidation of theophylline and cortisol in healthy men. *Journal of Pharmacology and Experimental Therapeutics, 245,* 513–523.

Cumming, R. G. (1988). Epidemiology of medication-related falls and fractures in the elderly. *Drugs and Aging, 12,* 43–53.

George, J., Byth, K., & Farrel, G. C. (1995). Age but not gender selectivity affects expression of individual cytochrome P450 proteins in human liver. *Biochemical Pharmacology, 50,* 727–730.

Greenblatt, D. J., Abernethy, D. R., Locniskar, A., Harmatz, J. S., Limjuco, R. A, & Shader, R. I. (1984). Effect of age, gender, and obesity on midazolam kinetics. *Anesthesiology, 61,* 27–35.

Greenblatt, D. J., Harmatz, J. S., Shapiro, L., Engelhardt, N., Gouthro, T. A, & Shader, R. I. (1991). Sensitivity to triazolam in the elderly. *New England Journal of Medicine, 324,* 1691–1698.

Greenblatt D. J., Harmatz J. S., & Shader R. I. (1991). Clinical pharmacokinetics of anxiolytics and hypnotics in the elderly: Therapeutic considerations. *Clinical Pharmacokinetics, 21,* 165–177, 262–273.

Greenblatt, D. J., von Moltke, L. L., Harmatz, J. S., & Shader, R. I. (1998). Drug interactions with newer antidepressants: Role of human Cytochromes P450. *Journal of Clinical Psychiatry, 59* (Supp. 15), 19–27.

Greenblatt, D. J., von Moltke, L. L., & Shader R. I. (1998). Pharmacokinetics of psychotropic drugs. In J. C. Nelson (Ed.), *Geriatric Psychopharmacology.* (pp. 27–41) New York: Marcel Dekker.

Greenblatt, D. J., & Wright, C. E. (1993). Clinical pharmacokinetics of alprazolam: Therapeutic implications. *Clinical Pharmacokinetics, 24,* 453–471.

Gupta, S. (1995). P-glycoprotein expression and regulation: Age-related changes and potential effects on drug therapy. *Drugs and Aging, 7,* 19–29.

Holladay, J. W., Dewey M. J., & Yoo, S. D. (1996). Steady-state kinetics of imipramine in transgenic mice with elevated serum AAG levels. *Pharmacy Research, 13,* 1313–1316.

Holladay, J. W., Dewey, M. J., & Yoo, S. D. (1998b). Pharmacokinetics and antidepressant activity of fluoxetine in transgenic mice with elevated serum alpha-1-acid glycoprotein levels. *Drug Metabolism Disposition, 26,* 20–24.

Holladay, J. W., Dewey, M. J., & Yoo, S. D. (1998a). Kinetic interaction between fluoxetine and imipramine as a function of elevated serum alpha-1-acid glycoprotein levels. *Journal of Pharmacy & Pharmacology, 50,* 419–424.

Houston, J. B. (1994). Relevance of in vitro kinetic parameters to in vivo metabolism of xenobiotics. *Toxicology in Vitro, 8,* 507–512.

Hunt, C. M., Westerkam, W. R., & Stave, G. M. (1992). Effect of age and gender on the activity of human hepatic CYP3A. *Biochemical Pharmacology, 44,* 275–283.

Ito, K., Iwatsubo, T., Kanamitsu, S., Nakajima, Y., & Sugiyama, Y. (1998). Quantitative prediction of in vivo drug clearance and drug interactions from in vitro data on metabolism., together with binding and transport. *Annual Review of Pharmacology and Toxicology, 38,* 461–499.

Iwatsubo, T., Hirota, N., Ooie, T., Suzuki, H., & Sugiyama, Y. (1996). Prediction of in vivo drug disposition from in vitro data based on physiological pharmacokinetics. *Biopharmaceutics and Drug Disposition, 17,* 273–310.

Kaye, C. M., Haddock, R. E., Langley, P. F., Mellows, G., Tasker, T. C. G., Zussman, B. D., & Greb, W. H. (1980). A review of the metabolism and pharmacokinetics of paroxetine in man. *Acta Psychiatrica Scandinavica, 80* (supp. 350), 60–75.

Klamerus K. J., Parker V. D., Rudolph R. L., Derivan, A. T, & Chiang, S. T. (1996). Effects of age and gender on venlafaxine and O-desmethylvenlafaxine pharmacokinetics. *Pharmacotherapy, 16,* 915–923.

Kroboth, P. D., McAuley, J. W., Kroboth, F. J., Bertz, R. J., & Smith, R. B. (1995). Triazolam pharmacokinetics after intravenous, oral and sublingual administration. *Journal of Clinical Psychopharmacology, 15,* 259–262.

Le Couteur, D. G, & McLean, A. J. (1998). The aging liver: Drug clearance and oxygen diffusion barrier hypothesis. *Clinical Pharmacokinetics, 34,* 359–373.

Lebowitz, B. D., Pearson, J. L., Schneider, L. S., Reynolds, C. F. 3rd, Alexopoulos, G. S., Bruce M. L. Conwell, Y., Katz, I. R., Meyers, B. S., Morrison, M. F., Massey, J., Niederehe, G., & Parmelle, P. (1997). Diagnosis and treatment of depression in late life. *Journal of the American Medical Association, 278,* 1186–1190.

Lebowitz, B. D., Pearson, P. L., & Cohen, G. D. (1998). Older Americans and Their Illnesses. In C. Salzman, (Ed.) *Clinical Geriatric Psychopharmacology.* (pp. 3–20) Baltimore: Williams & Wilkins.

Lemberger, L., Bergstrom, R. F., Wolen R. L., Farid, N. A., Enas, G. G., & Aronoff, G. R. (1985). Fluoxetine, Clinical pharmacology and physiologic disposition. *Journal of Clinical Psychiatry, 46,* [3, Sec. 2], 14–19.

Maes, M., Delange, J., Ranjan, R., Meltzer, H. Y., Desnyder, R., Cooremans, W., & Scharpe, S. (1997). Acute phase proteins in schizophrenia, mania and major depression: Modulation by psychotropic drugs. *Psychiatry Research, 66,* 1–11.

Manni A., Pardridge, W. M., Cefalu, W., Nisula, B. C., Bardin, C. W., Santner, S. J., & Santen, R. J. (1985). Bioavailability of albumin-bound testosterone. *Journal of Clinical Endocrinology & Metabolism, 61,* 705–710.

Maurel, P. (1996). The CYP3A family. In C. Ionnides (Ed.) *Cytochromes P450.* (pp. 241–270) Boca Raton, FL: CRC Press.

Nahoul, K., & Roger, M. (1990). Age-related decline of plasma bioavailable testosterone in adult men. *Journal of Steroid Biochemistry, 35,* 293–299.

Nikaido, A. M., Ellinwood, E. H., Heatherly, D. G., & Gupta, S. K. (1990). Age-related increase in CNS sensitivity to benzodiazepines as assessed by task difficulty. *Psychopharmacology, 100,* 90–97.

Obach, R. S., Baxter, J. G., Liston, T. E., Silber, B. M., Jones, B. C., MacIntyre, F., Rance, D. J., & Wastall, P. (1997). The prediction of human pharmacokinetic parameters from preclinical and in vitro metobolism data. *Journal of Pharmacology and Experimental Therapeutics, 283,* 46–58.

Overo, K. F., Toft, B., Christophersen, B., & Gylding-Sabroe, J. P. (1985). Kinetics of citalopram in elderly patients. *Psychopharmacology, 86,* 253–257.

Preskorn, S., Shad, M., Alderman, J., & Lane, R. (1998). Fluoxetine: Age and dose dependent pharmacokinetics and CYP 2C19 inhibition (abstract). *Clinical Pharmacology and Therapeutics, 63,* 166.

Preskorn, S. H. (1993). Recent pharmacologic advances in antidepressant therapy for the elderly. *American Journal of Medicine, 94* (suppl.5A), 2S–12S.

Richelson, E. (1997). Pharmacokinetic drug interactions of new antidepressants: A review of the effects on the metabolism of other drugs. *Mayo Clinic Proceedings, 72,* 835–847.

Rolan, P. E. (1994). Plasma protein binding displacement interactions: Why are they still regarded as clinically important? *British Journal of Clinical Pharmacology, 37,* 125–128.

Ronfeld, R. A., Tremaine, L. M., & Wilner, K. D. (1997). Pharmacokinetics of sertraline and its N-demethyl metabolite in elderly and young male and female volunteers. *Clinical Pharmacokinetics, 32* (Supp 1), 22–30.

Rudorfer, M. V, & Potter, W. Z. (1997). The role of metabolites of antidepressants in the treatment of depression. *CNS Drugs, 7,* 273–312.

Salem, S. A. M., Rajjayabun, P., Shepherd, A. M. M., & Stevenson, I. H. (1978). Reduced induction of drug metabolism in the elderly. *Age and Aging, 7,* 68–73.

Sansom, L. N., & Evans, A. M. (1995). What is the true clinical significance of plasma protein binding displacement interactions? *Drug Safety, 12,* 227–233.

Schinkel, A. H., Wagenaar, E., van Deemter, L., Mol C. A. A. M, & Borst, P. (1995). Absence of the mdr1a p-glycoprotein in mice affects tissue distribution and pharmacokinetics of dexamethasone, digoxin, and cyclosporin A. *Journal of Clinical Investigations, 96,* 1698–1705.

Shand, D. G. (1984). alpha 1-Acid glycoprotein and plasma lidocaine binding. *Clinical Pharmacokinetics, 9* Suppl 1, 27–31.

Sluzewska, A., Rybakowski, J., Bosmans, E., Sobieska, M., Berghmans, R., Maes, M,, & Wiktorowicz, K. (1996). Indicators of immune activation in major depression. *Psychiatry Research, 64,* 161–167.

Song, C., Dinan, T., & Leonard, B. E. (1994). Changes in immunoglobulin., complement and acute phase protein levels in the depressed patients and normal controls. *Journal of Affective Disorders, 30,* 283–288.

Sotaniemi, E. A., Arranto, A. J., Pelkonen, O., & Pasanen, M. (1997). Age and cytochrome P450-linked drug metabolism in humans: An analysis of 226 subjects with equal histopathologic conditions. *Clinical Pharmacology and Therapeutics, 61,* 331–339.

Thummel, K. E, & Wilkinson, G. R. (1998). In vitro and in vivo drug interactions involving human CYP3A. *Annual Review of Pharmacology and Toxicology, 38,* 389–430.

Transon, C., Lecoeur, S., Leeman, T., Beaune, P., & Dayer, P. (1996). Interindividual variability in catalytic activity and immunoreactivity of three major human liver cytochrome P450 isozymes. *European Journal of Clinical Pharmacology, 51,* 79–85.

Tucker, G. T. (1992). The rational selection of drug interaction studies: Implications of recent advances in drug metabolism. *International Journal of Clinical Pharmacology, Therapy, and Toxicology, 30,* 550–553.

von Moltke, L. L., Greenblatt, D. J., Harmatz, J. S., & Shader R. I. (1995). Psychotropic drug metabolism in old age: Principles and problems of assessment. In F. E. Bloom, & D. J. Kupfer, (Ed.), *Psychopharmacology: The Fourth Generation of Progress.* (pp. 1461–1469) New York: Raven Press.

von Moltke, L. L., Greenblatt, D. J., & Shader, R. I. (1993). Clinical pharmacokinetics of antidepressants in the elderly: Therapeutic implications. *Clinical Pharmacokinetics, 24,* 141–160.

von Moltke, L. L., Abernethy, D. R., & Greenblatt, D. J. (1998). Kinetics and dynamics of psychotropic drugs in the elderly. In C. Salzman, (Ed.), *Clinical Geriatric Psychopharmacology.* (pp. 70–93) Baltimore, MD: Williams & Wilkins.

Wacher, V. J., Wu, C. -Y, & Benet, L. Z. (1995). Overlapping substrate specificities and tissue distribution of cytochrome P450 3A and P-glycoprotein: Implications for drug delivery and activity in cancer chemotherapy. *Molecular Carcinogenesis, 13,* 129–134.

CHAPTER 5

Ethical Issues in Geriatric Psychopharmacologic Research

JASON H. T. KARLAWISH & BRYAN JAMES
DIVISION OF GERIATRIC MEDICINE, CENTER FOR BIOETHICS
AND ALZHEIMER'S DISEASE RESEARCH CENTER
UNIVERSITY OF PENNSYLVANIA

INTRODUCTION

The focus of this chapter is the ethics of research that involves elderly patients with neurodegenerative and psychiatric diseases. Society allows geropsychiatric research because it believes that research is among the best ways to improve the standard of care for elderly persons who have conditions such as anxiety, delerium, dementia, depression, and psychosis. This is scientific progressivism.

But this progressivism faces two challenges. First, some geropsychiatric patients are "vulnerable" because they have relative or even absolute impairments in their abilities to formulate and express their preferences and to make choices that protect their interests (Levine, 1986). Vulnerability can be the result of the patients' cognitive or emotional impairments, or their residence in a "total institution" such as a nursing home or psychiatric hospital. Like prisons, monasteries, and boarding schools, these are institutions where the residents must conform to routines and authorities (Goffman, 1961). Vulnerability is a challenge because it can limit a geropsychiatric patient's capacity to engage in a rational and uncoerced informed consent and to express his or her goals and risk tolerance for the development of the standard of care.

The second challenge to the ethical conduct of geropsychiatric research is how researchers design, analyze, and review research in order to make credible claims that a new treatment is both safe and effective. This challenge includes design issues such as the choice of comparison group, measures of safety and efficacy, and eligibility criteria. Particularly challenging designs include those that use a "wash-out" period when subjects stop an effective or partially effective medication (Horowitz, 1994), that "challenge" a subject to experience psychiatric symptoms (Miller & Rosenstein, 1997), and that compare a new drug to a placebo instead of a known safe and effective treatment for the disease under study (Farlow, 1998; Karlawish & Whitehouse, 1998; Knopman, Kahn, & Miles, 1998). These issues engage the often highly technical principles of rational trial design. But this does not mean that they are purely objective issues with one "right" answer. Instead, these issues are inherently moral because they engage matters of appropriate thresholds of risks and benefits that will determine progress in changing the standard of care.

We will address these challenges using the principles of research ethics developed in the 1979 *Belmont Report:* justice, beneficence and respect for persons (National Commission for the Protection of Human Subjects of Biomedical and Behavioral Research, 1979). The *Belmont Report* served as the normative foundation for the National Commission that drafted guidelines for human subjects research involving the general class of human subjects as well as separate guidelines for four vulnerable populations: children, prisoners, pregnant women, and the cognitively impaired. The moral force of the principles articulated in the *Report* endures today. Its content remains unaltered, and no new principles have been adopted.

But in the case of geropsychiatric research, we need to apply these principles with caution. All of the Commission's recommendations were ultimately adopted as federal research regulations except for the recommendations governing research that involves the cognitively impaired (Department of Health, Education, and Welfare). Recent scholarship shows that this occurred because the communities of researchers (particularly the leadership at the National Institutes of Mental Health) and research regulators at the then Department of Health, Education and Welfare disagreed sharply (Bonnie, 1997). On the one side, researchers argued that the regulations were too restrictive for the design and conduct of research that could produce evidence to improve the lives of patients with psychiatric and neurodegenerative diseases. On the other side, research regulators sought to protect vulnerable patients from participating in research that might benefit others but harm the subjects. This disagreement was never resolved. In this decade, efforts to disseminate guidelines for psychiatric research (American College of Physicians, 1989; Fletcher, Dommell, & Cowell, 1985; Keyserlingk, Glass, Kogan, & Gauthier, 1995; Melnick, Dubler, Weisbard, & Butler, 1985), write regulations (Schwartz, 1998) and resolve court cases (T. D. et al. vs. New York State Office of Mental Health, 1985) suggest that this disagreement endures. The most recent federal effort led by the National Bioethics Advisory Commission has met with the same disagreement as did the unfinished work of the

National Commission (Wadman, 1998). This history shows that while investigators and society have multiple guides to design and conduct ethical geropsychiatric research, none of them enjoy a consensus of wide support in the communities of researchers or subjects.

The continued inability to achieve consensus reflects significant disagreement upon how to address the challenges of subject vulnerability and the proper design, analysis, and review of research in order to make credible claims that a new treatment is safe and effective. The point of this chapter is to suggest ways that researchers can design and conduct geropsychiatric research that is both ethically and scientifically sound. To achieve these aims, the principles of research ethics need to be applied in context with two interrelated observations made by bioethicists, sociologists and historians of science: 1) the design and conduct of clinical research are a process grounded upon consensus within a community about what is the standard of care and how clinical research ought to change that standard (Freedman, 1987; Marks, 1997; Moreno, 1995); and 2) the ethical paradigm of clinical research is changing from the protection of subjects from research risks to the promotion of subjects' rights and interests in clinical research (Kahn, Mastroianni, & Sugarman, 1998; Karlawish & Lantos, 1997; McNeill, 1993). Our thesis is that consensus in the new ethical paradigm requires a transformation in the model of clinical research from one that separates science and ethics (a biomedical model) to one that integrates them in a community that includes investigators and subjects (a biopsychosocial model). To develop this thesis, we will examine two key issues: 1) enrolling geropsychiatric patients into research, and 2) assessing research risks and potential benefits.

ENROLLING GEROPSYCHIATRIC PATIENTS INTO RESEARCH

Geropsychiatric patients may be a vulnerable subject population because they may reside in a total institution or have impaired abilities to rationally manipulate information and express their preferences. These qualities can impair their ability to engage in an informed consent. In this section, we will examine how researchers should decide whether a person can grant an informed consent, and we will review various techniques that allow researchers to enroll ethically a subject who cannot grant an informed consent.

Tables 5.1-5.3 summarize the current consensus upon the components of informed consent, and steps to obtain it from the potential subject, or, if the subject lacks decision-making capacity, from the potential subject's proxy. The discussion here will focus upon two significant challenges in

TABLE 5.1 The Components of Informed Consent*

Disclosure:	Clear statements that this is research with descriptions of its purpose, risks, benefits and alternatives to participating in the research.
Voluntariness:	A condition marked by the absence of coercion. This is created by the researcher.
Competency:	The subject's ability to achieve at least one of four standards: 1) making a decision, 2) appreciating the consequences of the decision, 3) rationally manipulating the information, and 4) understanding the decision.
Authorization:	The subject clearly states whether he agrees to enroll.
Documentation:	The subject signs a document that contains the information disclosed (in certain kinds of low risk research, an IRB can waive this requirement).

*Adapted from Faden and Beauchamp, 1986; Grisso and Appelbaum, 1998.

geropsychiatric research: competency assessment and the enrollment of incompetent patients.

All adults are presumed competent until shown otherwise, and a competent person has the right to choose whether to enroll in clinical research. But how does an investigator assess competency? This question is critically important to the conduct of geropsychiatric research because the subjects may have impairments in their affect or cognition that prevent them from choosing competently whether to enroll in research. Unfortunately, there is no consensus upon the appropriate way to assess competency. This lack of consensus has caused significant controversy. The New York court that overturned regulations for research that involves cognitively impaired persons decided that the regulations were inadequate in part because they did not specify the standards or qualifications of the persons who assess a potential subject's competency (Anonymous, 1996). The same criticisms kept the State of Maryland from seeking legislative approval of its proposed regulations governing research that involves the decisionally impaired (Schwartz, 1998).

There is agreement that four standards exist for defining that a person has decision-making capacity and thus that person is competent:

1. Making a decision;
2. Appreciating the consequences of the decision;
3. Rationally manipulating the information; and
4. Understanding the decision (Grisso & Appelbuam, 1998).

A key controversy is which of these standards constitutes "decision-making capacity." Should a patient possess all four standards, or only

TABLE 5.2 The Steps to Obtain Informed Consent from the Subject*

STEP 1:

Verify that the person has the ability to communicate. If the person has the ability to communicate, proceed according to the structure described in Table 5.1. If the person does not have the ability to communicate and the research allows informed consent by a proxy, consult Table 5.3.

⇩

STEP 2:

Structure the process of informed consent as a dialogue. Allow the person the opportunity to include other people in the dialogue—such as a family member or trusted health care professional. For particularly complex disclosures, additional meetings may be useful.

⇩

STEP 3:

Conduct the informed consent dialogue to achieve the following goals:

Goal 1: Teach the person: (1) what is the purpose of the conversation: "I'd like to discuss this research project with you. After we talk about it, we'll go over whether you'd like to participate;" and (2) the purpose, risks, and benefits of the research.

Goal 2: Verify that the person is competent by assessing his decision-making capacity.

⇩

STEP 4:

Decision-making capacity includes: making a decision; and appreciating, recalling and rationally manipulating and understanding the information a person needs to make that decision. It is both a cognitive and moral condition. In many cases, the person's capacity is obvious. The investigator can determine whether the person has capacity by:

(1) Asking the person, "Do you have any questions about what we've discussed?"
(2) Reviewing the disclosure, e.g. "I'd like to go over some of the key points with you . . ."
(3) Having the person manipulate the information, e.g. raise the risk or change the benefits; "What would it mean of the chance of receiving a placebo control is 50% instead of 33%?"
(4) If the investigator doubts the person's capacity, he should employ a predetermined method for assessing it.
(5) A cut-off score on a measure of cognition or affect can serve to signal a patient in need of more thorough competency assessment, but it cannot serve as the assessment method.

⇩

STEP 5:

If the person does not have decision-making capacity, he or she does not have the competency to grant an informed consent. If the research allows proxy consent, proceed to Table 5.3

*Adapted from Department of Health and Human Services, 1991; Faden and Beauchamp, 1986; Grisso and Appelbaum, 1998.

TABLE 5.3 The Steps to Obtain Informed Consent from the Proxy*

STEP 1:

The research protocol should have a clear method for identifying a proxy. A key element of this is to start with the person who you determined lacks decision-making capacity. Ask the person if he can name someone who can help make the decision.

⇩

STEP 2:

Clearly inform the proxy that you determined the person lacks the capacity to make the decision.

⇩

STEP 3:

The proxy should follow the steps in Table 5.2. In addition, the proxy should be informed of the standards for proxy decision making: substituted judgment and best interests. The proxy should be encouraged to use a substituted judgment (e.g., "Try and think about this as you think your relative would."). If the proxy cannot exercise a substituted judgment, then clearly guide him through a best interests standard (e.g., "What do you think would be best for your relative?").

⇩

STEP 4:

Although the subject is not capable of an informed consent, the subject may be capable of an assent and this should be sought after proxy informed consent.

*Adapted from Department of Health, Education and Welfare, 1978; American College of Physicians, 1989; Fletcher et al., 1985; Keyserlingk et al., 1995; Melnick et al., 1985.

some combination? Furthermore, are these standards "hierarchical?" In other words, does standard 4 (understanding) follow from a patient having standards 1 thru 3? Research suggests that the answer to these questions depends upon the patient's disease. For example, affective disorders such as depression, cause emotional more than cognitive impairments. This suggests that a depressed person might be incompetent because while he retains the ability to manipulate information rationally, he does not care about or appreciate research risks (Elliott, 1997; Hirschfeld, Winslade, & Krause, 1997).

This hypothesis is supported by findings from a study that employed a capacity assessment instrument that compares the scores of healthy persons to hospitalized patients with angina, depression, or schizophrenia (Grisso & Applebaum, 1995). Using the scores of healthy persons as measures of construct validity for competency, the instrument effectively distinguished competent and noncompetent patients. In addition, the results showed that patients' competency did not obey the hierarchy of standards. Instead, a patient's competency varied depending upon the standard employed (understanding, reasoning, or appreciation). In particular, patients with depression scored as well as healthy persons and patients with angina on measures of understanding and reasoning, but, when compared to these same patients, patients with depression performed significantly worse on measures of appreciation. In contrast to these findings in patients with affective disorders, research shows that cognitive impairments caused by dementing disorders such as Alzheimer's disease can impair a person's competency in a manner that follows the hierarchy of standards (Marson, Ingram, Cody, & Harrell, 1995). These studies suggest that an investigator cannot simply assess whether a subject understands the information as a criteria for capacity assessment. Instead, a study protocol should include a clear statement of the kinds of information and standard of decision-making capacity that a subject will need to have in order to be assessed competent.

Including a method for competency assessment into a research protocol assures that the subjects are given a fair and unbiased assessment. The method should specify which of the four standards will be used and how they will be assessed. This will improve upon the current practices which use a variety of instruments or the judgment of an expert physician. Both of these practices are suboptimal. While instruments are appealing because they can standardize competency judgements, the claim that an instrument is standard is only as good as the criteria against which it is validated, and most studies validate instruments using a clinician's judgement of the patient's competence (Bean, Nishisato, Rector, & Glancy, 1996; Holzer, Gansler, Moczynski, & Folstein, 1997; Kaufman & Zun, 1995; Pruchno, Smyer, Rose, Harman-Stein, & Henderson-Laribee, 1995). This criterion has poor validity as shown by its poor inter-rater reliability (Marson, McInturff, Hawkins, Bartolucci, & Harrell, 1997) and significant disparities in physician's knowledge about competency assessment (Markson, Kern, Annas, & Glantz, 1994). In effect, an instrument that is valid based on its performance relative to a clinician's judgment can introduce contamination bias. Moreover, most instruments are validated for a particular decision by a particular kind of patient, such as whether an elderly person is competent to execute an advance directive. They cannot be used for other decisions involving other kinds of patients or decisions. A sensible approach for an investigator is to set a cut-off on a decision specific instrument as a signal to then apply the protocol's competency assessment method.

What if the subject lacks capacity to make a decision whether to enroll in the research? Three proposed solutions to address this are proxy consent from a person who is familiar with the patient and does not have a geropsychiatric illness, informed consent monitors, and research advance directives. We will address each of these solutions in turn.

Proxy Consent

Proxy consent describes informed consent from someone other than the subject, most commonly a family member. Provided the proxy adheres to standards for decision making (see Table 5.3), it is widely recommended as a means to assure that a noncompetent patient's enrollment in a study is ethical (Department of Health, Education, and Welfare, 1978; American College of Physicians, 1989; Fletcher et al., 1985; Keyserlingk et al., 1995; Melnick et al., 1985). Consensus exists on the standards that proxies should use to make a decision: substituted judgment (that is, what the patient would decide if he could decide) and best interests (that is, what a reasonable person would decide). But research shows that proxies typically do not use these standards. Proxies who claim to know what the subject would choose may act contrary to that knowledge (Sachs et al., 1994; Warren et al., 1986). No research exists that explains this. It may reflect either that researchers ineffectively communicate or enforce the standards of proxy decision making, or that proxies choose not to use the standards. To address this risk of proxies exposing noncompetent subjects to unwanted risks or benefits, standards suggest two measures. First, that the investigator seek the noncompetent subject's assent. Second, that proxies can only enroll a noncompetent subject if the IRB finds the research is either "minimal risk" or achieves a standard of benefit (Department of Health, Education, and Welfare, 1978; American College of Physicians, 1989; Fletcher et al., 1985; Keyserlingk et al., 1995; Melnick et al., 1985). In effect, the research risk and benefit assessment constrains the choices available to proxies. We will discuss the principles that should guide this assessment in the next section.

Informed Consent Monitors

Informed consent monitors (or auditors) are people other than the researchers who can determine whether the patient has decision-making capacity, obtain the subject's informed consent, assess whether a subject's informed consent endures over the course of the research, or perform all these activities (Department of Health, Education, and Welfare 1978; *T. D. et al. vs. NY State Office of Mental Health,* 1996). Monitors are widely recommended as a means to assure that a subject's or proxy's informed consent is competent and uncoerced (Dresser, 1996; High, Whitehouse, Post, & Berg, 1994). Federal regulations do allow for the use of monitors, but in practice, they are rarely employed (Department of Health and Human Services, 1991). Monitors were featured in the never-adopted federal regulations for research involving cognitively impaired adults, and are one of the chief reasons the regulations were never promulgated (Bonnie, 1997).

Recognizing that a monitor is only as good as the method used to assess decision-making capacity, a monitor can address the challenge of enrolling vulnerable patients into research. First, a monitor can address the investigator's conflict of interest. This conflict is the investigator's dual roles. In one role, the investigator seeks to protect the subject, but in the other role, the investigator wants to promote the research by enrolling subjects. Of course, this assumes that the monitor is not paid by the research budget and therefore does not have a commitment similar to the researcher to enroll subjects. A monitor can also improve subjects' performance on key elements of informed consent, such as the standard for decision-making capacity (Applebaum, Roth, Lidz, Benson, & Winslade, 1987). Finally, a monitor may be useful in the conduct of risky research that entails few benefits, or in research that involves institutionalized subjects who may experience coercive influences.

Research Advance Directives

Another means to mitigate the problems with assessing decision-making capacity is research advance directives (Sachs, 1994). Much like advance directives for clinical care, a patient can designate a proxy decision maker for research (similar to a durable power of attorney for health care decision making) and indicate what kinds of research he would or would not want to enroll in (similar to a living will for health care planning). Research advance directives feature in the proposed Maryland regulations and proposals from the National Bioethics Advisory Commission as a means to address the limits of informed consent in research that involves the cognitively impaired (Attorney General's Working Group, 1998; National Bioethics Advisory Commission, 1988). In these proposals, a research advance directive is the only legal means for a noncompetent patient to enroll in more than "minimal risk" research that does not achieve a standard of benefit.

The potential strength of research advance directives is that they introduce useful information about potential subjects' preferences that can guide the often ambiguous process of proxy informed consent. This guidance is also a potential weakness. Research on the use of clinical advance directives shows that patients vary in how closely they want the document followed (Sehgal et al, 1992). This ranges from using it as a general guide that can be set aside in light of present concerns, to a "letter of the law" obedience to it. Of course, this "strength of interpretation" could be written into the advance directive.

Another weakness is the content of the advance directive. Permissible research that involves noncompetent subjects is often described using terms such as "minimal risk" and some standard of potential benefit.

But the meanings of these terms are highly controversial. How can patients indicate the permissible kinds of research they wish to be involved in when consensus does not exist upon the meaning of the words they will use?

In summary, informed consent is an important procedural ethic to assure that a subject's decision to enroll in research respects his or her autonomous choice. However, the difficulties in assessing a person's decision making capacity, and the limitations of proxy consent, consent monitors, and research advance directives demonstrate that as important as informed consent is, it cannot assure that a person's enrollment respects his or her autonomous choice. Moreover, even if there is general consensus upon instruments available to researchers, monitors to assess decision making capacity and wide use of clearly designed research advance directives, informed consent would not address important ethical issues in clinical research that determine subjects' choices.

This chapter began with the point that society allows geropsychiatric research because it believes that it is among the best ways to improve the standard of care for these patients. This assumes that consensus exists upon the issues of what is the standard of care and how a clinical trial ought to change it. There is no reason to expect that informed consent substantively contributes to these important issues. It is a procedural ethic practiced on a subject-by-subject basis that does not address the ethical issues raised by the second challenge in geropsychiatric research: how researchers design, analyze, and review research in order to make credible claims that a new treatment is both safe and effective. To address this challenge, we must turn to the standards used to assess the risks and benefits of clinical research.

ASSESSING RESEARCH RISKS AND POTENTIAL BENEFITS

While informed consent allows an individual patient to make a personal risk and benefit assessment, the design and review of research requires a risk and benefit assessment about how to treat a collective of patients. This assessment determines the kinds of research subjects can participate in and how medicine will develop the standard of care. It serves as a critical determinant of the safety and efficacy standards for new therapies and the nature of medical progress. The principles that guide this assessment are the principles of beneficence (the risks should be minimized and the benefits maximized), and justice (the research risks and benefits should be distributed fairly among the populations that will participate in the research and benefit from its products) (National Commission, 1979).

In the case of geropsychiatric research, these principles are further specified by research risk and benefit standards. The standards describe a level of risk called "minimal risk"[1] and a level of benefit called, variously, "direct benefit" (Keyserlingk et al, 1995), "therapeutic" (American College of Physicians, 1989), "realistic prospect of direct benefit to the subject" (Melnick et al, 1985), or "reasonable prospect of direct medical benefit to the subjects" (Attorney General's Working Group, 1998a).[2] These standards are then combined with the subjects' decision-making capacity into a kind of algorithm. The normative structure is that a proxy can enroll a noncompetent subject in a clinical trial if the potential benefits of the research achieve a certain level (such as "direct benefit") or the risks are "minimal."

These standards are not part of research regulations. The most recent federal effort to use these standards has generated great controversy for the failure to include a middle strata of risk called "a minor increment above minimal risk" (Wadman, 1998). However, regardless of whether a researcher uses these standards, they reflect the consensus for the general conduct of clinical research that as the risks to subjects increase, there should be a commensurate increase in the degree of anticipated benefits (National Commission, 1979; Department of Health and Human Services, 1991).[3] This means that research reviewers must always weigh uncertain information to determine thresholds when risks become tolerable ("minimal") and benefits acceptable ("potentially beneficial"). How can the reviewers achieve this?

To begin to answer this question we need to articulate the nature of the uncertainty that justifies a clinical trial: a condition called "equipoise."

---

[1]Minimal risk is defined in federal regulations as: "The probability and magnitude of harm or discomfort anticipated in the research are not greater in and of themselves than those ordinarily encountered in daily life or the performance of routine physical or psychological examinations or tests." Department of Health and Human Services, (1991). This definition has a controversial interpretation (Karlawish & Hall, 1996). The definition of minimal risk does have a quantitative tone, "the probability and magnitude," but the claim that something is "minimal risk" is a qualitative judgment (Freedman, Fuks, & Weijer, 1993). The Belmont Report recognized this essential qualitative nature of research risk benefit assessment: "Only on rare occasions will quantitative techniques be available for the scrutiny of research protocols." (National Commission, 1979).

[2]Depending on the guidelines, there is either no definition of a standard of benefit (American College of Physicians, 1989; Fletcher et al., 1985; Melnick et al., 1985) or the following: "Reasonable prospect of direct medical benefit means that, on the basis of scientific evidence, a realistic possibility exists; that an individual's medical condition would be improved as a direct result of participation in research, including ameliorating symptoms or avoiding side effects of standard therapy." *Attorney General's Working Group,* (1998).

[3]The federal research regulations require that the IRB must ensure that "risks to subjects are reasonable in relation to anticipated benefits, if any, to subjects, and *the importance of the knowledge that may reasonably be expected to result* (46.111(a)(2)" (Department of Health and Human Services, 1991).

The term describes "a state of genuine uncertainty" whether the intervention under study is equal to, worse, or better than the standard of care, and the agreement that the design will settle that uncertainty (Freedman, 1987). In this state, beneficence dictates that a clinical trial ought to be done. In the state of equipoise, the benefits are worth the risks.

Equipoise is a consensus position. It means that agreement exists upon what is the standard of care, what research methods will change it, and the tolerable risks and acceptable benefits to achieve that change. By assigning value to the research design (i.e. "tolerable risks"), equipoise effectively links the ethical and scientific aspects of clinical care and research. The research risk and benefit standards simply formalize this consensus. How can research reviewers achieve consensus upon what design will ethically develop better therapies? Two ways to achieve this are: assessing the research risks and benefits according to the logic of clinical purpose, and addressing the ethics of peer review.

Assessing the Research Risks and Benefits According to the Logic of Clinical Purpose

The logic of clinical purpose describes a philosophic and scientific view that human subjects research should be logically based in and ethically justified by how it reflects and contributes to clinical practice (Freedman, 1990). It builds upon the axioms that the point of a clinical trial is to change clinical practice and that a good clinical trial is one whose methods are the best able to achieve this. This approach differs from one that separates the ethics and design of clinical research. An example of this separatist view is the argument that the use of a placebo control is a matter of scientific strategy with the ethics confined to the informed consent of the subject (Hirschfeld et al., 1997). This view portrays science as an objective enterprise and that scientists arrive at the design of a clinical trial without engaging in value choices such as risk and benefit tradeoffs. In fact, scientists typically do balance the risks and benefits of competing ways to arrive at a consensus position of what is the "best" design to answer the research question and to change clinical practice (Freedman, 1987; Marks, 1997; Moreno, 1995). Scientists achieve this position by answering three key value-laden questions: 1) Who is eligible for a trial? 2) What are a clinical trial's proper endpoints to measure safety and efficacy? and 3) What is a clinical trial's proper comparison group to measure efficacy and safety? We will address each of these questions in turn.

1. *Who is eligible for a trial?* Eligibility criteria determine what patients will have access to a potential new therapy and, at the close of the trial, the validity and generalizability of the trial's results. Because criteria determine who has access to research and is likely to benefit

by its results, the criteria operationalize the principle of distributive justice (that is: the research risks and benefits should be distributed fairly among the populations that will participate in the research and benefit from its products). Criteria that enroll patients who have only the disease under study and no other comorbidities may maximize the validity of the claim that the drug did or did not work to treat the disease, but they achieve this at the expense of patient access to the promising new drug and the generalizability of the study's results. Eligibility criteria create obvious trade-offs among issues of patient access, validity and generalizability.

Unfortunately, in geropsychiatric research, these trade-offs are often overlooked and criteria may seem plainly unfair. Access and generalizability are sacrificed to validity. Reviews of geropsychiatric research practice criticize the absence of well-designed trials that enroll a clinically relevant geriatric population (Baldwin, 1995; Kelly, Harvey, & Cayton, 1997; Schneider, Olin, Lyness, & Chui, 1997; Yastrubetskaya, Chiu, & O'Connell, 1997). For instance, Schneider has shown that no more than 7.9% of patients with Alzheimer's disease diagnosed at 9 Alzheimer's disease centers in California would be eligible for a clinical trial (Schneider, Olin, Lyness, et al., 1997). It is particularly concerning that although women are at greater risk to develop Alzheimer's disease, these criteria favor the enrollment of men with at least a college education. Yastrubetskaya has reported that of the 188 elderly patients referred for a phase III clinical trial of an antidepressant, 171 were depressed, but only 8 met the criteria for enrollment (Yastrubetskaya et al., 1997). Such fastidious enrollment criteria not only hinder interpreting and applying research results to the clinical setting, but they are unfair. True efficacy becomes the clinician's anecdotal experience with the new drug, a situation that can be as risky and uncertain as research itself.

The logic of clinical purpose can rationally guide the balancing of these tradeoffs by requiring that the results of a trial should be expected to change clinical practice. This is particularly true in the case of trials that will be used to substantiate claims of a drug's clinical safety and efficacy, such as phase III trials. In geropsychiatric research, this means that the trial's subjects should include a geriatric subject population that has comorbidities that resemble the kinds of patients who will use the drugs.

Criteria that select for an exclusive minority of eligible subjects do not make scientific or ethical sense, either in terms of shaping clinical practice or of providing fair access to patients whom might wish to participate in clinical trials. Such criteria make sense early in drug development when the goal is to establish whether a new drug works at all. But if the goal of a clinical trial is to promote the claim that the drug should be used in clinical practice, then that trial's eligibility criteria should reflect the clinical reality of geropsychiatric care. Patients with common medical diseases should be eligible for trials as long as there is a reasonable assurance that the patients are using medications that are unlikely to interact with the study drug. This is the among the best ways to gather credible evidence to determine whether a new drug actually works in clinical practice. It is also among the issues that substantiate the claim that a trial is "potentially beneficial." Eligibility criteria that enroll a subject population that resembles the clinical population will achieve the ends of both good science and good clinical practice.

2. *What are a clinical trial's proper endpoints to measure safety and efficacy?* Eligibility criteria engage the principle of justice in order to settle trade-offs in access and fairness. The choice of endpoints to measure safety and efficacy engages this principle as well as beneficence. To patients and clinicians, endpoints are measures of clinical practice that allow informed decision making to minimize the risks and maximize benefits of a treatment (beneficence). To clinical investigators, endpoints establish whether a drug works to treat patients with a disease (justice). In order to make these claims, the primary endpoints should show that a drug works to treat a disease by measuring a "clinically significant" change in a measure. Unfortunately, in geropsychiatric research, endpoints can be chosen to measure whether a drug works to treat a disease but not necessarily whether it works to treat patients with a disease. For example, the standard criterion for measuring the efficacy of a new antidepressant is a 50% change in the subjects' Hamilton Depression scores (HAM-D). Although this measure is preferred because it is a responsive scale that is portrayed as an "objective" measure that a drug works to treat depression, even after a 50% change in the HAM-D, a patient may still be symptomatic (Baldwin, 1995; Nemeroff, 1996). This means that measuring a "significant" change in subjects' HAM-D scores does not mean they experienced a clinically meaningful benefit.

The logic of clinical purpose guides the choice of the endpoints because it unifies the languages of clinical practice and clinical research. If what is measured in a clinical trial resembles what matters in the clinic, that trial can begin to be described as "potentially beneficial." For example, to address the clinical shortcoming of the HAM-D, recent trials of antidepressants incorporate "global measures of change." Research to develop new therapies for Alzheimer's disease use similar measures (Schneider et al,. 1997). Global measures are particularly useful in the study of chronic diseases where the goal is relief of symptoms and maximization of quality of life. They allow subjects and patients to make an overall and multi-attribute assessment of the effects of a therapy upon their illness. This kind of endpoint can bridge the gap between the languages of the clinic and clinical trials (Doody, 1988). A clinical trial that uses global measures as a primary endpoint can better achieve the principles of beneficence and justice.

3. *What is a clinical trial's proper comparison group to measure efficacy and safety?* The basic point of a clinical trial is to compare two or more interventions. This requires a control group that serves as the baseline for comparison. The control group can be a placebo or an active therapy. In clinical research, a common controversy is whether a placebo control is appropriate when a known effective treatment exists for the disease under study. For example, in Alzheimer's Disease clinical research, the development of cholinesterase inhibitor therapies such as donepezil (Rogers, Farlow, Doody, Mohs, & Friedhoff, 1998) and the NIH-funded trial that showed vitamin E slows the progression of Alzheimer's disease (Sano et al., 1997) raise the issue of whether the continued use of a placebo control is appropriate in future studies of potential therapies (Farlow, 1998; Karlawish & Whitehouse, 1998; Knopman et al., 1998). The availability of safe and effective treatments for depression raises similar issues (Baldwin, 1995).

   Three common reasons to support the use of a placebo control when an effective treatment exists are: a placebo response rate must be explicitly measured; showing superiority in an active control study often requires a large number of subjects for the study to have an acceptably low chance of false negative results, and the benefits of current therapies are sufficiently modest that they can be forgone for the study of new medications (Farlow, 1998; Lever, 1986, 1989). But these reasons have less to do with the design of scientifically sound clinical trials and more to do with judgments about acceptable benefits (beneficence), concerns about the efficient use of research resources (justice), and the need for marketing claims to state that a drug works by comparing it to a placebo control.

   The logic of clinical purpose reduces these issues to a scientifically and ethically relevant question: For the kinds of patients who will be subjects of this research, what are their current therapeutic options? The answer to this question begins to describe the choice of

> the proper control. This means that if patients have access to an effective treatment, the use of a placebo control is presumed to be scientifically and ethically invalid. According to the logic of clinical purpose, a placebo control is scientifically and ethically justified in the setting of an effective treatment if the patients with the disease would be willing to forgo the benefits of that treatment or are eligible if they have failed to respond to or cannot take standard therapy. This suggests that as the patient's perception of disease severity and the benefits of available therapies decrease, the acceptability of a placebo control design can increase.

The choices of eligibility criteria, endpoints, and comparison group are all scientific and ethical issues that engage values about tolerable risks and acceptable benefits for the individual patient (beneficence) and collective of patients (justice). Clinical researchers are quite familiar with the tradeoffs inherent in design, such as during sample size calculation, when the number of subjects (as determined by a trial's duration, endpoints and their effect sizes, number of comparison groups, and frequency of interim data analyses) must be balanced against the number of available subjects. The logic of clinical purpose can serve as an epistemic guide for investigators to work through these tradeoffs by applying the principles of justice and beneficence. But what process should they follow as they weigh these benefits, risks, and costs? The answer to this question requires addressing the ethics of peer review.

Addressing the Ethics of Peer Review

The design of clinical research is ethical if the risks are in a favorable balance with both the potential benefits and the value of the knowledge to be gained from the research (Department of Health and Human Services, 1991). Consensus upon these risk-benefit and risk-knowledge balances is largely overseen by the process of "peer review." This term describes investigators' assessment of the validity and value of a clinical trial. Validity and value are the features of ethical research. Peer review operates in quality assurance throughout the process of clinical research because it is one of the chief means to decide what kinds of research should be funded and approved and what kinds of completed research should be published.

There are several ways that peer review can influence the ethics of clinical research. At the funding end, when research priorities are set by government or industry, peer review should include a broad range of views in the committee that assesses the value of the research goals. The principle that guides these goals is the principle of justice: the research risks and benefits should be distributed fairly among the populations that will participate in the research and benefit from its products (National Commission, 1979). To assure that this principle reflects the population's interests, the review should have a democratic representation. For example, clinician and patient representatives can interject the perspectives of the clinic and the disease experience. Researchers from outside the discipline of geropsychiatry can interject innovative methodologic perspectives. Democratic representation relies upon the various members recognizing not only the strength of their unique views but their limits as well. A clinician should not be expected to contribute nuanced points on the pharmacodynamics of a new drug. This concept of democratic representation can be useful, too, in the review of particular research designs.

Presently, research designs are assessed by researchers and IRBs. Unfortunately, the interests of subjects are not well represented on these boards. Although representation from the subject community is suggested in federal research regulations (Department of Health and Human Services, 1991), IRB membership is largely composed of members of the research community. This means that the expertise of science is well represented in the research review but the patient's expertise about the disease experience is not (McNeill, 1993). Scientific expertise is necessary in order to rationally address issues such as the numbers of potential subjects, sample size, and the available valid and reliable instruments to measure endpoints. Subject expertise can add to the assessment of benefits and risks from a patient perspective. Together, the groups can achieve a democratic deliberation upon what are appropriate research risks and benefits.

Subject expertise is being incorporated into the design and review of clinical research in large part because subjects have lobbied to be part of the process (Epstein, 1996). This reflects how the paradigm of research ethics is moving from protecting subjects from research risks to representing subjects' interests in the design and conduct of research (Karlawish & Lantos, 1997; McNeill, 1993). For example, requirements for the approval of new cancer drugs have been modified to reflect the changing interests of patients with cancer. In the mid-1980s, the FDA initiated the requirement that all phase III trials of new oncologic drugs should show efficacy in either survival or quality of life (Johnson & Temple, 1985). The goal was to approve drugs that achieved documented patient needs. In 1996, the agency noted that patients wanted more rapid access to new therapies. The agency modified these requirements to allow approval on the basis of a change in a surrogate endpoint with subsequent post-approval research devoted to showing improvement in survival or quality of life (U.S. Food and Drug Administration, 1996). The issue here is that a decision that is essentially one of values—what is the measure of benefit for the approval of treatments for chronic and often incurable diseases—was resolved in a manner that tried to incorporate the biological facts with the experiences of subjects.

Democratic deliberation can be useful for addressing controversial kinds of geropsychiatric research, such as studies that evoke psychiatric symptoms in patients—the so-called "challenge studies." In this kind of study, a patient will likely not benefit, and may actually experience harm (Miller & Rosenstein, 1997). The assurance that a subject's enrollment in a study is ethical is granted by the subject's informed consent (arguably following assessment of competency according to all four standards described above and in Tables 5.1 and 5.2). But this cannot assure that the study is ethical. This relies upon weighing the risks of the study against the value of the knowledge to be gained. A favorable risk-knowledge balance is essential to justify such a study. What counts as "valuable knowledge" requires a consensus among investigators and subjects upon the kinds of knowledge that will serve useful for improving the standard of care. This consensus should be achieved by incorporating the preferences of subjects into the peer review of clinical research.

Peer review can also influence the ethics of research during the process of reviewing completed research. The approval of a clinical trial demonstrates a commitment to the value of the knowledge to be gained. That commitment should be followed through when the research is completed. Investigators should plan to publish their results, even negative results, and peer reviewers should not view negative results as less valuable than positive results. This commitment by investigators and peer reviewers is faithful to the theories of frequentist statistics that justify the design of clinical trials. "Every experiment may be said to exist only in order to give the facts a *chance* of disproving the null hypothesis" (Fisher, 1937, p. 19; emphasis ours). The point here is that a "negative trial" does not mean "useless knowledge." Instead, a negative trial means that the null hypothesis cannot be rejected with a predetermined probability of error. This may be valuable knowledge for researchers who will design subsequent trials. The failure to publish this knowledge inappropriately suppresses that knowledge from the community. This commitment to publishing data means that investigators should avoid commitments where data is owned by a third party who can suppress publication of undesirable results.

Another way that peer review can address the ethics of clinical research is if the reviewer scrutinizes the quality of the ethics of the research, in particular the reporting of IRB review and informed consent, in the same manner that the reviewer scrutinizes the science. Researchers that fail to obtain IRB review or waive a subject's informed consent without IRB approval should not be published.

In summary, researchers who adhere to the logic of clinical purpose and address the ethics of peer review can help to assure that research is ethical. This will assure that the research review will more effectively link the ethical and scientific aspects of clinical care and research. Greater confidence can be applied to the claims that the benefits outweigh the risks and that the knowledge to be gained is valuable. This is particularly important in the conduct of geropsychiatric research which faces the challenges that some subjects are vulnerable and there are competing ways to make credible claims that a new treatment is both safe and effective.

CONCLUSION

Geropsychiatric research includes a number of interrelated scientific and ethical challenges for the enrollment of subjects and the assessment of research risks and potential benefits. Recent efforts by the National Bioethics Advisory Commission to resolve these challenges have recapitulated many of the disagreements that scuttled previous national efforts (Wadman, 1998).

Researchers can begin to address these disagreements if they recognize that they are the result of difficulties in achieving consensus upon how to assess decision-making capacity, settle trade-offs in the risks and benefits of possible clinical trial designs, and address the ethical aspects of peer review. Consensus over these issues begins with the recognition that the point of a clinical trial is to change clinical practice and that clinical practice should be the result of a consensus among patients and physicians about what is the standard of care and how it ought to be changed. Human subjects research should be logically based in and ethically justified by how it reflects and contributes to this clinical practice.

Researchers should continue to adopt a biopsychosocial model that respects the simple fact that all successful clinical trials are the result of a consensus within a community about what is the standard of care and how clinical research ought to change that standard (Freedman, 1987; Marks, 1997; Moreno, 1995). The ethical paradigm that guides this consensus does not emphasize simply protecting subjects from research risks, but promoting subjects' rights and interests in clinical research (Karlawish & Lantos, 1997; McNeill, 1993). This model unifies the biomedical and social sciences, and ethics because it requires that the research design is both the most valid and valued. The assessment of a study's value is informed by the principles of research ethics and by social science that can identify what endpoints and thresholds of risks patients value, how best to allocate resources, and cognitive models to improve the practice of informed consent. This unified model is the model that should guide scientific progressivism.

ACKNOWLEDGMENT

The authors thank David Casarett, MD, MA for his careful critique of this manuscript.

REFERENCES

American College of Physicians. (1989). Cognitively impaired subjects. *Annals of Internal Medicine, 111*(10), 843–848.

Applebaum, P., Roth, L., Lidz, C., Benson, P., & Winslade, W. (1987). False hopes and best data: Consent to research and the therapeutic misconception. *Hastings Center Report, 17*, 20–24.

Attorney General's Working Group, Office of the Maryland Attorney General. (1998). *Third report of the Attorney General's Research Working Group: Consent to research: Protection of decisionally incapacitated individuals* (p. A-6). Baltimore, MD: Office of the Maryland Attorney General.

Baldwin, R. C. (1995). Antidepressants in geriatric depression: What difference have they made? *International Psychogeriatrics, 7*, 55–68.

Bean, G., Nishisato, S., Rector, N. A., & Glancy, G. (1996). The assessment of competence to make a treatment decision: An Empirical Approach. *Canadian Journal of Psychiatry, 41*,(2), 85–92.

Bonnie, R. J. (1997). Research with cognitively impaired subjects: Unfinished business in the regulation of human subject research. *Archives of General Psychiatry, 54, 105–111.*

Department of Health, Education and Welfare (1978). Protection of human subjects: Proposed regulations on research involving those institutionalized as mentally disabled. *Federal Register*, 43, 53950–53956.

Department of Health and Human Services. (1991). Federal policy for the protection of human subjects: Notices and rules. *Federal Register, 56*, 28003–28032.

Doody, R. S. (1998). Test scores in clinical trials vs performance in real life: Can clinical global assessments bridge the gap? In A. Wimo, B. Jonsson, G. Karlsson, & B. Winblad (Eds.), *Health Economics of Dementia* (pp. 311–325) New York: John Wiley and Sons.

Dresser, R. (1996). Mentally disabled research subjects: The enduring policy issues. *Journal of the American Medical Association, 276*(1), 67–72.

Elliott, C. (1997). Caring about risks: Are severely depressed patients competent to consent to research? *Archives of General Psychiatry, 54,* 113–116.

Epstein, S. (1996). *Impure science: AIDS, activism, and the politics of knowledge.* Berkeley: University of California Press.

Faden, R. R., & Beauchamp, T. L. (1986). *A history and theory of informed consent.* New York: Oxford University Press.

Farlow, M. R. (1998). New treatments in Alzheimer Disease and the continued need for placebo-controlled trials. *Archives of Neurology, 55,* 1396–1398.

Fisher, R. (1937). *The design of experiments.* London: Olivera and Boyd.

Fletcher, J. C., Dommell, W., Jr., & Cowell, D. D. (1985). Consent to research with impaired human subjects. *IRB: A Review of Human Subjects Research, 7*(6), 1–6.

Freedman, B. (1987). Equipoise and the ethics of clinical research. *New England Journal of Medicine, 317,* 141–145.

Freedman, B. (1990). Placebo-controlled trials and the local of clinical purpose. *IRB: A Review of Human Subjects Research, 12*(6), 1–6.

Freedman, B., Fuks, A., & Weijer, C. (1993) In loco parentis minimal risk as an ethical threshold for research upon children. *Hastings Center Report, 23,* 13–19.

Goffman, E. (1961). *Asylums: Essays on the social situation of mental patients and other inmates.* Chicago: Aldine.

Grisso, T., & Applebaum, P. S. (1995). Comparisons of standards for assessing patients' capacities to make treatment decision. *American Journal of Psychiatry, 152*(7), 1033–1037.

Grisso, T., & Applebaum, P. S. (19998). Abilities related to competence. *Assessing competence to consent to treatment: A guide for physicians and other health professionals* (pp. 31–60). New York: Oxford University Press.

High, D. M., Whitehouse, P. J., Post, S. G., & Berg, L. (1994). Guidelines for addressing ethical and legal issues in Alzheimer Disease research: A position paper. *Alzheimer Disease and Associated Disorders, 8*(Suppl 4), 66–74.

Hirschfeld, R. M. A., Winslade, W., & Krause, T. L. (1997). Protecting subjects and fostering research: Striking the proper balance (commentary). *Archives of General Psychiatry, 54,* 121–123.

Holzer, J. C., Gansler, D. A., Moczynski, N. P., & Folstein, M. F. (1997). Cognitive functions in the informed consent evaluation process: A pilot study. *Journal of American Academic Psychiatry Law, 25*(4), 531–540.

Horowitz, J. (1994, September 11). For the sake of science: When Tony Lamadrid, a schizophrenic patient and a research subject committed suicide, it set off a national debate: what is acceptable in human experimentation and who decides? *Los Angles Times,* p. 16.

Johnson, J. R., & Temple, R. (1985). Food and Drug Administration requirements for approval of new anticancer drugs. *Cancer Treatment Reports, 69*(10), 1155–1159.

Kahn, J. P., Mastroianni, A. C., & Sugarman, J. (1998). Implementing justice in a changing research environment. In J. P. Kahn, A. C. Mastroianni, & J. Sugarman (Eds.), *Beyond consent: Seeking justice in research* (pp. 166–173). New York: Oxford University Press.

Karlawish, J. H. T., & Landos, J. (1997). Community equipoise and the architecture of clinical research. *Cambridge Quarterly of Healthcase Ethics, 6*, 385–396.

Karlawish, J. H. T., & Whitehouse, P. J. (1998). Is the placebo control obsolete in a world after donepezil and vitamin E? *Archives of Neurology, 55*, 1420–456.

Kaufman, D. M., & Zun. L. (1995). A quantifiable, brief mental status examination for emergency patients. *The Journal of Emergency Medicine, 13*(4), 449–456.

Kelly, C. A., Harvey, R. J., & Cayton, H. (1997). Drug treatments for Alzheimer's disease. *British Medical Journal, 314*, 693–694.

Keyserlingk, E. W., Glass, K., Kogan, S., & Gauthier, S. 91995). Proposed guidelines for the participation of persons with dementia as research subjects. *Perspectives in Biology and Medicine, 38*(2), 319–362.

Knopman, D., Kahn, J., & Miles, S. (1998). Clinical research designs for emerging treatments for Alzheimer Disease: Moving beyond placebo-controlled trials. *Archives of Neurology, 55*, 1425–1429.

Leber, P. (1986). The placebo control in clinical trials (A view from the FDA). *Psychopharmacology Bulletin, 22*(1), 30–32.

Leber, P. D. (1989). Hazards of inference: The active control investigation. *Epilepsia, 30*(Suppl 1), 557–563.

Levine, R. J. (1986). *Ethics and regulation of clinical research* (2nd ed.). Baltimore: Urban & Schwarzenberg.

Marks, H. M. (1997). *The progress of experiment: Science and therapeutic reform in the United States, 1900–1990.* Cambridge: Cambridge University Press.

Markson, L., Kern, D., Annas, G., & Glantz, L. (1994). Physician assessment of patient competence. *Journal of American Geriatrics Society, 42*(10), 1074–1080.

Marson, D. C., Ingram, K. K., Cody, H. A., & Harrell, L. E. (1995). Assessing the competency of patients with Alzheimer's Disease under different legal standards. *Archives of Neurology, 52*, 949–954.

Marson, D. C., McInturff, B., Hawkins, L., Bartolucci, A., & Harrell, L. E. (1997). Consistency of physician judgements of capacity to consent in mild Alzheimer's Disease. *Journal of the American Geriatrics Society, 45*(4), 453–457.

McNeill, P. (1993). *The ethics and politics of human experimentation.* Cambridge, England: Cambridge University Press.

Melnick, V. L., Dubler, N., Wiesbard, A., & Butler, R. N. (1985). Clinical research in senile dementia of the Alzheimer's type: Suggested guidelines addressing the ethical and legal issues. *Alzheimer's Dementia: Dilemmas in Clinical Research,* 295 –310.

Miller, F., & Rosenstein, D. (1997). Psychiatric symptom-provoking studies: An ethical appraisal. *Biological Psychiatry, 42,* 403–409.

Moreno, J. D. (1995). *Deciding together: Bioethics and moral consensus.* New York: Oxford University Press.

National Bioethics Advisory Commission. *Research involving subjects with mental disorders that may affect decision-making capacity.* Rockville, MD: Department of Health and Human Services.

National Commission for the Protection of Human Subjects of Biomedical and Behavioral Research. (1979). The Belmont report: Ethical principles and guidelines for the protection of human subjects of research. *Federal Register, 44,* 23192–23197.

Nemeroff, C. B. (1996). Incentive bias? (letter to the editor). *Journal of Clinical Psychiatry, 57,* 267–269.

Pruchno, R. A., Smyer, M. A., Rose, M. S., Harman-Stein, P. E., & Henderson-Laribee, D. L. (1995). Competence of long-term care residents to participate in decisions about their medical care: A brief, objective assessment. *The Gerontologist, 35*(5), 622–629.

Rogers, S., Farlow, M., Doody, R., Mohs, R., & Freidhoff, L. (1998). A 24-week, double-blind, placebo-controlled trial of donepezil in patients with Alzheimer's Disease. *Neurology, 50,* 136–45.

Sachs, G. A., Stocking, C. B., Stern, R., Cox, D. M. (1994). Advance consent for dementia research. *Alzheimer Disease and Associated Disorders, 8*(Suppl 4), 19–27.

Sano, M., Ernesto, C., Thomas, R. G., Klauber, M. R., Schafer, K., Grundman, M., Woodbury, P., Growdon, J., Cottman, C. W., Pfeiffer, E., Schneider, L. S., & Thal, L. F. (1997). A controlled trial of selegiline, alpha-tocopherol, or both as treatment for Alzheimer's disease. *The New England Journal of Medicine, 336,* 1216–1222.

Schneider, L., Olin, J., Doody, R., Clark, C., Morris, J., Reisberg, B., Schmitt, F., Grundman, M., Thomas, R., & Ferris. S. (1997). Validity and reliability of the Alzheimer's Disease Cooperative Study: Clinical global impression of change. The Alzheimer's Disease cooperative study. *Alzheimer Disease and Associated Disorders, 11S,* S22–S32.

Schneider, L. S., Olin, J. T., Lyness, S. A., & Chui, H. C. (1997). Eligibility of Alzheimer's Disease clinic patients for clinical trials. *Journal of American Geriatrics Society, 45*, 923–928.

Schwartz, J. (1998, January). *Update on Maryland Attorney General's Working Group*. Paper presented at the National Bioethics Advisory Commission, Arlington, Virginia.

Sehgal, A., Galbraith, A., Chesney, M., Schoenfeld, P., Charles, G., & Lo, B. (1992). How strictly do dialysis patients want their advance directive followed? *Journal of American Medical Association, 267*, 59–63.

T. D. v. New York State Office of Mental Health, 650 N.Y.S. 2d 173 (App. Div., 1st Dept, 1996).

U.S. Food and Drug Administration (1996). *Reinventing the regulation of cancer drugs: Accelerating approval and expanding access*. Rockville, MD.

Wadman, M. (1998). Ethical protection for subjects "could stifle psychiatric research." *Nature, 394*, 713.

Warren, J. W., Sobal, J., Tenney, J. H., Hopes, J. M., Damron, P. D. D., Levenson, S., DeForge, B. R., & Muncie, H. L. (1986). Informed consent by proxy (An issue in research with elderly patients). *The New England Journal of Medicine, 315*, 1124–1128.

Yastrubetskaya, O., Chiu, E., & O'Connell, S. (19997). Is good clinical research practice for clinical trials good clinical practice? *International Journal of Geriatric Psychiatry, 12*, 227–231.

CHAPTER 6

Psychotropic Drug Use in Home Health Care: Problems and Directions for Research

SARAH MEREDITH & WAYNE A. RAY
DEPARTMENT OF PREVENTIVE MEDICINE
VANDERBILT UNIVERSITY SCHOOL OF MEDICINE

INTRODUCTION

Elderly people receive professional health care in a variety of settings—hospitals, clinics, doctor's offices, skilled nursing facilities, assisted living complexes and in their own homes. Each setting differs both in terms of the morbidity of the population and the opportunities to improve patient care. Thus, studies to define and improve quality of care for older people need to take into consideration the setting in which the care is provided.

In recent years, there has been growing recognition of the clinical and economic consequences of suboptimal pharmacotherapy,[1–3] to which older people are particularly vulnerable. Inappropriate medication use has been documented in the elderly noninstitutionalized population,[4, 5] as well as in long-term care[6–11] and inpatient settings,[12] leading to the development of programs to improve the quality and economy of prescribing. Approaches have included provider education programs in outpatient care,[13, 14] nursing homes,[15, 16] and hospitals,[17] and a variety of policy changes such as mandated drug utilization review for Medicaid,[18] explicit criteria for use of psychotropic drugs in long-term care,[19] and prior authorization requirements.[20]

One clinically important setting in which there has been little research regarding medication use is in home health care settings. Home health care agencies provide professional nursing, physical therapy, and other services to patients with acute and chronic health care needs in their homes. Home health care serves predominantly elderly patients who receive coverage for visiting nurse services from Medicare. It is preferred by patients to institutional alternatives,[21, 22] and can be more cost-effective.[21] Medicare utilization and expenditures for home health care are growing rapidly.[23] The increasing number of community-dwelling older persons with functional limitations is likely to further increase the demand for home health services.

Suboptimal use of medications is likely in home health care patients. Such patients are frequent medication users, and advanced age and frailty may increase their susceptibility to adverse medication effects. For the large number of patients who enter home health following a hospital stay, either the change of medications that frequently occurs in hospital[24] or deterioration of health may increase the risk of medication problems. The home care setting also offers great opportunities to improve medication use. Unlike most community residents, patients who receive home health care are closely monitored by nurses, whose role includes clinical assessment and medication education. A medication review capacity could become a valuable component of home care provider services.

THE HOME CARE SETTING

The use of home health services in the United States has increased dramatically, largely due to liberalization of the requirements for Medicare coverage in the 1970s and 1980s.[25] In 1974, just under 400 thousand Medicare enrollees received home health care services (less than 2% of enrollees); in 1984, 1.5 million, and in 1995, nearly 3.5 million Medicare enrollees received services at home, 10% of the total.[26] Not only have the number of people served increased, but so have the numbers of visits, from 21 per person served in 1974 to 72 in 1995 (see Figure 6.1).

Over half of the people who receive home health care services in the United States are 65 or over,[27] and among that population, the majority are women. In a 1994 survey of home health care users aged 65 years or older, 70% were over the age of 74 and 71% were female.[28] Among Medicare enrollees, 14% of those aged 75–84 and 24% of those 85 years or over had home health care services in 1995.[26] Compared with Medicare enrollees who did not have services, those who did were poorer, more likely to live alone, and required more help with Activities of Daily Living (ADLs) and Instrumental Activities of Daily Living (IADLs).[29]

Medicare limits home health care benefits to those who are homebound and in need of intermittent skilled nursing care or physical, occupational or speech therapy, which must be prescribed by a physician.[25] Although Medicare home health services were intended to facilitate earlier discharge from hospital and originally limited to patients who had been in hospital,[23] only about half of all Medicare home health admissions and less than a quarter of all visits are within 30 days of hospital discharge.[29, 30] Thus a great deal of the home health care currently provided is long-term community care for the frail elderly population.

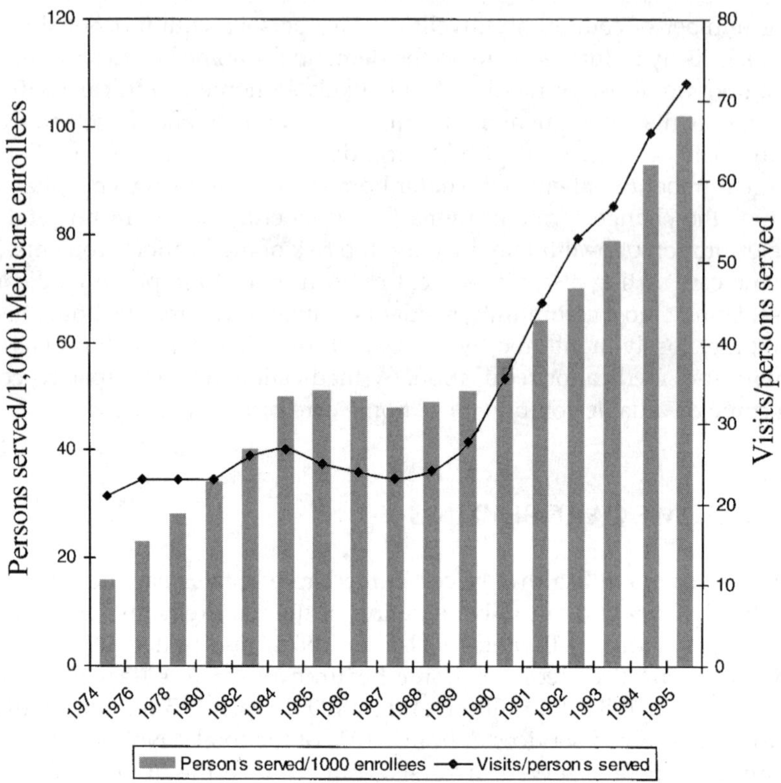

FIGURE 6.1 Medicare home health service use by year, 1974–95.
Note. From "Medicare and Medicaid Statistical Supplement," 1997, *Health Care Financing Review,* 1997 Statistical Supplement, p. 132.

Over 80% of home health care patients receive skilled nursing services,[28] mainly for chronic diseases such as heart failure, diabetes, cerebrovascular disease and musculoskeletal disorders.[26] Very few patients (<2%) have a primary psychiatric diagnosis,[28, 29] however, comorbidity in this population is common: in a 1986 survey of Medicare home health admissions, 18% were categorized as having mental functional limitations;[31] and in 1992, 16% of Medicare home health care users had a history of Alzheimer's disease or another mental disorder.[29] A study of elderly patients admitted to a home health agency found that, based on the Mini-Mental State Examination, 60% were cognitively impaired.[32] These figures are consistent with the high prevalence of both cognitive impairment and symptoms of anxiety and depression found in surveys of homebound elderly people.[33, 34]

The growing use of assisted living, adult day care, and other alternatives to long-term care provided by nursing homes may further increase the use of home health services. These alternatives to nursing homes are increasingly popular with older persons and their families, as they are perceived as providing a higher quality of life with greater autonomy. However, most do not have sufficient staff to meet the needs of people with the level of functional impairment requiring long-term care. Home health agencies are frequently used for this purpose, and if this trend continues, it will change the case mix of the home care population, increasing the levels of comorbidity and functional impairment. It will also result in greater use of home health services for chronic rather than acute conditions.

While the use of home health care has increased, physician involvement in that care appears to have decreased.[35] Certainly, the number of physicians who see patients in their homes has declined over time, and whereas nearly half of Medicare beneficiaries who received house calls in 1993 were also in receipt of home health agency services, they accounted for less than 5% of all Medicare home health care patients.[36] Although most people who have home health care services paid for by Medicare have a physician office visit in the same year,[29] their disabilities and homebound status are likely both to limit their access to their doctors and impede comprehensive medical assessment.

The high levels of psychiatric morbidity among patients with limited contact with mental health care professionals are grounds for concern. Important treatable morbidities, such as depression, may be unrecognized, or, if recognized, be treated suboptimally. Treatment may be provided for symptoms such as sleep problems or agitation, but with failure to recognize an underlying problem such as major depression. Medical conditions, such as infections or endocrine imbalances that cause psychiatric symptoms, may be unrecognized.

There have been numerous calls for increased physician involvement in home health care, including from the American Medical Association and the Health Care Financing Administration.[23,35,37,38] The physician is a vital member of the multidisciplinary home care team, and important aspects of patient assessment, such as functional status and psychosocial circumstances, are better judged in the home than in the doctor's office or hospital. However, physicians can still take an active part in home health care without making house calls, provided there is easy and effective communication between them and the home care staff, in particular with the attending nurse. Unfortunately, difficulty in contacting physicians is a common complaint among visiting nurses, and the frequent use by physicians of office staff to act as intermediaries, and the itinerate nature of home care nursing mean that direct communication may be less frequent than is desirable.[39]

Physicians have a particular role in medication assessment because it is they who prescribe drugs. Considerable discrepancy has been observed between medication histories taken in the home and those taken in an outpatient setting,[40] and it seems likely that the former is the more accurate. Inappropriate drug combinations or duplications are a particular hazard when more than one physician is prescribing medications for a patient.[41]

MEDICATION USE

Most elderly people take drugs, both prescribed by a physician and not. Between 60% and 80% of community-dwelling older people in the United States take at least one prescribed medication and a similar proportion take non-prescription drugs.[42–44] The older the individual, the more likely they are to have medications prescribed and the greater the number of different medications they are likely to take.[42, 43] Home health care patients, as might be expected of a frail elderly population, are very frequent users of medication. All but a few take at least one prescription drug, and the majority take four or more.[31, 45] In a survey of medication use in an elderly rural population in Pennsylvania, home health care within the past year was the strongest risk factor for increasing medication use, even after adjustment for demographic variables and other health service use.[43]

Psychotropic medications are used frequently by older people prevalence estimates from cross-sectional surveys range from 9 to 25%.[42–44] Benzodiazepines are the most commonly prescribed class of psychotropic medication, but antidepressants and, to a lesser extent, antipsychotic drugs are also frequently used (see Table 6.1). The prevalence of psychotropic drug use is highest in the oldest age groups, in which it is estimated that over 10% take benzodiazepines. Of particular concern are the long-acting benzodiazepines, considered inappropriate in the elderly because of their associated psychomotor effects (see below). Recent surveys found that 5 to 6% of community dwelling-elderly people were taking long-acting benzodiazepines.[4, 5] Cognitive impairment, which is common in home health patients, has been found to be associated with generally lower levels of drug use, but increased use of psychotropic medications.[46] Although some of the increased use may be attributed to increased psychiatric morbidity, the prevalence of benzodiazepine use found in this population gives cause for concern.

The frequency of psychotropic drug use in home health patients is unknown, but likely to be greater than for community-dwelling elderly people as a whole. The medication database of one home care agency included among the list of the 50 most common drugs taken by patients admitted in 1994 several benzodiazepines, including longer-acting preparations such as

TABLE 6.1 Psychotropic Medication Use in Community-Dwelling Elderly People from Cross-Sectional Surveys

<table>
<tr><th>Population</th><th>No.</th><th>Age</th><th>Drug Class</th><th colspan="7">Percentage Who Were Taking Medications of That Class</th></tr>
<tr><th></th><th></th><th></th><th></th><th>All</th><th>Female</th><th>Male</th><th>65–74</th><th>75–79</th><th>80–84</th><th>≥85</th></tr>
<tr><td>Rural Pennsylvania, 1987–89[43]</td><td>1360</td><td>≥65</td><td>Benzodiazepines</td><td>5.9</td><td>7.0</td><td>4.5</td><td>5.5</td><td colspan="2">5.9</td><td>10.8</td></tr>
<tr><td></td><td></td><td></td><td>Antidepressants</td><td>2.4</td><td>3.5</td><td>1.0</td><td>1.7</td><td colspan="2">3.3</td><td>4.6</td></tr>
<tr><td></td><td></td><td></td><td>Antipsychotics</td><td>1.3</td><td>1.3</td><td>1.3</td><td>1.1</td><td colspan="2">1.7</td><td>1.5</td></tr>
<tr><td>Santa Monica, California</td><td>414</td><td>≥75</td><td>Benzodiazepines</td><td>11.1</td><td>13.1</td><td>6.5</td><td>–</td><td>10.2</td><td colspan="2">11.9</td></tr>
<tr><td></td><td></td><td></td><td>Antidepressants</td><td>3.4</td><td>4.1</td><td>1.6</td><td>–</td><td>5.9</td><td colspan="2">1.3</td></tr>
<tr><td></td><td></td><td></td><td>Antipsychotics</td><td>1.7</td><td>1.4</td><td>2.4</td><td>–</td><td>2.1</td><td colspan="2">1.3</td></tr>
</table>

flurazepam and diazepam, SSRIs, and haloperidol (D. Frey, personal communication, September 1998).

PSYCHOTROPIC DRUGS: HAZARDS AND WAYS TO REDUCE THEIR FREQUENCY

The widespread use of psychotropic medications by the generally frail patients who receive home health care services raises several concerns. Most presently used psychotropic drugs have substantial potential to cause adverse effects, which requires the clinician to balance carefully the potential benefit of the drug versus the risks of side effects. The therapeutic goals of psychotropic medication are sometimes imprecise or outdated.[47] Thus, a hypnotic started in hospital may be continued after the patient returns home with minimal evaluation.

The psychotropic drug regimen may not have been well tailored to the needs of the older patient. Age-related changes in pharmacokinetics and pharmacodynamics may increase the central nervous system (CNS) effects of medications. Reduced hepatic circulation may increase blood concentrations of compounds with high first-pass extraction or clearance. Loss of efficiency of oxidative metabolism and renal function may prolong elimination half-lives. The increase in fat-to-lean body mass ratio can increase volume of distribution for lipophilic compounds and the decrease in serum albumin can increase free concentrations of protein-bound drugs. For some drugs, there is evidence that receptor sensitivity increases with age. Thus, it is prudent to start with very low doses and to increase cautiously. Reevaluation of patients often reveals that adequate symptom control is possible at lower doses. Whenever possible, compounds with long-elimination half-life or for which metabolism is impaired with age should be avoided.

Adverse effects of a medication, of which the original prescriber may be unaware, could change the risk:benefit assessment. Reevaluation may be appropriate for patients taking benzodiazepines who fall or who become confused, or for patients taking a cyclic antidepressant who are afraid to get up because of severe orthostasis.

Use of multiple psychotropic medications will almost certainly increase the risk of adverse effects, so it is important to assure that such use is indicated. In older persons, concurrent use of multiple sedative medications is sufficiently common[48, 49] that additive or other synergistic CNS effects may increase the risk of adverse psychomotor effects. Use of multiple psychotropic medicines has been linked with increased risk of falls[50] and is one of the more common causes of hospitalization for delirium.[51] Similarly, use of multiple medications with anticholinergic activity,[52] including antidepressants, antihistamines, antiparkinsonian drugs, and antipsychotics, may impair psychomotor function.

Benzodiazepines

Because of their well-established short-term efficacy and high safety relative to older sedative agents, benzodiazepines currently are the most frequently prescribed drugs for the management of anxiety and insomnia in the elderly. Although zolpidem is not a benzodiazepine, its pharmacodynamic properties are comparable to those of benzodiazepines.[53] Benzodiazepines also are useful as anticonvulsants, muscle relaxants, adjuncts to general anesthesia, and in the management of alcohol withdrawal, although fewer than 5% of prescriptions are for these indications.[54, 55] Among the elderly, 85% or more of total benzodiazepine use is for more than 30 days,[54, 56] despite limited data supporting long-term efficacy.[57]

All benzodiazepines bind to high-affinity receptors on the widely distributed γ-aminobutyric acid (GABA) receptor complex,[58] which is thought to underlie both their therapeutic and adverse effects. The primary differences in the clinical effects of currently available compounds are determined by pharmacokinetic characteristics. The elimination half-lives of benzodiazepines and their active metabolites range from under 2 hours for midazolam to 96 or more hours for desalkylflurazepam,[58] the active metabolite of flurazepam and quazepam. Long half-life drugs are most likely to accumulate and to produce residual sedation, whereas those with very short half-lives are more likely to produce rebound insomnia or other withdrawal effects when drug is stopped.

Benzodiazepines impair psychomotor function in a dose-related manner,[59] and there are considerable data that impairment increases with age.[59, 60] Epidemiologic studies have found that in older populations benzodiazepines are associated with increased risk of falls[61–69], fall-related injuries[54, 70–74], and motor vehicle crashes[56, 75]. Other adverse effects of benzodiazepines directly related to their pharmacologic properties include impairment of short-term memory, confusion, and habituation.[76]

Reevaluation of a home-health patient taking a benzodiazepine thus may provide several benefits. Concurrent use of more than one benzodiazepine is not uncommon[41] and rarely, if ever, is clinically justified. Patients taking both a benzodiazepine and another CNS-active medication are at higher risk of adverse effects; it often is possible to stop at least one of these. For elderly patients, doses commonly used may be too high; thus, a trial of dose reduction may find a lower dose that provides adequate control of symptoms. Long-acting compounds such as diazepam, quazepam, or flurazepam should generally be avoided; intermediate or short-acting compounds, such as lorazepam or temazepam are preferred. For patients with evidence of a serious adverse benzodiazepine effect, such as acute confusion or a recent fall, the patient may benefit by trial of a tapered withdrawal,[77] although this process is likely to be difficult.

Antidepressants

Although depression has been treated with a variety of pharmacologic agents, three classes of medication now account for nearly all antidepressant use in clinical practice, namely heterocyclic compounds, selective serotonin reuptake inhibitors (SSRIs), and trazodone. Tricyclic and other heterocyclic antidepressants (TCAs), particularly nortriptyline, have been the recommended pharmacologic treatment for depression in older patients.[78] The therapeutic effects of these agents are thought to result from the inhibition of the reuptake of serotonin (5HT) and norepinephrine at the presynaptic nerve ending.[79] These effects produce psychomotor impairment[59] and orthostasis,[80–83] particularly among patients with concomitant cardiac disease,[84] which have been thought to increase risk falls[85, 86] and other unintentional injuries.[59] Because frail home-care residents are very susceptible to falls and related injuries, this possible adverse effect is of major concern. The anticholinergic effects of cyclic antidepressants also may increase the risk of confusion or delirium and adversely affect memory.[50] Susceptibility to TCA adverse effects is thought to increase with age.[87]

SSRIs lack the sedative, anticholinergic, and cardiovascular side effects of cyclic antidepressants. Fluoxetine was the first widely used agent in this class in the U.S.; several others now are available in the U.S. However, among older patients, these drugs can produce agitation, insomnia, and weight loss.[88] SSRI antidepressants also are considerably more expensive than TCAs,[89] and, among nursing home patients, recent evidence shows that these drugs are associated with a similar risk of falling to that of TCAs.[90]

Trazodone is an atypical antidepressant that has pronounced sedative effects.[89] Although trazodone is not thought to be a highly effective antidepressant,[89] it is commonly prescribed for agitation or insomnia.[91]

For home health patients being treated with antidepressants, there are several opportunities to improve therapy. Those taking TCAs who have severe orthostasis and a recent history of fall or other unintentional injury or who show confusion, memory impairment, or other evidence of anticholinergic toxicity may be reevaluated to consider changing to an SSRI antidepressant.[77] This may be particularly important for patients on multiple drugs with CNS, adrenergic, or anticholinergic effects. For all patients, the response to therapy may be evaluated, as failure to achieve adequate doses is a common reason for therapeutic failures.[89]

Because mood disorders are common in elderly patients, particularly those with medical comorbidities,[92] and are often unrecognized,[93] it is likely that many home-health patients will have untreated major depression. Because untreated major depression confers substantial excess morbidity and mortality[94–100] and because depression is eminently treatable, even in the frail elderly,[93] bringing such patients to medical attention should have high priority. Home health care providers, who visit patients in their homes and often interact with relatives or other care givers, may have a unique opportunity to perform this function.

Antipsychotics

A major contemporary trend is the shift of care for functionally impaired older patients away from nursing homes and other institutional settings. Home-health providers often are used to provide essential services formerly provided by nursing home staff, either in the patient's home or in an assisted living facility. In the past, dementia was a common reason for admission to the nursing home. The trend away from nursing homes is thus likely to increase the number of home-health patients with dementia and its behavioral manifestations.

Antipsychotic medications are commonly used for treatment of behavioral manifestations of dementia. Indeed, among noninstitutionalized elderly patients, this is probably the most common reason for antipsychotic use. Although there is substantial clinical experience that antipsychotics calm acutely agitated patients,[101, 102] their efficacy for long-term behavior management is less certain.[101–103] The frequent and serious adverse effects of antipsychotics[104] include tardive dyskinesia and other movement disorders,[105] dystonia,[104] peripheral and central anticholinergic toxicity,[6] postural hypotension,[104] impaired alertness,[104] affective blunting,[104] social withdrawal,[101] and an association with increased risk of falls[106, 107] and hip fractures.[1]

Management of behavior due to dementia may be an important component of maintaining a patient in a community setting. However, reevaluation of patients taking antipsychotics may permit achieving this goal in ways that reduce medication-associated risks to the patient.[8] For such patients, home-health providers can evaluate use of nonpharmacological modalities and consider trial of a gradual reduction of dose. Indeed, federally mandated guidelines for such reevalulation in nursing home residents reduced antipsychotic use in this population by approximately one quarter.[19] Home-health providers also can minimize the exposure of patients taking antipsychotics to other medications with CNS, adrenergic, or anticholinergic effects.

IMPROVING PSYCHOTROPIC DRUG USE IN HOME HEALTH CARE: OPTIONS AND OBSTACLES

Medicare has mandated that certified home health agencies identify all of the patient's medications and screen for ineffective drug therapy, adverse reactions and allergies, and contraindicated drugs. However, there is no process (or reimbursement) specified for achieving these goals. Although many agencies have developed standardized approaches to medication inventory and teaching, there are no procedures specified to resolve problems that are identified by screening, and there is little research either documenting or seeking to improve medication use in this setting.[108]

As we have described, there are many ways to improve psychotropic drug use in older people that would be particularly appropriate to the home health setting. Unlike most community patients, those receiving home health care are visited by registered nurses, who can gather information on both medication use and determinants of appropriateness. Nurses have the clinical training and skills to evaluate patients, coordinate the procedures needed to change regimens and to monitor the effects of medication change or withdrawal. Thus home health provides excellent opportunities to improve drug treatment, whether by monitoring the patient and supporting them during reduction of a potentially hazardous drug, such as a long-acting benzodiazepine, or helping to identify unmet needs for treatment, such as unrecognized depression. However, the structure needed to make the most of the opportunities afforded by home health care is currently lacking.

A medication review capacity could become a valuable component of home care provider services. It may be particularly appropriate for those who use home health for extended periods of time. Medication use and length of stay are closely related. A recent study found that those with no medications received an average of 13 visits in the course of an admission compared with 26 visits for those with 7 or more drugs.[31] Thus, long stayers use more medications, and will be more likely to have suboptimal medication use, but the greater number of visits also provides more time for visiting care providers to identify medication problems and coordinate changes.

Improving suboptimal medication use in home care settings could also have substantial economic as well as clinical benefits. Although we are not aware of studies of the costs of inappropriate drug use in the home care setting, estimates from the Health Care Financing Administration[31] and from the National Medical Care Expenditures Survey[109] suggest that home care patients spend $4 billion annually on medications. Other data suggest it is reasonable to assume that an equal volume of health care expenditures is generated by adverse medication effects.[110, 111] Although better studies are needed to quantify the benefits of more rational drug use in the home care setting, these approximate estimates suggest that even a 10% reduction in suboptimal use potentially could generate $800 million in annual savings.

Although there are considerable opportunities and potential benefits, there are also a number of obstacles to medication improvement in the home care setting. Perhaps the most important of these is the lack of physician involvement and the barriers to communication discussed above. Any modification to a patient's drug regimen must, quite rightly, be agreed to by the responsible physician. However, without open channels of communication, it may be difficult for the nurse to discuss medication issues with the physician. The nurse may also lack the confidence or pharmacological knowledge to feel comfortable initiating a discussion of possible medication changes with a doctor, and the line of least resistance must be tempting, particularly as it is the physician and not the nurse who is responsible for drug prescribing. Elderly home care patients often have a combination of physical and mental medical problems. The nurses and physicians looking after them may lack the psychogeriatric training to manage some of the more complex problems. In addition, reimbursement pressures have resulted in shorter lengths of stay and more focused treatment plans, which have reduced the opportunities for intervention. Finally, the information systems and the accuracy of medication recording in many home care agencies may be inadequate for the purposes of medication review. We found frequent errors in the recording of drugs in a study which used the computerized records of two large home care agencies to screen for possible medication problems. Accurate drug histories are an essential prerequisite for any medication review program.

Previous research in long-term care settings, many with similarly functionally impaired patients, has provided models of medication regimen improvement that could be applied to the home care setting.

Academic Detailing

Focused provider education can result in reduction of potentially inappropriate psychotropic use, improvement in patient function, and no deterioration of psychiatric symptoms.[15, 16, 112, 113] Mark Beers extended this model to other types of drugs and effectively utilized computerized pharmacy records to reduce the labor costs of medication review[114]. The success of these projects has led to national dissemination of their guidelines and to initiatives within the Health Care Financing Administration to encourage all nursing homes in the U.S. to conduct this type of provider educational program. However, although this is a useful approach and such initiatives should be continued, it does not take full advantage of the involvement of a visiting nurse provided in the home care setting.

Computerized Drug Utilization Review (DUR)

Computerized DUR is widely used, but has been criticized for lack of evidence of benefit, for producing clinically irrelevant alerts, and for failure to consider under-use of effective medication.[115] Furthermore, commercially available DUR systems (usually operated by chain pharmacies and prescription benefit managers) have not been designed to screen for problems in this vulnerable patient population.

Community Pharmacist

Clinical pharmacists working in hospital inpatient[116] and outpatient[117] settings have been shown in randomized controlled trials to reduce inappropriate prescribing for elderly patients. Unfortunately, evidence is lacking of similar efficacy in community practice.[118, 119] Community pharmacists recognize many potential drug-related problems,[45, 119] and educational programs can improve their identification rate[120] but to our knowledge, this has not been shown to have reduced the frequency of medication problems in their elderly clients. Possible explanations for the difference in outcomes for hospital-based compared with community pharmacists include easier communication between pharmacists and physicians, and greater familiarity with and therefore greater respect for pharmacists in the hospital setting.

Nurse-Pharmacist Collaboration

We are currently testing the efficacy of an intervention model for home health in which drug histories and clinical information collected by the visiting nurse are screened for specific medication problems. When a potential problem is identified, the attending nurse consults with a pharmacist about ways to resolve the identified problem using guidelines provided.[77] The role of the pharmacist is to educate the nurse about the medications and the guidelines for problem resolution, to provide clinical consultation for difficult cases, and to give the nurse sufficient confidence to be able to discuss the problem with the physician. We have yet to determine whether this model will be successful in reducing medication-related problems in home health. However, a major obstacle we have encountered has been difficulty in communication between the nurses, pharmacists, and physicians. Some home care agencies employ a pharmacy consultant, and it may be that such a model may work better in this situation.

Fully Integrated Care

There are examples of programs in the United States in which multidisciplinary teams, which include a physician, care for frail elderly patients at home, however, they are the exception rather than the rule. Although such programs have not been designed primarily for the reduction of medication-related problems, and may be no more effective in that respect than the more fragmented care usually provided, it would seem likely that interventions to improve medication use in that setting would have a better chance of success.

CONCLUSION

There are both considerable needs and good opportunities to improve medication use in home health care. The frequent use, attendant hazards, and potential benefits of psychotropic medication make these drugs prime candidates for attention. However, effective models for patient assessment, medication review, and intervention in the home care setting are lacking. Research in this area is sorely needed if we are to provide good quality care for frail elderly people in their own homes. Clearly, to meet the multiple physical and psychosocial health care needs of this population requires a multidisciplinary approach that is difficult to achieve within the fragmented health care system available to most Americans.

REFERENCES

1. Ray WA, Griffin MR, Schaffner W, Baugh DK, Melton LJ. Psychotropic drug use and the risk of hip fracture. *N Engl J Med* 1987; 316:363–369.
2. Shalat L, True LD, Fleming LE, Pace P. Kidney cancer in utility workers exposed to polychlorinated biphenyls (PCBs). *Br J Ind Med* 1989; 46:823–824.
3. Schondelmeyer SW, Thomas J, III. Data watch: Trends in retail prescription expenditures. *Health Aff* (Millwood) 1990; 9:131–145.
4. Wilcox SM, Himmelstein DU, Woolhandler S. Inappropriate drug prescribing for the community-dwelling elderly. *JAMA* 1994; 272:292-296.
5. Stuck AE, Beers MH, Steiner A, Aronow HU, Rubenstein LZ, Beck JC. Inappropriate medication use in community-residing older persons. *Arch Intern Med* 1994; 154:2195–2200.

6. Blazer DG, Federspiel CF, Ray WA, Schaffner W. The risk of anticholinergic toxicity in the elderly: A study of prescribing practices in two populations. *J Gerontol* 1983; 38:31–35.
7. Ray WA, Federspiel CF, Schaffner W. A study of antipsychotic drug use in nursing homes: Epidemiologic evidence suggesting misuse. *Am J Pub Health* 1980; 70:485–491.
8. Ray WA, Taylor JA, Meador KG, Lichtenstein MJ, Griffin MR, Fought R, et al. Reducing antipsychotic drug use in nursing homes: A controlled trial of provider education. *Arch Intern Med* 1993; 153:713–721.
9. Beers M, Avorn J, Soumerai SB, Daniel EE, Sherman DS, Salem S. Psychoactive medication use in intermediate-care facility residents. *JAMA* 1988; 260:3016–3020.
10. Avorn J, Dreyer P, Connelly K, Soumerai SB. Use of psychoactive medication and the quality of care in rest homes. *N Engl J Med* 1989; 320:227–232.
11. Gurwitz JH, Soumerai SB, Avorn J. Improving medication prescribing and utilization in the nursing home. *J Am Geriatr Soc* 1990; 38:542–552.
12. Avorn J, Soumerai SB, Taylor W, Wessels MR, Janousek J, Weiner M. Reduction of incorrect antibiotic dosing through a structured educational order form. *Arch Intern Med* 1988; 148:1720–1724.
13. Avorn J, Soumerai SB. Improving drug-therapy decisions through educational outreach. A randomized controlled trial of academically based "detailing". *N Engl J Med* 1983; 308:1457–1463.
14. Ray WA, Schaffner W, Federspiel CF. Persistence of improvement in antibiotic prescribing in office practice. *JAMA* 1985; 253:1774–1776.
15. Avorn J, Soumerai SB, Everitt DE, Ross-Degnan D, Beers MH, Sherman D, et al. A randomized trial of a program to reduce the use of psychoactive drugs in nursing homes. *N Engl J Med* 1992; 327:168–173.
16. Thapa PB, Meador KG, Gideon P, Fought RL, Ray WA. Effects of antipsychotic withdrawal on elderly nursing home residents. *J Am Geriatr Soc* 1994; 42:280–286.
17. Buchwals D, Soumerai SB, Vandevanter N, Wessels MR, Avorn J. Effect of hospitalwide change in clindamycin dosing schedule on clinical outcome. *Rev Infect Dis* 1989; 11:619–624.
18. Feinberg JL. OBRA '90: Remnants of the Medicaid Prudent Pharmaceutical Purchasing Act become law. *The Consultant Pharmacist* 1991; 6:6–11.
19. Shorr RI, Fought RL, Ray WA. Changes in the use of antipsychotic drugs in nursing homes following implementation of OBRA-87. *JAMA* 1994; 271:358–362.

20. Smalley WE, Griffin MR, Fought RL, Sullivan L, Ray WA. Effect of a prior-authorization requirement on the use of nonsteroidal antiinflammatory drugs by Medicaid patients. *N Engl J Med* 1995; 332:1612–1617.
21. Cummings JE, Hughes SL, Weaver FM, Manheim LM, Conrad KJ, Nash K, et al. Cost-effectiveness of veterans administration hospital-based home care. *Arch Intern Med* 1990; 150:1274–1280.
22. Jones EW, Densen PM, Brown SD. Posthospital needs of elderly people at home: Findings from an eight-month follow-up study. *Health Serv Res* 1989; 24:643–664.
23. Welch HG, Wennberg DE, Welch WP. The use of Medicare home health care services. *N Engl J Med* 1996; 335:324–329.
24. Burns JMA, Sneddon I, Lovell M, McLean A, Martin BJ. Elderly patients and their medication: a post-discharge follow-up study. *Age and Ageing* 1992; 21:178–181.
25. Vladeck BC, Miller NA. The Medicare home health initiative. *Health Care Financ Rev* 1994; 16:7–16.
26. Medicare and Medicaid statistical supplement, 1997. *Health Care Financ Rev* 1997; 1997 Statistical Supplement:126–141.
27. Agency for Health Care Policy and Research. Home health care: *Use, expenditures, and sources of payment.* U.S.Department of Health and Human Services 1998; *Research Findings* 15:2–19.
28. Dey AN. Characteristics of elderly home health care users: data from the 1994 national home and hospice care survey. *Adv Data* 1996; 279:1–12.
29. Mauser E, Miller NA. A profile of home health users in 1992. *Health Care Financ Rev* 1994; 16:17–33.
30. Neutel CI. Risk of traffic accident injury after a prescription for a benzodiazepine. *Ann Epidemiol* 1995; 5:239–244.
31. Branch LG, Goldberg HB, Cheh VA, Williams J. Medicare home health: A description of total episodes of care. *Health Care Financ Rev* 1993; 14:59–74.
32. Dellasega C, Dansky K, King L, Stricklin ML. Use of home health services by elderly persons with cognitive impairment. *JONA* 1994; 24:20–25.
33. Ganguli M, Fox A, Gilby J, Belle S. Characteristics of rural homebound older adults: A community-Based study. *J Am Geriatr Soc* 1996; 44:363–370.
34. Bruce ML, McNamara R. Psychiatric status among the homebound elderly: An epidemiologic perspective. *J Am Geriatr Soc* 1992; 40:561–566.
35. Council on Scientific Affairs. Educating physicians in home health care. *JAMA* 1991; 265:769–771.

36. Meyer GS, Gibbons RV. House calls to the elderly—a vanishing practice among physicians. *N Engl J Med* 1997; 337:1815–1820.
37. Health Care Financing Administration. Physician involvement with Medicaid's home and community based services waiver program. *JAMA* 1994; 272:1569
38. Keenan JM, Hepburn KW. The role of physicians in home health care. *Clinics in Geriatric Medicine* 1991; 7:665–675.
39. Gray LK, Cozmin L, Esenwine J. Improving home care. A survey on physician and nurses communication. *Home Care Prov* 1998; 3:100–103.
40. Jackson JE, Ramsdell JW, Renvall M, Swart J, Ward H. Reliability of drug histories in a specialized geriatric outpatient clinic. *J Gen Intern Med* 1989; 4:39–43.
41. Tamblyn RM, McLeod PJ, Abrahamowicz M, Laprise R. Do too many cooks spoil the broth? Multiple physician involvement in medical management of elderly patients and potentially inappropriate drug combinations. *Can Med Assoc J* 1996; 154:1177–1184.
42. Chrischilles EA, Foley DJ, Wallace RB, Lemke JH, Semla TP, Hanon JT, et al. Use of medications by persons 65 and over: Data from the established populations for epidemiologic studies of the elderly. *J Gerontol* 1992; 47:M137–M144
43. Lassila HC, Stoehr GP, Ganguli M, Seaberg EC, Gilby JE, Belle SH, et al. Use of prescription medications in an elderly rural population: The MoVIEW project. *Ann Pharmacother* 1996; 30:589–595.
44. Ostrom JR, Hammarlund ER, Christensen DB, Plein JB, Kethley AJ. Medication usage in an elderly population. *Med Care* 1985; 23:157–164.
45. Rupp MT, DeYoung M, Schondelmeyer SW. Prescribing problems and pharmacist interventions in community practice. *Med Care* 1992; 30:926–940.
46. Hanlon JT, Landerman LR, Wall WE, Horner RD, Fillenbaum GG, Dawson DV, et al. Is medication use by community-dwelling elderly people influenced by cognitive function? *Age Ageing* 1996; 25:190–196.
47. Avorn J. Drug prescribing, drug taking, adverse reactions, and compliance in elderly patients. In: Salzman C, editor. *Clinical geriatric psychopharmacology* (3rd ed.) Boston: Williams & Wilkins, 1998:21–47.
48. Kroenke LTCK, Pinholt EM. Reducing polypharmacy in the elderly: A controlled trial of physician feedback. *J Am Geriatr Soc* 1990; 38:31–36.
49. Kurfees JF, Dotson RL. Drug interactions in the elderly. *J Fam Prac* 1987; 25:477–488.
50. Ray WA, Thapa P, Shorr RI. Medications and the older driver. *Clinics in Geriatric Medicine* 1993; 9:413–438.

51. Francis J, Martin D, Kapoor WN. A prospective study of delirium in hospitalized elderly. *JAMA* 1990; 263:1097–1101.
52. Peters NL. Snipping the thread of life: Antimuscarinic side effects of medications in the elderly. *Arch Intern Med* 1989; 149:2414
53. Lobo BL, Greene WL. Zolpidem: Distinct from Triazolam? *Ann Pharmacother* 1997; 31:625–632.
54. Ray WA, Griffin MR, Downey W. Benzodiazepines of long and short elimination half-life and the risk of hip fracture. *JAMA* 1989; 262:3303–3307.
55. Potter WZ. Psychotropic medications and work performance. *J Occup Med* 1990; 32:355–361.
56. Ray WA, Fought RL, Decker MD. Psychoactive drugs and the risk of injurious motor vehicle crashes in elderly drivers. *Am J Epidemiol* 1992; 136:873–883.
57. Shorr RI, Robin DW. Rational use of benzodiazepines in the elderly. *Drugs & Aging* 1994; 4:9–20.
58. Greenblatt DJ, Miller LG, Shader RI. Neurochemical and pharmacokinetic correlates of the clinical action of benzodiazepine hypnotic drugs. *Am J Med* 1990; 88:18S–24S.
59. Ray WA. Psychotropic drugs and injuries among the elderly: a review. *J Clin Psychopharmacol* 1992; 12:386–396.
60. Greenblatt DJ, Harmatz JS, Shapiro L, Engelhardt N, Gouthro TA, Shader RI. Sensitivity to triazolam in the elderly. *N Engl J Med* 1991; 324:1691–1698.
61. Wells BG, Middleton B, Lawrence G, Lillard D, Safarik J. Factors associated with the elderly falling in intermediate care facilities. *Drug Intell Clin Pharm* 1985; 19:142–145.
62. Sorock GS, Shimkin EE. Benzodiazepine sedatives and the risk of falling in a community-dwelling elderly cohort. *Arch Intern Med* 1988; 148:2441–2444.
63. Cumming RG, Miller PJ, Kelsey JL, Davis P, Arfken CL, Birge SJ, et al. Medications and multiple falls in elderly people. The St. Louis OAISIS study. *Age Ageing* 1991; 20:455–461.
64. Gales BJ, Menard SM. Relationship between the administration of selected medications and falls in hospitalized elderly patients. *Ann Pharmacother* 1995; 29:354–358.
65. Tinetti ME, Doucette J, Claus E, Marottoli R. Risk factors for serious injury during falls by older persons in the community. *J Am Geriatr Soc* 1995; 43:1214–1221.
66. Thapa PB, Gideon P, Fought RL, Ray WA. Psychotropic drugs and the risk of recurrent falls in ambulatory nursing home residents. *Am J Epidemiol* 1995; 142:202–211.

67. Lord SR, Anstey KJ, Williams P, Ward JA. Psychoactive medication use, sensori-motor function and falls in older women. *Br J Clin Pharmac* 1995; 39:227–234.
68. Mendelson WB. The use of sedative/hypnotic medication and its correlation with falling down in the hospital. *Sleep* 1996; 19:698–701.
69. Ray, W. A., Thapa, P., and Gideon, P. Benzodiazepines and the risk of falls in nursing home residents. Submitted 1998. (GENERIC)
70. Cumming RG, Klineberg RJ. Psychotropics, thiazide diuretics and hip fractures in the elderly. *Med J Aust* 1993; 158:414–417.
71. Lichtenstein MJ, Griffin MR, Cornell JE, Malcolm E, Ray WA. Risk factors for hip fractures occurring in the hospital. *Am J Epidemiol* 1994; 140:830–838.
72. Herings RMC, Stricker BH, de Boer A, Bakker A, Sturmans F. Benzodiazepines and the risk of falling leading to femur fractures. *Arch Intern Med* 1995; 155:1801–1807.
73. Cummings SR, Nevitt MC, Browner WS, Stone K, Fox KM, Ensrud KE, et al. Risk factors for hip fracture in white women. *N Engl J Med* 1995; 332:767–773.
74. Neutel CI, Hirdes JP, Maxwell CJ, Patten SB. New evidence on benzodiazepine use and falls: The time factor. *Age & Ageing* 1996; 25:273–278.
75. Hemmelgarn B, Suissa S, Huang A, Francois Boivin J, Pinard G. Benzodiazepine use and the risk of motor vehicle crash in the elderly. *JAMA* 1997; 278:27–31.
76. Bixler EO, Kales A, Manfredi RL, Vgontzas AN, Tyson KL, Kales JD. Next-day memory impairment with triazolam use. *Lancet* 1991; 337:827–831.
77. Brown NJ, Griffin MR, Ray WA, Meredith S, Beers MH, Marren J, et al. A model for improving medication use in home health care patients. *J Am Pharm Assoc* 1998; 38:696–702.
78. Blazer D. Current concepts: Depression in the elderly. *N Engl J Med* 1989; 320:164–166.
79. Richelson E. Pharmacology of antidepressants in use in the United States. *J Clin Psychiatry* 1982; 43:4–11.
80. Glassman AH, Bigger JT, Jr. Cardiovascular effects of therapeutic doses of tricyclic antidepressants. *Arch Gen Psychiatry* 1981; 38:815–820.
81. Glassman AH, Giardina EV, Perel JM, Bigger JT, Jr., Kantor SJ, Davies M. Clinical characteristics of imipramine-induced orthostatic hypotension. *Lancet* 1979; March 3:468–472.
82. Glassman AH, Walsh BT, Roose SP, Rosenfeld R, Bruno RL, Bigger JT, Jr., et al. Factors related to orthostatic hypotension associated with tricyclic antidepressants. *J Clin Psychiatry* 1982; 43:35–38.

83. Roose SP, Glassman AH, Giardina EGV, Walsh T, Woodring S, Bigger JT, Jr. Tricyclic antidepressants in depressed patients with cardiac conduction disease. *Arch Gen Psychiatry* 1987; 44:273–275.
84. Roose SP, Glassman AH, Giardina EGV, Johnson LL, Walsh BT, Bigger JT, Jr. Cardiovascular effects of imipramine and bupropion in depressed patients with congestive heart failure. *J Clin Psychopharmacol* 1987; 7:247–251.
85. Thapa PB, Gideon P, Brockman KG, Fought RL, Ray WA. Clinical and biomechanical measures of balance as fall predictors in ambulatory nursing home residents. *J Gerontol* 1996; 51A:M239–M246
86. Monane M, Avorn J. Medications and falls. Causation, correlation, and prevention. *Clinics in Geriatric Medicine* 1996; 12:847–858.
87. Salzman C. Geriatric psychopharmacology. *Ann Rev Med* 1985; 36:217–228.
88. Cohn CK, Shrivastava R, Mendels J, Cohn JB, Fabre LF, Claghorn JL, et al. Double-blind, multicenter comparison of sertraline and amitriptyline in elderly depressed patients. *J Clin Psychiatry* 1990; 51[12, Suppl B]:28–33.
89. Small GW, Salzman C. Treatment of depression with new and atypical antidepressants. In: Salzman C, editor. *Clinical geriatric psychopharmacology.* 3rd. ed. Boston: Williams & Wilkins, 1998:245–261.
90. Thapa PB, Gideon P, Cost TW, Milam AB, Ray WA. Antidepressants and the risk of falls among nursing home residents. *N Engl J Med* 1998; 339:875–882.
91. Reynolds CF, III, Regestein Q., Nowell PD, Neylan TC. Treatment of insomnia in the elderly. In: Salzman C, editor. *Clinical geriatric psychopharmacology.* 3rd. ed. Boston: Williams & Wilkins, 1998:395–416.
92. Koenig HG, Meador KG, Cohen HJ, Blazer DG. Depression in elderly hospitalized patients with medical illness. *Arch Intern Med* 1988; 148:1929–1936.
93. NIH Consensus Development Panel on Depression in Late Life. Diagnosis and treatment of depression in late life. *JAMA* 1992; 268:1018–1024.
94. Wells KB, Stewart A, Hays RD, Burnam MA, Rogers W, Daniels M, et al. The functioning and well-being of depressed patients: Results from the medical outcomes study. *JAMA* 1989; 262:914–919.
95. Broadhead WE, Blazer DG, George LK, Tse CK. Depression, disability days, and days lost from work in a prospective epidemiologic survey. *JAMA* 1990; 264:2524–2528.
96. Parmelee PA, Katz IR, Lawton MP. Depression and mortality among institutionalized aged. *J Gerontol* 1992; 47:P3–10.
97. Mossey JM, Murtran E, Knott K, Craik R. Determinants of recovery 12 months after hip fracture: The importance of psychosocial factors. *Am J Public Health* 1989; 79:279–286.

98. Fredman L, Schoenbach VJ, Kaplan BH, Blazer DG, James SA, Kleinbaum DG, et al. The association between depressive symptoms and mortality among older participants in the epidemiologic catchment area-Piedmont health survey. *J Gerontol* 1989; 44:S149–156.
99. Murphy E, Smith R, Lindesay J, Slattery J. Increased mortality rates in late-life depression. *Br J Psychiatry* 1988; 152:347–353.
100. Rovner BW, German PS, Brant LJ, Clark R, Burton L, Folstein MF. Depression and mortality in nursing homes. *JAMA* 1991; 265:993–996.
101. Risse SC, Barnes R. Pharmacologic treatment of agitation associated with dementia. *J Am Geriatr Soc* 1986; 39:368–376.
102. Helms PM. Efficacy of antipsychotics in the treatment of the behavioral complications of dementia: A review of the literature. *J Am Geriatr Soc* 1985; 33:206–209.
103. Schneider LS, Pollock VE, Lyness SA. A metaanalysis of controlled trials of neuroleptic treatment in dementia. *J Am Geriatr Soc* 1990; 38:553–563.
104. Baldessarini RJ. Drugs and the Treatment of Psychiatric Disorders. In: Gilman AG, Goodman LS, Rall TW, Murad F, editors. *The pharmacologic basis of therapeutics.* New York: MacMillan Publishing Company, 1985:387
105. Toenniessen LM, Casey DE, McFarland BH. Tardive dyskinesia in the aged. *Arch Gen Psychiatry* 1985; 42:278–284.
106. Tinetti ME, Williams TF, Mayewski R. Fall risk index for elderly patients based on number of chronic disabilities. *Am J Med* 1986; 80:429–434.
107. Granek E, Baker SP, Abbey H, Robinson E, Myers AH, Samkoff JS, et al. Medications and diagnoses in relation to falls in a long-term care facility. *J Am Geriatr Soc* 1987; 35:503–511.
108. Pesznecker BL, Patsdaughter C, Moody KA, Albert M. Medication regimens and the home care client: a challenge for health care providers. *Home Health Care Serv Q* 1990; 11:9–68.
109. Berk ML, Schur CL, Mohr P. Using survey data to estimate prescription drug costs. *Health Aff* 1990; 9:146–156.
110. Stolley PD, Lasagna L. Prescribing patterns of physicians. *J Chron Dis* 1969; 22:395–405.
111. Stolley PD, Strom BL. Evaluating and monitoring the safety and efficacy of drug therapy and surgery. *J Chron Dis* 1986; 39:1145–1155.
112. Ray WA, Meador KG, Taylor JA, Thapa PB. Improving nursing home quality of care through provider education. *Ann Rev Gerontol Geriatr* 1992; 12:183–204.

113. Smith DH, Christensen DB, Stergachis A, Holmes G. A randomized controlled trial of a drug use review intervention for sedative hypnotic medications. *Med Care* 1998; 36:1013–1021.
114. Beers MH, Fingold SF, Ouslander JG. A computerized system for identifying and informing physicians about problematic drug use in nursing homes. *J Med Syst* 1992; 16:237–245.
115. Soumerai SB, Lipton HL. Computer-based drug-utilization review—risk, benefit, or boondoggle? *N Engl J Med* 1995; 332:1641–1645.
116. Lipton HL, Bero LA, Bird JA, McPhee SJ. The impact of clinical pharmacists' consultations on physicians' geriatric drug prescribing. *Med Care* 1992; 30:646–658.
117. Hanlon JT, Weinberger M, Samsa GP, Schmader KE, Uttech KM, Lewis IK, et al. A randomized, controlled trial of a clinical pharmacist intervention to improve inappropriate prescribing in elderly outpatients with polypharmacy. *Am J Med* 1996; 100:428–437.
118. Tett SE, Higgins GM, Armour CL. Impact of pharmacist interventions on medication management by the elderly: A review of the literature. *Ann Pharmacother* 1993; 27:80–86.
119. Kimberlin CL, Berardo DH, Pendergast JF, McKenzie LC. Effects of an education program for community pharmacists on detecting drug-related problems in elderly patients. *Med Care* 1993; 31:451–468.
120. Currie JD, Chrischilles EA, Kuehl AK, Buser RA. Effect of a training program on community pharmacists' detection of and intervention in drug-related problems. *J Am Pharm Assoc* 1997; NS 37:182–191.

PART II

Review of Selected Diseases and Syndromes

CHAPTER 7

Treatment of Alzheimer's Disease

LON S. SCHNEIDER
DEPARTMENT OF PSYCHIATRY AND THE BEHAVIORAL SCIENCES
UNIVERSITY OF SOUTHERN CALIFORNIA

INTRODUCTION

Therapeutic approaches to the cognitive impairment of dementia are making their way into clinical practice, albeit more slowly than previously anticipated. Clinical pharmacological approaches toward improvement of cognitive symptoms will be discussed, with an emphasis on cholinergic approaches since they are most developed, and additional cholinesterase inhibitors may soon be available for prescribing. The cholinergic deficit—although by no means the only deficit in an illness characterized by progressive nerve cell damage and death—occurs early in the disease and perhaps to a much greater and denser degree than deficits to other neuronal systems. Table 7.2 outlines pharmacologic therapies considered in this chapter. Pharmacologic agents that increase cholinergic function in the central nervous system (CNS) have shown efficacy in improving cognitive symptoms, and remain an intensively researched area. As more knowledge is gained about dosing, side effects, and mechanisms of action, these drugs can be prescribed with greater deliberation.

Drugs that improve cognition also may have effects on behavioral symptoms, severe dementia, and non-Alzheimer's dementia, although the evidence for this is limited.

Current clinical and research approaches to slowing symptomatic or clinical progression have yet to be fully conceptually developed, but pharmacological candidates include antioxidants, monoamine oxidase-B inhibitors, and cholinesterase inhibitors, based on evidence that their use may prolong the time until institutionalization is required. Psychosocial interventions also may contribute to prolonging the time to institutionalization, and, indeed their potentially considerable effect has been underappreciated. Clinical approaches to prevent or delay the onset of the dementia of Alzheimer's disease (AD) are just now being tested.

PHARMACOLOGIC APPROACHES FOR TREATING COGNITIVE SYMPTOMS

Cholinergic agents are currently the most immediately promising and frequently used experimental treatment for cognitive impairment associated with AD. The rationale behind the use of these drugs is the cholinergic hypothesis, which proposes an association between cognitive decline and cholinergic cell loss in the cortex and other areas of the brains of patients with AD (Bartus, Dean, Beer, & Lippa, 1982) (Perry, Gibson, Blessed, Perry, & Tomlinson, 1977). Any augmentation of cholinergic function would be expected to enhance cognition. The classes of cholinergic agents include muscarinic and nicotinic agonists, cholinesterase inhibitors (ChEIs), and indirect modifiers of acetylcholine release.

Precursor Loading

Acetylcholine precursors such as choline and phosphatidyl choline (lecithin) have been used in attempts to augment acetylcholine synthesis but have not worked. Early trials in which lecithin was combined with the cholinesterase inhibitor tacrine did not reveal any added benefit (Jorm, 1986).

Cholinergic Agonists

If this review had been written 2 years ago, it would have waxed optimistically on the potential for cholinergic agonists to improve cognitive symptoms of AD. The range of medications being tested was broad, the drugs differing from each other largely on the basis of muscarinic receptor subtype sensitivity. Unfortunately, thus far, the cholinergic agonists that have entered phase III clinical trials, including xanomeline (Bodick et al., 1997), SB 202026, AF102B, and LU 25-109, have not proven to be adequately efficacious and safe, and are not being further developed. Despite these results, the direct cholinergic approach remains potentially promising, although it would be fair to comment that there is relatively little current commercial interest in cholinergic agonists for AD. Therefore, at present, one would not want to prematurely predict their eventual success.

Cholinesterase Inhibitors

Much of the more immediately promising research, more likely to result in imminent clinical use, is with cholinesterase inhibitors (ChEI's). The ChEI's include a number of agents: tacrine (Farlow et al., 1992; Knapp et al., 1994); physostigmine and donepezil (Rogers, Doody, Mohs, & Friedhoff, 1998; Rogers, 1998); rivastigmine (Corey-Bloom, Anand, &

Veach, 1998; Rosler, Anand, Gharabawi, and the International Exelon Investigators, 1998); metrifonate (Cummings et al., 1998; Morris et al., 1998); and galantamine (Dal-Bianco et al., 1991), eptastigmine, and others.

Newer ChEIs tend to be longer-acting and more predictable in their pharmacokinetics. ChEIs differ among themselves in their specificity toward inhibiting acetylcholinesterase (AChE) compared to butyrl cholinesterase and other peripheral cholinesterases. It is theoretically possible that those ChEIs that relatively selectively inhibit AChE may produce fewer peripheral side effects than are associated with other agents, but this remains to be formally assessed.

Furthermore, ChEIs may have more profound effects than were originally anticipated. Initially, the rationale for ChEI treatment focused on improvement of cognitive symptoms through the intra-synaptic effects of increasing acetylcholine. It was hypothesized that inhibition of acetylcholine degradation led to a greater amount of acetylcholine at muscarinic and nicotinic receptors, resulting in improved cognitive functioning. Preclinical evidence now indicates that ChEIs may provide neuroprotective effects as well, perhaps through the activation of nicotinic receptors (Nordberg, Lilja, Lundqvist, & Harting, 1992); appear to enhance neurotrophic regeneration, perhaps through direct muscarinic receptor stimulation; and may regulate processing and secretion of amyloid precursor protein (APP) and the production of β-amyloid (Buxbaum et al., 1992; Nitsch, Slack, Wurtman, & Growdon, 1992). One hypothesis is that long-term AChE inhibition, by increasing acetylcholine concentrations in the surviving AD brain synapses, may activate normal APP processing in such a manner as to slow down or preclude formation of amyloidogenic APP fragments or ß-amyloid.

Of course, much of this is theoretical, based on pre-clinical research, and adequately designed and controlled clinical trials have not been carried out. Rather, the clinical trials undertaken for drug development and FDA regulatory approval are only 12 weeks to 6 months in duration, and assess only symptomatic cognitive change.

In late 1997, it seemed virtually certain that within the next year at least four cholinesterase inhibitors would be available for prescribing. As of this writing, however, in January 1999, only two are available in the United States: tacrine (Cognex) and donepezil (Aricept). The delays in approving rivastigmine (Exelon) and metrifonate have to do with issues of safety awaiting clarification. Recently, the FDA disapproved the new drug application for sustained-release physotigmine, and eptastigmine has been withdrawn from further development, both largely because of safety concerns.

The following is a brief review of several cholinesterase inhibitors available, or possibly likely to become available in 1999.

Tacrine (Cognex)

Tacrine became the first agent approved for the treatment of AD in September 1993. It is a centrally and peripherally active, reversible, acridine-based ChEI with a duration of action of 4 to 6 hours. It is nonspecific in that it inhibits AChE, butyrl cholinesterases, and other cholinesterases (Schneider, 1993). Tacrine is characterized by variable absorption, extensive distribution, good CNS penetration, and nonlinear pharmacokinetics at therapeutic doses, with a high degree of dose-dependent activity. It has a therapeutic dosage range extending from 20 mg to 40 mg q.i.d. and therefore requires individualized titration (Knapp et al., 1994).

The efficacy of tacrine in the treatment of mild to moderate AD was established by a paradigmatic, double-blind, placebo-controlled, 30-week multicenter trial (Knapp et al., 1994) in addition to several other trials. This pivotal trial demonstrated that 160 mg/day of tacrine produced statistically significant, clinically observable improvement on cognitive tests (such as the Alzheimer's Disease Assessment Scale cognitive [ADAS-cog] subscale and the MMSE), clinician- and caregiver-rated global evaluations, and quality-of-life assessments.

The primary reason for the substantial withdrawal from the study among tacrine-treated subjects was a 28% occurrence of asymptomatic reversible liver transaminase elevations higher than three times the upper limit of normal. Over 90% of this was observed within the first 12 weeks of the 30-week study, and regular monitoring of serum transaminases is required during the initial prescribing periods. Gastrointestinal side effects associated with cholinergic excess such as nausea, vomiting, and diarrhea (occurring in approximately 16% of subjects) also were associated with withdrawal from treatment.

The characteristics of tacrine, including its titration scheme over 12 to 18 weeks, q.i.d. dosing, its pharmacokinetic profile, serum monitoring and side effects makes tacrine a difficult drug to use clinically, and certainly more difficult to use than donepezil, the cholinesterase inhibitor introduced subsequently.

Donepezil (Aricept)

Donepezil is a piperidine-based ChEI that has dose-dependent activity showing greater selectivity for AChE and a longer duration of cholinesterase inhibition than tacrine or physostigmine. It received marketing approval by the FDA in November 1997 and has been available for prescribing since January 1998. It is characterized by linear pharmacokinetics at therapeutic doses with a slow clearance and a 70-hour elimination half-life, allowing it to be given once a day.

Two phase III trials examined donepezil 5 and 10 mg/day vs. placebo for 12 and 24 weeks, respectively (Rogers, Doody et al., 1998; Rogers, Farlow et al., 1998). Over the course of the 24-week trial, patients receiving placebo declined as expected on the ADAS-cog and MMSE cognitive outcome measures, while patients receiving donepezil improved somewhat compared to baseline. Overall, results showed statistically significant benefit in both cognition and clinician-rated improvement when compared with placebo. There was a trend toward a greater effect of 10 mg/d vs. 5 mg/d early in the course of treatment but not at the end of 24 weeks.

As expected, the main adverse reactions were related to peripheral cholinergic effects and are more common with higher doses. Nausea, vomiting, and diarrhea occur in approximately 10% to 20% of patients and muscle cramping and fatigue in approximately 8% to 10%. As with other ChEIs, the effects, however, are generally mild in intensity, short-lived (lasting only a few days), and generally resolve with continued treatment. In this initial study, approximately 68% of patients completed the 10 mg/d dose, 85% the 5 mg/d dose, and 80% the placebo.

Since donepezil requires only once per day administration, little dosage titration, and is not associated with transaminase elevations, it has been prescribed far more frequently than tacrine, virtually displacing its use.

Rivastigmine (Exelon)

Rivastigmine (Exelon® Novartis) is a pseudo-irreversible carbamate selective acetylcholinesterase subtype inhibitor (Corey-Bloom et al., 1998; Rösler et al., 1998). It is characterized by its selective binding and inactivation of acetylcholinesterase subtypes in the cerebral cortex and hippocampus (areas that are more involved in AD) in preference to the pons and medulla. As with other ChEIs, it shows dose-dependent activity, with higher doses generally being associated with greater improvement. A new drug application was filed with the FDA in spring 1997 but the medication has yet to be approved by the FDA. It is, however, approved in several countries in Europe and South America.

Rivastigmine is not metabolized by the hepatic microsome system. Rather, after binding to AChE, the carbamate portion of rivastigmine is slowly hydrolyzed, cleaved, conjugated to a sulphate, and excreted. The duration of AChE inhibition by rivastigmine is approximately 10 hours.

Four placebo-controlled trials, 6 months in duration, using both fixed and adjustable doses involving 2800 patients, many with concomitant illnesses and taking multiple medications, showed significant effects on cognition, clinical global impression, and functional activities. Three of these trials have been systematically reviewed (see Table 7.1), and two have been published

TABLE 7.1 Changes in ADAS-Cog scores in Alzheimer's disease patients treated with tacrine, donepezil, rivastigmine, and metrifonate

Drug	Study	No. on Medication	Max. Daily Dose (mg)	Duration (Weeks)	Difference from Placebo
Tacrine	Davis et al., 1992	187	40/80	6	2.5
	Farlow et al., 1992	36	80	12	3.8
	Knapp et al., 1994	67	160	30	4.1
Donepezil	Rogers, Doody et al., 1998	150/150	5/10	24	2.8
					3.1
	Rogers, Farlow et al., 1998	150/150	5/10	12	2.7
					3.0
Rivastigmine	Corey-Bloom et al., 1998	231	6-12 mg	264.9	
	Rösler et al., 1998	243	6-12 mg	26	2.6
	Corey-Bloom, 1998	354	6 mg	26	1.8
			9 mg	26	1.7
Metrifonate	Morris et al., 1998	(234)	30–60 mg	25	2.8
	Cummings et al., 1998	(480)	10–60 mg	12	2.9

Note: Outcome effect sizes are drug-placebo and are based on the highest dose used in the trial and on the more conservative (modified) intent-to-treat analyses. All effects listed are statistically significant as reported by the authors. Differences in outcome are not strictly comparable among studies and should be used as a guide only, since actual differences depend on variances, statistical model, and type of analysis, and are not performed consistently from study to study. Mean difference scores are not to be taken as relative measures of effect size.

(Corey-Bloom et al., 1998; Rösler et al., 1998). If the drug is approved, the indicated dosage range will be within 3 mg and 6 mg b.i.d. As with other cholinesterase inhibitors, cholinergic side effects are generally mild to moderate in severity, dose-dependent, and generally seen during titration. The most frequent side effects are GI-related, such as nausea, vomiting, diarrhea, and weight loss. As with other cholinesterase inhibitors, about 65% of patients were able to complete the trials at the higher doses, compared to 85% on placebo, and there was dose-dependent activity, with higher doses generally associated with greater improvement and more cholinergic effects.

Metrifonate

Metrifonate is unique as a cholinesterase inhibitor in that it is a prodrug that is non-enzymatically transformed into its active metabolite 2,2-dimethyl dichlorovinyl phosphate (DDVP), an irreversible CNS ChEI with somewhat greater selectivity for AChE than for other cholinesterases (Hinz, Grewig, & Schmidt, 1996) (Nordgren, Bergstrom, Holmstedt, & Sandoz, 1978). Very low concentrations of DDVP steadily released from metrifonate lead to levels that are sufficient to inhibit cholinesterase. Historically, metrifonate had been used to treat schistosomiasis, and DDVP (brand name Dichlorvos®) is a widely used insecticide as well. Although metrifonate has linear pharmacokinetics, clinical response may be linked to levels of cholinesterase inhibition rather than to drug concentration, and because of its irreversibility it has a red blood cell AChE inhibition half-life of 50 days. Cholinergic side effects occur with relatively low frequency at levels of red blood cell cholinesterase inhibition of 75%.

Early metrifonate trials and observations tended to use weekly doses. In a 3-month, double-blind trial using a weekly dosing regimen, metrifonate-treated patients showed significant improvements on cognitive and clinical measures, and in an 18-month open follow-up deteriorated by only 1.68 points/year on the MMSE (Becker et al., 1996). Later trials used once-daily doses to reduce fluctuation between peak and trough inhibition levels, resulting in a more stable level of AChE inhibition, and to improve commercial application. The phase III studies tended to use single individualized dosages or a fixed dose, and the two currently published phase III clinical studies are summarized in Table 7.1.

Metrifonate at various doses was associated with significant cognitive improvement compared to placebo (Cummings et al., 1998; Morris et al., 1998). Higher doses were consistently more effective than lower doses on both cognitive and global assessments. In one trial (Morris et al., 1998) over the course of 6 months, patients who received metrifonate were rated as significantly better than placebo on both cognitive and global ratings. In addition to being rated better on a behavioral rating instrument, the

Neuropsychiatric Inventory, especially with respect to hallucinations, depression, apathy, and motor behavior.

A safety concern, however, is that approximately 20 patients out of 3000 in the metrifonate clinical studies developed "asthenia, myasthenia, and malaise" and "four patients with muscular weakness received respiratory support" (personal communication from Bayer Pharmaceuticals, September 18, 1998). Currently, medication has been withdrawn from subjects, and the development program temporarily halted by Bayer and the FDA in order to investigate this further.

PHARMACOLOGIC APPROACHES FOR SLOWING THE RATE OF CLINICAL DECLINE

One aspect of treatment gaining interest is the attempt to slow the rate of decline of both cognition and functional activities, thereby preserving patients' quality of life and autonomy. Methods that have been proposed for slowing the clinical progression of AD generally offer the rationale that the intervention is altering processes of neuronal death. Medications include antioxidants, monoamine oxidase inhibitors (MAOIs), antiinflammatory agents, cholinergic agents, estrogens, or neurotrophic factors.

Antioxidants and Monoamine Oxidase-B Inhibitors

Evidence from animal and human studies suggests that oxidative mechanisms may play a role in the loss of at least some neuronal systems (LeBel & Bondy, 1991; Volicer & Crino, 1990). The brain is known to be susceptible to oxidative stress, which can result in a "neurodegenerative" cascade involving disruption of DNA, damage to membranes, and neuronal death (Tariot, Scheider, & Patel, 1993). Regional losses of glutamine synthetase activity, an enzyme particularly sensitive to mixed-function oxidation, were observed in dying patients with AD but not in control subjects, suggesting a specific brain vulnerability to age-related oxidation and an excess of oxygen-based free radicals or a decrease in endogenous antioxidant activity (Smith et al., 1991).

Among the antioxidants considered to have a potential neuroprotective effect are selegiline, vitamin E, ascorbic acid, coenzyme Q, and idebenone (a proprietary co-enzyme Q analog, Takeda Pharmaceuticals). It had been proposed that a low-dose, chronic administration of selegiline, a selective MAOI type B, would reduce the concentrations of free radicals and other neurotoxins (Cohen & Spina, 1989) and has been shown in vitro to reduce the oxidative stress associated with the catabolism of dopamine (Cohen & Spina, 1989).

The Alzheimer's Disease Cooperative Study (ADCS), a consortium funded by the National Institute on Aging, conducted the only large study of antioxidant agents: a doubleblind, placebocontrolled, randomized, multicenter trial comparing selegiline (5 mg b.i.d), alpha-tocopherol (1000 IU b.i.d.), the combination, and placebo for 2 years in 341 patients with moderately severe Alzheimer's disease (Sano et al., 1997). The primary outcome was the time to the occurrence of one of the following endpoints: death, institutionalization, loss of the ability to perform basic activities of daily living, or operationally defined severe dementia. There were significant delays in the time to the primary outcome (principally nursing home placement) for patients treated with selegiline (median time 655 days), alpha-tocopherol (670 days), or combination therapy (585 days), as compared with the placebo group (440 days). The major impact appeared to be reduced progression in functional impairments over time, with no beneficial effect on cognition.

Idebenone

Idebenone is a benzoquinone synthetic compound structurally similar to coenzyme Q (ubiquinone). In addition to other actions, there is considerable evidence to support its effects as an "electron trapper" and oxygen free radical scavenger. Three randomized, parallel group trials comparing idebenone with placebo and other agents have been conducted in patients with Alzheimer's disease or cognitive impairment (Bergamasco, Villardite, & Copri, 1992; Senin et al., 1992; Weyer, Babej-Dole, Hadler, Hofmann, & Herrmann, 1997). In the 4-month study by Senin and colleagues (1992) idebenone was associated with a statistically significant improvement in memory and attention. In the study by Weyer and colleagues (1997) patients were randomly assigned to receive one of two doses of idebenone or placebo for 6 months with the idebenone patients showing a significant benefit on the ADAS cog, the global rating of change and on measures of noncognitive functions.

Based on these results, an ambitious and ill-conceived development program was initiated with three phase III clinical trials. Unfortunately, idebenone did not prove to be efficacious in the first trial, so the subsequent trials were discontinued and the development program stopped.

Cholinesterase Inhibitors

The rate of cognitive decline in patients with AD also appears to be slowed by the use of ChEIs, which may have neuroprotective as well as other effects. Such long-term slowing of clinical decline has been suggested by data on subjects with AD who were treated with physostigmine (Stern, Sono, & Mayuex, 1988), and also with tacrine and monitored from the end of a 30-week, double-blind study for at least 2 years (Knopman, 1996). Time to institutionalization was longer for subjects maintained on higher therapeutic doses of tacrine compared with those receiving low-dose tacrine. Results from these studies suggest that cognitive deterioration in patients with AD who received a ChEI was slowed by several months to a year. But these observations must be considered with caution considering that they are based on historical comparisons.

Anti-inflammatory Agents

There is substantial evidence supporting the hypothesis that inflammatory processes and immune systems are implicated in the pathology of AD (Aisen & Davis 1994; McGeer & McGeer, 1996). Inflammatory and immune reactions are evidenced by observations of reactive microglial cells surrounding senile plaques and astrocytes, and the consequent production of inflammatory cytokines. Two of these cytokines, interleukin-1 and interleukin-6, promote the synthesis of APP, which then may be processed to potentially neurotoxic ß-amyloid. The unexpectedly low prevalence of AD in patients with rheumatoid arthritis, a condition treated with nonsteroidal antiinflammatory drugs (NSAIDs), supports the theory that NSAIDs confer protection against AD (McGeer & McGeer 1996). Case-control twin studies have also demonstrated that NSAIDs provide a protective effect (Breitner et al., 1994). The potential role of NSAIDs in AD is supported by results from a small, controlled trial that indicated stable cognitive function in the indomethacin-treated group and declining function in the placebo group (Rogers, 1993). A long-term treatment trial with low-dose prednisone (10 mg/day) is underway, sponsored by the NIA/ADCS and results should be available by the middle of 1999 (Aisen et al., 1996).

Cyclooxygenase 2 inhibitors have recently become available for treating arthritis. They are associated with less gastrointestinal side effects than are the conventional NSAIDs. Studies are underway assessing their symptomatic effects over 1 year and in possibly delaying the onset of dementia in people with mild cognitive impairment.

PHARMACOLOGIC APPROACHES TO TREATING OTHER SYMPTOMS IN DEMENTIA

Drugs that improve cognition also may be efficacious in treating behavioral symptoms, severe dementia, and non-Alzheimer dementia. For

TABLE 7.2 Available or Soon-to-be Available Medications for Alzheimer's Disease

Cholinesterase Inhibitors
FDA-approved for AD
Tacrine
Donepezil
NDA-filed (approval expected)
Rivastigmine (ENA 713)
Metrifonate
In Late Stages of Research
Galantamine
Cholinergic Agonists
None
Other medications available on the US market (not indicated for AD)
Anti-inflammatories
e.g., Ibuprofen, naprozyn, celecoxib
Estrogens
Premarino®
Estradiol and others
Vitamin E
Selegiline

Note: Only tacrine and donepezil are approved for use in AD. Other medications are listed for informational purposes only.

example, there is evidence from open-case series that tacrine improved behavioral symptoms in patients with AD (Kaufer, Cummings, & Christine, 1996). Findings from other studies suggest that ChEIs or a cholinergic agnonist improve behavioral symptoms in patients enrolled in such trials (Bodick et al., 1997; Morris et al., 1998; Raskind, Sadowsky, Sigmund, Beitler, & Auster, 1997). However, these patients were selected precisely because they had few behavioral symptoms at baseline, hence the significance of a drug-placebo difference in this population is unclear. Prospectively designed clinical trials, assessing the efficacy of cholinesterase inhibitors in patients with delusions, hallucinations, and agitation are required.

PSYCHOSOCIAL INTERVENTIONS

In addition to drug therapy, psychosocial intervention has been shown to postpone the institutionalization of patients with AD. Mittelman and colleagues (Mittelman, Ferris, Shulman, Steinberg, & Levin, 1996) reported a randomized clinical trial in which a structured psychosocial intervention directed toward the caregiver, and involving a total of six individual and family counseling sessions over a 16-week period, delayed the time until the patients with AD needed to be institutionalized by their caregivers compared with usual clinical care. In this study, 206 caregivers were randomly assigned either to the treatment group, that received individual and family counseling; to support-group participation, and consultation as needed; or to the comparison group, that received routine clinical care.

"PREVENTION" STUDIES

There is a new paradigm for the design of clinical trials in AD, referred to as "prevention" studies, or "mild cognitive impairment" (MCI) studies. Essentially, patients who have impairments in delayed recall, but who do not fulfill criteria for dementia are randomized to drug or placebo and followed for several years. Approximately 50-60% of subjects with MCI "convert" to Alzheimer's dementia within 3 years. In these trials, it is expected that the active medication will delay the time to onset of dementia. Clinical trials are underway comparing a cyclooxygenase 2 inhibitor antiinflammatory, Vioxx with placebo (funded by Merck), comparing vitamin E and donepezil with placebo (NIA Alzheimer's Cooperative Study), and rivastigmine with placebo (funded by Novartis).

SUMMARY

Current therapeutic approaches to treating patients with AD focus on improving symptomatology over approximately a 6-month period and on slowing clinical or symptom progression. Treatment with ChEIs is currently the most clearly proven symptomatic therapy over the short term. The efficacy of antioxidant therapy has been demonstrated in only one clinical trial. Theoretically, ChEIs may have disease-modifying effects, but this remains to be demonstrated in controlled clinical trials. The most important predictors of response to ChEIs appear to be adequate dosages, plasma drug concentrations, and degree of cholinesterase inhibition. Current multicenter studies are assessing the efficacy of vitamin E, cholinesterase inhibitors, or the new cyclooxygenase-2-inhibitor antiinflammatories to delay the onset of dementia in people with mild cognitive impairment.

ACKNOWLEDGEMENTS

NIH, University of Southern California, Alzheimer's Disease Research Center, NIH Alzheimer's Disease Cooperative Study.

REFERENCES

Aisen, P. S., Davis, K. L. (1994) Inflammatory mechanisms in Alzheimer's disease: Implications for therapy. *American Journal of Psychiatry, 151,* 1105–13.

Aisen, P. S., Marin, D., Altstiel, L., Goodwin, C., Baroch, B., Jacobson, R., Ryan, T. & Davis, K. L. (1996) A pilot study of prednisone in Alzheimer's disease. *Dementia, 7,* 201–6.

Bartus, R. T., Dean, R. L., Beer, B., Lippa, A. S. (1982) The cholinergic hypothesis of geriatric memory dysfunction. *Science, 217,* 408–14.

Becker, R. E., Colliver, J. A., Markwell, S. J., Moriearty, P. L., Unni, L. K., Vicari, S. (1996) Double-blind, placebo-controlled study of metrifonate, an acetylcholinesterase inhibitor, for Alzheimer disease. *Alzheimer Disease & Associated Disorders, 10,* 124–31.

Bergamasco, B, Villardite, C., & Copri, R. (1992) Effects of idebenone in elderly subjects with cognitive decline. Results of a multicentre clinical trial. *Archives of Gerontology and Geriatrics, 15,* 279–286.

Bodick, N. C., Offen, W. W., Levey, A. I., Cutter, N. R., Gauthier, S. G., Satlin, A., Shannon, H. E., Tollefson, G. D., Rasmussen, K., Bymaster, F. P., Hurley, D. J., Potter, W. Z., & Paul, S. M. (1997) Effects of xanomeline, a selective muscarinic receptor agonist, on cognitive function and behavioral symptoms in Alzheimer disease. *Archives of Neurology, 54,* 465–73.

Breitner, J. C., Gau, B. A., Welsh, K. A., Plassman, B. L., MCDonald, W. M., Hohms, M. J., & Anthony, J. C. (1994) Inverse association of anti-inflammatory treatments and Alzheimer's disease: Initial results of a co-twin control study. *Neurology, 44,* 227–32.

Buxbaum, J. D, Oishi. M., Chen, H. I., Pinkas-Kramarski, R., Jaffe, E. A., Gawly, S. E., & Greengard, P. (1992) Cholinergic agonists and interleukin 1 regulate processing and secretion of the Alzheimer beta/A4 amyloid protein precursor. *Proceedings of the National Academy of Sciences of the United States of America, 89,* 10075–8.

Cohen, G., Spina, M. B. (1989) Deprenyl suppresses the oxidant stress associated with increased dopamine turnover. *Annals of Neurology, 26,* 689–90.

Corey-Bloom, J. (1998). The efficacy and safety of ENA-713 in patients with mild to mederately sever Alzheimer's disease. *Journal of the American Geriatrics Society, 46,* A19.

Corey-Bloom, J., Anand, R., Veach, M. S. for the ENA713 (rivastigmine tartrate) B352 Study Group. (1998). A randomised trial evaluating the efficacy and safety of ENA713, a new acetylcholinesterase inhibitor in patients with mild to moderately severe Alzheimer's disease. *International Journal of Geriatric Psychopharmacol,* in press.

Cummings, J. L., Cyrus, P. A., Bieber, F., Mas, J., Orazem, J., & Gulanski, B. (1998) Metrifonate treatment of the cognitive deficits of Alzheimer's disease. [published erratum appears in Neurology 1998 Jul;51(1), 332]. *Neurology, 50,* 1214–21.

Dal-Bianco, P., Maly, J., Wober, C., Lind, C., Kock, G., Hofgard, J., Marschall, J. Mraz, M., & Deecke, L. (1991) Galanthamine treatment in Alzheimer's disease. *Journal of Neural Transmission. Supplementum, 33,* 59–63.

Davis, K. L., Thal, L. J., Gamzu, E. R., Davis, C. S., Woolson, R. F., Gracon, S. I., Drachman, D. A., Schneider, L. S., Whitehouse, P. J., Hoover, T. M., Morris, J. C., Kawas, C. H., Knopman, D. S., Earl, N. L., Kumar, V., Doody, R. S. (1992) A double-blind, placebo-controlled multicenter study of tacrine for Alzheimer's disease. *New England Journal of Medicine, 327,* 1253–9.

Farlow, M., Gracon, S. I., Hershey, L. A., Lewis, K. W., Sadowsky, C. H., & Dolan-Ureno, J. (1992) A controlled trial of tacrine in Alzheimer's disease. The Tacrine Study Group [see comments]. *JAMA, 268,* 2523–9.

Hinz, V. C., Grewig, S., & Schmidt, B. H. (1996) Metrifonate induces cholinesterase inhibition exclusively via slow release of dichlorvos. *Neurochemical Research, 21,* 331–7.

Jorm, A. F. (1986) Effects of cholinergic enhancement therapies on memory function in Alzheimer's disease: A meta-analysis of the literature. *Australian & New Zealand Journal of Psychiatry, 20,* 237–40.

Kaufer, D. I., Cummings, J. L., & Christine, D. (1996) Effect of tacrine on behavioral symptoms in Alzheimer's disease: An open-label study. *Journal of Geriatric Psychiatry & Neurology, 9,* 1–6.

Knapp, M. J., Knopman, D. S., Solomon, P. R., Pendlebury, W. W., Davis, C. S., Gracon, S. I., Apter, J. T., Lazarus, C. N., et al. (1994) A 30-week randomized controlled trial of high-dose tacrine in patients with Alzheimer's disease. *JAMA, 271,* 985–91.

Knopman, D., Schneider, L., Davis, K., Talwalker, S., Smith, F., Hoover, T., & Gracon, S. (1996) Long-term tacrine (Cognex) treatment: Effects on nursing home placement and mortality, *Neurology, 47,* 166–77.

LeBel, C. P., & Bondy, S. C. (1991) Oxygen radicals: Common mediators of neurotoxicity. *Neurotoxicology & Teratology, 13,* 341–6.

McGeer, P. L., & McGeer, E. G. (1996) Anti-inflammatory drugs in the fight against Alzheimer's disease. *Annals of the New York Academy of Sciences, 777,* 213–20.

Mittelman, M. S., Ferris, S. H., Shulman, E., Steinberg, G., & Levin, B. (1996) A family intervention to delay nursing home placement of patients with Alzheimer disease. A randomized controlled trial [see comments]. *JAMA, 276,* 1725–31.

Morris, J. C., Cyrus, P. A., Orazem, J., Mas, J., Bieber, F., Ruzicka, B. B., & Gulguski, B. (1998) Metrifonate benefits cognitive, behavioral, and global function in patients with Alzheimer's disease [see comments]. *Neurology, 50,* 1222–30.

Nitsch, R. M., Slack, B. E., Wurtman, R. J., & Growdon, J. H. (1992) Release of Alzheimer amyloid precursor derivatives stimulated by activation of muscarinic acetylcholine receptors. *Science, 258,* 304–7.

Nordberg, A., Lilja, A., Lundqvist, H., & Harting, P. (1992) Tacrine restores cholinergic nicotinic receptors and glucose metabolism in Alzheimer patients as visualized by positron emission tomography. *Neurobiology of Aging, 13,* 747–58.

Nordgren, I., Bergstrom, M., Holmstedt, B., & Sandoz, M. (1978) Transformation and action of metrifonate. *Archives of Toxicology, 41,* 31–41.

Perry, E. K., Gibson, P. H., Blessed, G., Perry, R. H., & Tomlinson, B. E. (1977) Neurotransmitter enzyme abnormalities in senile dementia. Choline acetyltransferase and glutamic acid decarboxylase activities in necropsy brain tissue. *Journal of the Neurological Sciences, 34,* 247–65.

Raskind, M. A., Sadowsky, C. H., Sigmund, W. R., Beitler, P. J., & Auster, S. B. (1997) Effect of tacrine on language, praxis, and noncognitive behavioral problems in Alzheimer disease. *Archives of Neurology, 54,* 836–40.

Rogers,J., Kirby, L. C., Hempelman, S. R., Bernz, P. L., McGear, P. L., Kosniak, A. W., Zalinski, J., Cofield, H., Mansokhani, L., & Allson, P. (1993) Clinical trial of indomethacin in Alzheimer's disease. *Neurology, 43,* 1609–11.

Rogers, S. L., Doody, R. S., Mohs, R. C., & Friedhoff, L. T. (1998) Donepezil improves cognition and global function in Alzheimer disease: A 15-week, double-blind, placebo-controlled study. *Archives of Internal Medicine, 158,* 1021–31.

Rogers, S. L., Farlow, M. R., Doody, R. S., Mohs, R., & Friedhoff, L. T. (1998) A 24-week, double-blind, placebo-controlled trial of donepezil in patients with Alzheimer's disease. *Neurology, 50,* 136–45.

Rösler, M., Anand, R., Gcin-Sain, A., Gaotheier, S., Agid, Y., Dal-Bianoc, P., Stahelin, H. B., Hartman, R., Gharabawi, G. (1999). Efficacy and safety of rivastigmine in patients with Alzheimer's disease: International randomized controlled trial. *Br Med J, 318,* 633–638.

Sano, M., Ernesto, C., Thomas, R. G., Klauber, M. R., Schafer, K., Grundman, M., Woodbury, P., Growdon, J., Cotman, C. W., Pfeifer, E., Schneider, L. S., & Thal, L. J. (1997) A controlled trial of selegiline, alpha-tocopherol, or both as treatment for Alzheimer's disease. *New England Journal of Medicine, 336,* 1216–22.

Schneider, L. S. (1993) Clinical pharmacology of aminoacridines in Alzheimer's disease. *Neurology, 43*(suppl 4), S64–S79.

Senin, U., Parnetti, L., Barbagallosangiorgi, G., Bartorelli, L., Bocola, V. Capunso, A., Cussupoli, M., Denaro, M. Marigliano, V., Tammaro, A. E., & Fioravanti, M. (1992) Idebenone in senile dementia of Alzheimer type: A multicentre study. *Archives of Gerontology and Geraitrics, 15,* 249–260.

Smith, C. D., Carney, J. M., Starke-Reed, P. E., Oliver, C. N., Stadtman, E. R., Floyd, R. A., & Markesbery, W. R. (1991) Excess brain protein oxidation and enzyme dysfunction in normal aging and in Alzheimer disease. *Proceedings of the National Academy of Sciences of the United States of America, 88,* 10540–3.

Stern, Y., Sano, M., & Mayeux, R. (1988) Long-term administration of oral physostigmine in Alzheimer's disease. *Neurology, 38,* 1837–41.

Tariot, P. N., Schneider, L. S., & Patel, S. V. (1993). Alzheimer's disease and l-deprenyl: Rationales and findings. In: I. Szelenyi, (Ed.), *Inhibitors of monoamine oxidase B: Pharmacology and clinical use in neurodegenerative disorders.* (pp. 301–317). Basel, Switzerland: Birkhauser Verlag.

Volicer, L., & Crino, P. B. (1990) Involvement of free radicals in dementia of the Alzheimer type: A hypothesis. *Neurobiology of Aging, 11,* 567–71.

Weyer, G., Babej-Dolle, R. M., Hadler, D., Hofmann, S., & Herrmann, W. M. (1997) A controlled study of 2 doses of idebenone in the treatment of Alzheimer's disease. *Neuropsychobiology, 36,* 73–82.

CHAPTER 8

Alzheimer's Disease: Behavioral Management

REBEKAH LOY, PIERRE N. TARIOT,* & KLARA ROSENQUIST
DEPARTMENTS OF PSYCHIATRY AND NEUROLOGY
UNIVERSITY OF ROCHESTER MEDICAL CENTER, AND
PROGRAM IN NEUROBEHAVIORAL THERAPEUTICS
MONROE COMMUNITY HOSPITAL

INTRODUCTION

No medication has been approved by the U.S. Food and Drug Administration for treatment of agitation or aggression associated with dementia, or any diagnosis for that matter. Further, the Omnibus Budget Reconciliation Act (OBRA) guidelines of 1987 restrict the use of psychotropics in patients with dementia who reside in nursing homes. However, absent regulatory approval, clinicians attempt to deal the best they can with agitation on a case-by-case basis. They are guided by consensus statements regarding this issue, which support the use of psychotropics when other approaches fail, and by clinical trials data, which are rapidly emerging and can influence clinical decision making. In 1997, the American Psychiatric Association issued practice guidelines for the management of patients with dementia and behavior problems (American Psychiatric Association, 1997). This evidence-based consensus process rested on the assumption that selection of medication hinged on matching target symptoms to relevant drug classes. Traditional antipsychotics were featured most prominently in these guidelines, reflecting the fact that they had been studied most extensively by the time this review occurred. In a sep-

*Corresponding author

arate consensus procedure, experienced clinicians were queried regarding use of any form of psychotropic for "agitation", even those not extensively studied (Alexopoulous, Silver, Kahn, Frances, & Carpenter, 1998). This process also relied on the assumption that it was important to match target symptoms to drug class. The reader is referred to both of these interesting publications for further details regarding the actual consensus processes.

The approach offered in this chapter deliberately goes beyond regulatory guidelines, and more or less reflects the consensus statements with respect to the use of target symptoms to guide selection of drug class. We select the medication class relevant to the dominant behavioral target symptoms, one with at least some empirical evidence of efficacy, and with the highest likelihood of safety and tolerability. The choice is sometimes influenced by the likelihood of particular desired side effects. The remainder of the chapter will summarize available evidence regarding the major psychotropic agents that have been studied for the treatment of agitation in dementia. The emphasis will be on information in the last 5 years, as prior reviews have provided comprehensive surveys previously. Table 8.1 provides an overview of individual agents and typical starting doses. Some of the doses suggested are based partially upon anecdote and clinical experience; they should be viewed with a certain degree of caution. The chapter will rely on the use of summary tables, which will be elaborated on in the text. We will close with an overview of new directions that may influence the field in the coming decade.

TABLE 8.1 Current Pharmacological Treatments for Agitation in Dementia

Drug and Class	Suggested Starting* and (Maximal) Daily Dose (mg/day)
Antipsychotics	
Traditional:	
haloperidol	0.25-0.5 (2-4)
thioridazine	12.5-25 (50-100)
Atypical:	
clozapine	6.25-12.5 (25-100)
risperidone	0.5 (1-2)
quetiapine	25 (100-200)
olanzapine	2.5 (5-10)
Antidepressants	
citalopram	10 (20)
fluoxetine	10 (20)
sertraline	25-50 (100-200)
trazodone	25-50 (200-300)

Continued

TABLE 8.1 Continued

Drug and Class	Suggested Starting* and (Maximal) Daily Dose (mg/day)
Anticonvulsants	
carbamazepine	50-100 (300-500)
valproate	125-375 (1000-1500)
Anxiolytics	
Benzodiazepines:	
alprazolam	0.5 (1-2)
lorazepam	1 (2-4)
Non-benzodiazepines:	
buspirone	10 (40-60)
zolpidem	2.5 (5)
β-blockers	
propranolol	20 (50-100)
Others	
selegiline	10
estradiol/progesterone	0.625/2.5

**Note.* Suggestions based on published data as well as anecdotal experience, and should be regarded accordingly

CONVENTIONAL ANTIPSYCHOTICS

According to the approach adopted in this chapter, antipsychotics would be chosen first for agitation that included psychotic features. Historically, however, antipsychotics have been used for virtually all forms of behavioral disturbance in dementia, especially agitation, aggression, and psychosis, and the evidence supports efficacy for these target symptoms in many cases. Antipsychotics can be grouped into two main categories: conventional antipsychotics and newer atypical antipsychotics. Conventional antipsychotics tend to block dopamine D2 receptors in particular, including those in brain regions linked to control of motor function. Reports since 1994 are summarized in Table 8.2. Haloperidol and thioridazine have been studied the most extensively. Wragg and Jeste (1988) previously reviewed controlled studies of typical agents for agitation and concluded that the effects of these drugs were modest and consistent, and that no single agent was better than another. The magnitude of the effect varied from patient to patient, and low doses were often effective. Although many of the older studies surveyed did not specify target symptoms being treated, some did. When psychotic features were present, such as hallucinations, delusions, paranoia, or excessive suspiciousness, such symptoms tended to respond (reviewed in Tariot, 1996; see also Barnes, Veith, Okimoto, Raskind, & Gumbrecht, 1982; Devanand et al.,

TABLE 8.2 Conventional Antipsychotics

Study	Diagnosis	*N*	Design	Dose (mg/day) Duration	Response	Adverse Effects
HALOPERIDOL						
Dysken, et al. 1994	AD	29	Open	1–4, 3 weeks	Good response on BEHAVE-AD in 55% of patients	EPS, sedation
Hayashi, Yamawaki, Nishikamo, & Jeste, 1995	AD, mixed, vascular dementia	51	Chart review comparison with other neuroleptics	Mean 1.8, duration variable	Improvement 77% for hallucinations, 67% delusions, 66% aggression	EPS (3/7 with haloperidol only)
Cantillon, Brunswick, Molina, & Bahro, 1996	AD	26	DB, parallel group vs. buspirone	1.5, duration variable	Overall no group differences, buspirone caused greater decrease in tension and anxiety on BPRS (10.9% vs. 1.6%)	None reported
Auchus & Bissey-Black, 1997	AD	15	DB, parallel group vs. fluoxetine or placebo	3, 6 weeks	Neither more effective than placebo for agitation	Sedation, EPS, gait disturbance, anxiety, depression in haloperidol group
Sultzer, Gray, Gunay, Berisford, & Mahler, 1997	Dementia	28	Randomized DB, parallel trazodone	1–5, 9 weeks	Decreased agitation in both; haloperidol better for excessive motor activity and paranoia	Sedation, balance, coordination problems, rigidity, weakness, rash, (50% of haloperidol group), akathisia (2)

Continued

TABLE 8.2 Continued

Study	Diagnosis	*N*	Design	Dose (mg/day) Duration	Response	Adverse Effects
Frenchman & Prince, 1997	AD, dementia NOS, organic brain syndrome	186	Chart review (83 on haloperidol)	Mean 2.0, duration variable	Decreased violence, delusions, shouting, paranoia, pacing (65% haloperidol vs. 94% risperidone)	EPS 22% haloperidol group
Devanand et al., 1998	AD	71	Randomized DB, PC, parallel group	2–3 or 0.5–0.75, 6 weeks	Decreased psychosis, aggression, agitation with higher dose only, 55–60% response vs. 25–35% low dose response vs. 25–30% placebo	Moderate-severe EPS at high dose (20%)
Christensen & Benfield, 1998	Organic mental syndrome	48	Randomized crossover to alprazolam	Mean 0.64, 6 weeks	No difference between treatments on CGI, SCAG	None seen at this low dose
DeDeyn et al., 1999	AD, vascular, mixed	344	Randomized MC, DB, parallel group risperidone or placebo	Mean 1.2, 13 weeks	Significantly greater improvement for haloperidol vs. placebo on BEHAVE-AD and CMAI, decreased physical and verbal aggression (72% risperidone vs. 69% haloperidol vs. 61% placebo on BEHAVE-AD)	EPS 22%, solmnolence (18% haloperidol vs. 4% placebo)

TABLE 8.2 Continued

Study	Diagnosis	*N*	Design	Dose (mg/day) Duration	Response	Adverse Effects
THIORIDAZINE						
Frenchman & Prince, 1997	AD, dementia NOS, organic brain syndrome	186	Chart review (43 on thicridazin)	Mean 33, 3 months	Decreased violence, delusions (67% thioridizine vs. 94% risperidone)	EPS (18% thioridazine)
THIOTHIXENE						
Finkel & Sheriell, 1995	Primary degenerative dementia	33	PC	0.25–18, 11 weeks	Improved on CMAI	EPS, sedation , lethargy (none significantly different from placebo)
TIAPRIDE						
Hayashi et al., 1995	AD, mixed, vascular dementia	51	Chart review comparison of neuroleptics	Tiapride mean 49, duration variable	Decreased hallucinations (77%), delusions (67%), aggression (66%)	Tiapride only (22): constipation (7), enuresis (2), EPS (6)
Gutzmann & Kuhl, Kanowski, & Khan-Boluki, 1997	Dementia	176	Randomized MC, DB, parallel vs. melperone		Identical response rate to melperone (74%)	Slightly higher on tiapride
ZUCLOPEN-THIXOL						
Nygaard, Bakke, Brudvik, Elgen, & Lien, 1994	Dementia	73	Randomized DE, parallel group	2–20, 4 weeks	Decreased physical aggression, agitation, verbal aggression, sleep disorder (except at 2 mg)	Few, mild
Myronuk, Geizer, & Ancill, 1997	Dementia	1	Case report	50, 3 days	Decreased aggression, more compliant	Sedation

Continued

TABLE 8.2 Continued

Abbreviations used in all tables:

AD	Alzheimer's disease
ADAS-noncog	Alzheimer's disease Assessment Scale—noncognitive subscale
BEHAVE-AD	Behavioral Pathology in Alzheimer's Disease Rating Scale
BPRS	Brief Psychiatric Rating Scale
BRSD	CERAD Behavioral Rating Scale for Dementia
CGI	Clinical Global Impression
CIBIC+	Clinician's Interview-Based Impression of Change
CMAI	Cohen–Mansfield Agitation Inventory
CRF	corticotropin releasing hormone
CSF	cerebrospinal fluid
DA	dopamine
DB	double blind
EPS	extrapyramidal symptoms
GBS	Gottfries-Bråne-Steen
GI	gastrointestinal
HD	Huntington's disease
HIAA	hydroxyindoleacetic acid
HVA	homovanillic acid
LBD	Lewy body disease
MC	multicenter
NE	norepinephrine
NOS	not otherwise specified
NR	not reported
NPI-NH	Neuropsychiatric Inventory—Nursing Home version
PC	placebo controlled
PD	Parkinson's disease
PRN	*pro re nata* (as needed)
SCAG	Sandoz Clinical Assessment-Geriatric Scale
SN	substantia nigra, pars compacta
5-HT	5-hydroxytryptamine (serotonin)

1998; Petrie et al., 1982; Reisberg et al., 1987; Sugerman, Williams, & Adlerstein, 1964; Tune, Steele, & Cooper, 1991). Increased psychosis was observed when antipsychotic therapy was withdrawn in some cases (Barton and Hurst, 1966; Devanand et al., 1998; Findlay et al., 1989).

Schneider, Pollock, & Lyness (1990) identified 33 clinical trials of these agents conducted in patients with dementia. Of these, 17 were placebo-controlled, and only 7 used a double-blind, parallel group design in patients with well-characterized dementia. These 7 trials were used in the meta-analysis and included 252 patients treated for up to 8 weeks. Antipsychotic treatment was typically associated with only a modest improvement in behavioral symptoms assessed by blinded experienced clinicians. Overall, improvement was observed in 59% of patients on antipsychotic versus 41% of patients taking placebo, an 18% difference. The paper noted that placebo response rates across these trials ranged from 20 to about 65%. A more recent meta-analysis including less rigorous studies as well as some more recent ones (Lanctot et al., 1998) came to roughly similar conclusions: type and potency of the agents did not influence response; the average therapeutic effect (antipsychotic vs. placebo) was 26%; and the placebo response rate ranged from 18–50%. Side effects were also examined in this report and found to occur more often on drug than placebo (mean difference 25%). In other words, efficacy rates are low and roughly equivalent to side effect rates.

Finally, Devanand and colleagues (1998) recently published results from a relatively large (n=71), methodologically sound placebo controlled study of haloperidol for psychosis and disruptive behaviors in Alzheimer's disease. They reported response rates of 55–60% for "standard" (2–3 mg/d) doses of haloperidol, 25–35% for "low" doses (0.50–0.75 mg/d), and 25–30% for placebo. However, a subgroup of the standard-dose group (20%) developed moderate to severe extrapyramidal signs, highlighting the relatively narrow therapeutic index of this agent in this disorder.

Significant side effects are common with conventional antipsychotics, including akathisia, parkinsonism, tardive dyskinesia, peripheral and central anticholinergic effects, cardiovascular toxicity including postural hypotension and conduction defects, sedation, and falls (Lanctot et al., 1998). For practical purposes, side effects dictate the selection of a particular typical antipsychotic in this population. It is because of these manifest side effects that safer agents are desired and needed. This issue is dramatically highlighted by the evidence of supersensitivity to antipsychotics that has been reported to occur in patients with dementia with Lewy bodies *vs.* patients with AD (Ballard, Grace, McKeith, & Holmes, 1998; Caligiuri, et al., 1998; Sweet, Mulsant, Pollock, Rosen, & Altieri, et al., 1996)

ATYPICAL ANTIPSYCHOTICS: GENERAL ISSUES

Atypical antipsychotics also block D2 dopamine receptors, but relatively less avidly than the conventional agents and they also generally block an array of receptors relevant to other neurotransmitter systems. There are considerable differences among the different atypical antipsychotics with respect to their selectivity for dopamine, serotonin, and other receptor subtypes. As a group they are less likely to be associated with toxicity, especially motor, than the conventional agents. This may reflect in part their relative selectivity for mesolimbic versus nigrostriatal dopamine receptors. Agents are summarized in Table 8.3 according to the order in which they appeared on the market in the United States.

Clozapine

There are only anecdotes and case reports regarding the efficacy, safety, and tolerability of this agent in patients with dementia (see Table 8.3). These indicate that some patients showed partial improvement in agitated or psychotic features, but many also experienced numerous side effects, including sedation and anticholinergic effects in particular. Agranulocytosis and seizures are also concerns when clozapine is used. The anecdotal evidence indicates that a wide range of doses is used by clinicians; we typically start at 6.25 or 12.5 mg/day. While clozapine may well be regarded as the most effective atypical antipsychotic for treatment of psychosis in other indications, the lack of information regarding dose response, the risk of side effects, particularly in the elderly, and the lack of controlled data may relegate it to a status as a medication selected only when other, safer, medications fail.

Risperidone

The literature includes a wide range of case reports and chart reviews suggesting that risperidone may decrease aggression, agitation, or psychosis. Side effects in these unstructured reports included dose-related extrapyramidal symptoms, sedation, and postural hypotension. While risperidone administration is sometimes associated with increased prolactin levels in other populations, the clinical significance of this in patients with dementia is uncertain.

Two large multicenter trials of risperidone have been conducted in nursing home patients. The first of these enrolled 625 patients at 40 sites in the United States, 73% of who were diagnosed as having probable AD and 15% with probable vascular dementia (Katz et al., 1999). The mean age was 83 years; 68% were women. Most patients were characterized as

TABLE 8.3 Atypical Antipsychotics

Study	Diagnosis	*N*	Design	Dose (mg/day) Duration	Response	Adverse Effects
CLOZAPINE						
Factor, Brown, Molho, & Podskalny, 1994	PD with dementia	17	Open	12.5–150, 3–24 months	Improved BPRS score (in all 17), mean 49% decrease BPRS at 3 months	Drooling (10), sedation (9), confusion (5)
Frankenburg & Kalunian 1994	Dementia	2	Case reports	>12.5, NR	No benefit	Ataxia, falls, confusion, drooling, sedation, incontinence
Salzman, Vaccan, Lieff, & Weiner, 1995	Psychosis with dementia (3), AD (1), Korsakoff (1)	5	Chart review	Modal 150, mean duration 20 days	Decreased agitation (3), delusions (1), aggression (1)	None reported
Pitner, Mintzer, Penny Packer, & Jackson 1995	AD (3), mild cognitive impairment (1)	4	Case reports	6.25–43.75, 2–16 days	Decreased hallucinations (2), aggression (1)	Sedation (2), falls (2), bradycardia (2), psychosis (1)
Wagner, Defilippi, Menza, & Sage, 1996	PD (28 with dementia)	49	Chart review	Mean 50, 3–18 months	Decreased psychotic symptoms (76% including non-demented PD)	Leukopenia (2), back pain (1), delirium (1), sedation (1), fever (1)
RISPERIDONE						
Lee, Cooney, & Lawler, 1994	LBD	1	Case report	1–5	Decreased agitation, psychosis	Sedation at higher doses

Continued

TABLE 8.3 Continued

Study	Diagnosis	*N*	Design	Dose (mg/day) Duration	Response	Adverse Effects
Allen, et al., 1995	LBD	3	Case reports	0.5–1	Decreased hallucinations (2), physical aggression (1), delusions (1)	Worsening dysarthria (1)
McKeith, Ballard, & Harrison, 1995	LBD	3	Case reports	1, 2–4 days	No benefit for hallucinations	Rigidity, stiffness, gait disturbance
Jeanblanc & Davis, 1995	AD, vascular dementia	5	Case reports	1.5–2.5, 10–31 days	Decreased (in all 5) agitation, violence	EPS (2)
Madhusoodanan, Brenner, Aranjo, & Abaza, 1995	Senile dementia, AD	2	Case reports	1.5–2, 10–14 days	Decreased psychosis	Somnolence (1), hypotension (1)
Goldberg & Goldberg, 1997	AD, mixed dementia	109	Open (concurrent psychotropics allowed)	0.5–1.0, 6 months	Decreased agitation (70%), verbal outbursts (68%); aggression, delusions, hallucinations (71%)	Sedation (9), hypotension (3), agitation (2), rash (1), urinary retention (1) EPS (1)
RISPERIDONE (Continued)						
Frenchman & Prince, 1997	AD, dementia NOS, organic brain syndrome	186	Chart review (risperidone in 60)	Mean 1.0, duration NR	Decreased violence, delusions, shouting, paranoia, pacing (94% risperidone vs. 65% haloperidol)	EPS 7%

TABLE 8.3 Continued

Study	Diagnosis	*N*	Design	Dose (mg/day) Duration	Response	Adverse Effects
Kopala & Honer, 1997	Mixed dementia	2	Open	1.5, 3 weeks	Decreased persistent vocalizations	None reported
Workman, Orengo, Bakey, Molinari, & Kunik 1997	PD dementia	9	Open (concurrent psychotropics allowed)	Mean 1.9, mean duration =37 days	Decreased psychosis, agitation (in all 9)	No worsening EPS
Hermann, 1998	Dementia	22	Case reports	"low"	Improvement in 50%	EPS (50%)
Lavretsky & Sultzer, 1998	AD, vascular, PD, PSP, mixed	15	Open (concurrent psychotropics allowed)	0.5–3, 9 weeks	Decreased agitation (in all 15)	Sedation (5), akathisia (1)
De Deyn et al., 1999	AD, vascular, mixed dementia	344	Randomized MC, DB, parallel group vs. placebo or haloperidol	Mean 1.1, 13 weeks	Decreased physical and verbal aggression (72% risperidone vs. 69% haloperidol vs. 61% for placebo)	EPS not different from placebo, somnolence (12% risperidone vs. 4% placebo)
Katz et al., 1999	AD, vascular, mixed dementia	625	Randomized MC, PC, DB, parallel group (lorazepam, benztropine & chloral hydrate allowed PRN)	0.5, 1.0, 2.0, 12 weeks	Dose-dependent decrease in aggression and psychosis, significant at 1 and 2 (but not 0.5 mg/day)	Somnolence, EPS 21% (on 2 mg/day, compared to 12% on placebo), mild peripheral edema in some

Continued

TABLE 8.3 Continued

Study	Diagnosis	*N*	Design	Dose (mg/day) Duration	Response	Adverse Effects
OLANZAPINE						
Satterlee et al., 1995	AD	238	Randomized, MC, PC, DB	1–8, 8 weeks	No benefit vs. placebo	None reported vs. placebo
Street et al., 1998	AD, moderate-severe	206	Randomized, MC, PC, DB, parallel group	5, 10 & 15, 6 weeks	Decreased agitation, delusions, hallucinations on NPI-NH at 5 and 10 (but not 15) mg/day vs. placebo	Dose-dependent sedation, abnormal gait
QUETIAPINE						
McManus et al., 1999	AD (75), vascular dementia (11)	151	Open (concurrent psycho-tropics and choral hydrate allowed PRN)	25–800, 52 week s (3 month interim report)	Improved total BPRS and positive and negative clusters	Somnolence (32%), dizziness (14%), hypotension (13%), EPS (6%)

Note: See Table 8.2 for abbreviations.

severely demented. Prior to being enrolled, patients had to experience agitation and/or psychotic features. Fixed daily doses (0.5, 1 mg, and 2 mg/day) were compared with placebo. Using an *a priori* definition of global response, roughly 52% of the placebo group improved, versus 60–65% of patients on 1 and 2 mg/day, respectively. Specific subscales indicated that, where present, psychosis tended to improve at the effective doses of 1 and 2 mg/day, as did agitated or aggressive behaviors. Risperidone was generally well-tolerated, with extrapyramidal features tending to emerge in about 22% of patients at 2 mg/day. In summary, risperidone was clearly shown to be efficacious, and generally well-tolerated (with the highest likelihood of efficacy combined with freedom from toxicity being at 1 mg/day, although some patients clearly benefited from and tolerated the higher dose). The high placebo response rate underscores the difficulty of conducting such studies and perhaps the evanescent nature of such behaviors in patients like this. It is interesting to note that this largest-ever study of medication for this problem found a drug/placebo difference analogous to that reported in the 1990 meta-analysis of Schneider, Pollock, & Lyness (1990).

Another study compared flexible doses of risperidone and haloperidol (up to 4 mg/day each) with placebo in 344 patients, with similar but less robust results (De Deyn et al., in press). The average doses were relatively low (mean dose for risperidone 1.1 mg; day, for haloperidol 1.2 mg/day), meaning that the likelihood of both efficacy and toxicity was likely to be reduced. All three conditions were equal with respect to treatment of psychotic features, while risperidone use was associated with reduction in some measures of aggression analyzed *a posteriori*. It will be important to review the full details of these two studies when they become available, in order to shed further light on the efficacy and safety of this medication.

Olanzapine

There are no published data regarding this agent in this population at present. One unpublished abstract (Satterlee et al., 1995) summarized a placebo-controlled pilot study in 238 outpatients with dementia and psychotic features which primarily addressed tolerability and preliminary dose ranging. Blinded investigators could select a dose between 1 and 10 mg/day, and eventually used a mean dose of 2.7 mg/day. At this dose, neither toxicity nor efficacy was demonstrated. At higher doses, clinical anecdotes suggest that beneficial effects can be seen, as can sedation and, less commonly, ataxia. Prolactin elevation can occur in younger patients, the clinical significance of which is uncertain. A follow-up study of olanzapine in patients with dementia has been completed using fixed doses, of 5, 10, and 15 mg/day (Street et al., 1998). The available information thus far suggests that there were reductions in measures of psychosis as well as agitation that were achieved with olanzepine 5 and 10 mg/d, with the greatest benefit as well as best tolerability at 5 mg/d. It will be important to review the details of this very recent study.

Quetiapine Fumarate

A relatively large (n = 151) 1-year open-label study of quetiapine for psychosis in elderly patients has recently been completed; 86 of these subjects had either vascular dementia or AD. The available data at this point come primarily from a manuscript in press regarding 3-month interval data and indicate reduction of psychotic features as well as agitation and aggression (McManus et al., in press). Starting doses were 25 mg/day, with a median dose of about 100 mg/day. The most common side effects reported included sedation in up to 30% of subjects, and orthostatic hypotension and dizziness in 10–15% of subjects. These typically occurred early in the course of treatment and were often characterized as mild and transient, although not always. The incidence of extrapyramidal signs and symptoms was very low, consistent with dose-ranging studies in other populations (McManus et al., in press) indicating that the incidence of extrapyramidal signs and symptoms is not different from placebo across the full dose range. This apparently low risk of motor toxicity may lead to special utility in patients with extrapyramidal disorders, although this advantage has not been proven as yet. The broad dose range in which this agent is effective makes individualization of the dosage clinically appropriate. One high-dose animal study has shown cataract formation (package insert). While a causal link in humans has not been shown, evaluation of possible cataract formation is recommended at present.

Early impressions of the atypical antipsychotics have been encouraging, and the details of these studies will bear close examination in order for us to be able to understand whether the apparent advantages in terms of efficacy compared to conventional antipsychotics (and toxicity) translate to improved effectiveness. There is every reason to believe that this is likely to be the case, although the point has not been proven as yet by published studies. If and when it is, consensus guidelines and clinical practice will both be altered in that the use of atypical agents very likely will be preferred over conventional agents. Although cost may be a constraining factor, this issue may be mitigated if cost-benefit analyses indicate that the more "expensive" agents are superior in terms of efficacy and tolerability and are associated with cost savings due to decreased side effects, improved compliance, and decreased need for hospitalization or physician contacts.

ANXIOLYTICS/SEDATIVES: BENZODIAZEPINES

Anxiolytics tend to be considered in agitated patients who also experienced prominent anxious features. Since anxious and depressive features co-occur so often in this population, many clinicians would be inclined to use an antidepressant first. This issue aside, anxiolytics have been widely used in practice for agitation and dementia, and several studies of benzodiazepines have been performed. Most of these are older and have been reviewed previously (Patel & Tariot, 1991; Tariot, 1996). While none of the small number of studies published in the last 10 years, including only one in the last 5 years, has been placebo-controlled, there may be a reduction in agitation in some patients during short-term therapy (Chesrow, Kaplitz, & Vetra, 1965; DeLemos, Clement, & Nickels, 1965).

The more recent studies will be reviewed briefly. The study of Christensen and Benfield (1998) compared very low doses of haloperidol (0.1–1.0 mg/d; mean 0.6 mg/d) to 0.5 mg alprazolam b.i.d., finding no difference between the two drugs with respect to efficacy or tolerability. This is not surprising, since the doses of medication were very low and unlikely to show benefit or toxicity. Small sample size and use of a crossover design limit interpretation of this study. Only anecdotes are available regarding clonazepam (Freinhar & Alvarez, 1986; Ginsburg 1991), and none from the last 5 years. It is typically started at 0.125 or 0.25 mg qd and increased slowly. Sedation was the major side effect reported. In the aggregate, available data suggest that agitation associated with anxiety, sleep problems, and tension might be most likely to respond (Beber, 1965; Coccaro et al., 1990). Some earlier studies in which benzodiazepines were compared to traditional antipsychotics suggested that antipsychotics might be superior.

Sedation is the most common side effect with this class of agents, along with ataxia, increased risk of falls, confusion, anterograde amnesia, lightheadedness, paradoxical agitation, and tolerance and withdrawal syndromes (Patel & Tariot, 1991). In a cognitive study examining single doses of lorazepam 0.5 mg in non-agitated patients with AD vs. controls, Sunderland and co-workers (1989) reported sedation-impaired attention, and disinhibition that was greater in patients than controls. These adverse effects argue against the use of benzodiazepines in patients with dementia except for situational disturbances (e.g., procedures), as-needed, or in instances where it is clear that routine use is not associated with toxicity. Because of age-associated changes in drug metabolism, drugs requiring simple metabolism and with relatively short half-lives tend to be preferred, e.g., lorazepam and oxazepam.

ANXIOLYTICS/SEDATIVES: NON-BENZODIAZEPINES

The literature contains modest evidence that buspirone, a non-benzodiazepine anxiolytic with partial 5HT 1A agonist effects, might be effective for agitation associated with dementia (Table 8.4). However, there have been no definitive studies and no randomized, placebo-controlled, double-blind pilot studies. Case reports and open trials suggest reduction of agitation in some patients, typically given in doses up to 30 mg/day. A single blind study of 30 mg/d versus placebo found improved aggression, but only 12/20 subjects completed the protocol (Levy et al., 1994). A small (n=10) crossover study with trazodone found no benefit of buspirone 30 mg/d (Lawlor, 1994). Finally, a study of low-dose buspirone (15 mg/d) versus low-dose haloperidol (mean = 1.3 mg/d) found no significant benefit of either (Cantillon et al., 1996). The medication is generally well-tolerated, with the most commonly reported side effects including headache, nervousness, and dizziness. It is unknown whether tolerance or paradoxical effects occur with this drug in this population.

There have been two case reports suggesting that zolpidem use (2.5–15 mg/d) was associated with improved agitation (Jackson, Pitner, & Mintzer, et al., 1996; Shelton & Hocking, 1997). This does not constitute adequate evidence to support its use.

ANTIDEPRESSANTS

This class of agents would have to be used first in patients with agitation accompanied by discernible depressive features. The serotonergic agents have attracted the most attention, most likely because of their widespread use in other clinical disorders, as well as some theoretical considerations linking impulsivity and aggression to serotonergic dysfunction (Coccaro et al., 1990).

Trazodone is a serotonergic antidepressant with alpha-2 adrenergic blocking activity that has been studied to a moderate extent. Most evidence comes from case reports or open studies; there have been no published double blind placebo-controlled studies (Table 8.5). One blinded study has been performed, comparing trazodone (mean dose about 220 mg/d) with haloperidol, which found equal improvement in agitation in both groups with better tolerability in the trazodone group (Sultzer et al., 1997); there was no placebo arm. Doses in the published reports generally range from 50 mg to 400 mg per day, sometimes higher. The available literature suggests that features of irritability, anxiety, restlessness and depressed affect might improve, along with sleep disturbance. Reported side effects, which are at least partially dose-related, include

TABLE 8.4 Non-Benzodiazepine Anxiolytics/Sedatives

Study	Diagnosis	*N*	Design	Dose (mg/day) Duration	Response	Adverse Effects
BUSPIRONE						None reported
Levy et al., 1994	AD	0	Single blind, PC	15–60, 8 weeks	Decreased delusions, aggression, anxiety subscales BEHAVE-AD, only 12 completed	
Lawlor, 1994	AD	10	DB crossover to trazodone	30, 4 weeks	No benefit with buspirone	None reported
Holzer, Gitelman, & Price, 1995	Mixed AD and vascular dementia	1	Case report	20, 3 months	Decreased aggression	None reported
Cantillon et al., 1996	AD	26	DB parallel haloperidol (mean =1.3)	Mean=15, 10 weeks	Overall no group differences, buspirone caused greater decrease in tension and anxiety on BPRS (10.9% buspirone vs. 1.6% haloperidol)	None reported

Continued

TABLE 8.4 Continued

Study	Diagnosis	*N*	Design	Dose (mg/day) Duration	Response	Adverse Effects
Hamner, Huber, & Gauthier, 1996	HD with dementia	1	Case report (concurrent haloperidol and lorazepam)	120, 8 weeks	Decreased anger, improved chorea	None reported
Bhandary & Masand, 1997	HD with dementia	1	Case report	30, 3 weeks	Decreased aggression	None reported
ZOLPIDEM						
Jackson et al., 1996	AD, history of alcohol abuse	2	Case report, concomitant haloperidol, lorazepam (1)	2.5, 5, through out hospital stay	Decreased labile mood, irritability, physical aggression (2); no change yelling (1)	Sedation (1)
Shelton & Hocking, 1997	Dementia	2	Case report	10–15, 3 months	Improved sleep, decreased wandering	None reported

Note: See Table 8.2 footnote for abbreviations.

TABLE 8.5 Antidepressants

Study	Diagnosis	*N*	Design	Dose (mg/day) Duration	Response	Adverse Effects
TRAZODONE					Decreased agitation (16)	Delirium (2), mild sedation
Houlihan et al., 1994	Dementia	22	Open	Mean 172, mean duration 20 days		
Lebert, Pasquier, & Petit, 1994	AD	13	Open	75, 10 weeks	Decreased irritability, anxiety, restlessness and affective disturbance	None reported
Lawlor, 1994	AD	10	Crossover to placebo, buspirone	Mean 120, 12 weeks	Small but significant reduction BPRS	Sedation at 150 mg
Sultzer, Gray, Gunay, Berisford, & Mahler, 1997	Dementia	28	Randomized DB parallel haloperidol	50–250, 9 weeks	Decreased agitation for both; trazodone better for verbal aggression, oppositional and repetitive behaviors	Sedation (1), imbalance (1); 1/3 fewer dropouts in trazodone group

Note: See Table 8.2 footnote for abbreviations.

sedation, orthostatic hypotension, and delirium. In the study of Sultzer and colleagues, trazodone appeared to be more effective for verbal aggression and oppositional behaviors, while haloperidol was better for repetitive motor behaviors and excessive suspiciousness.

Evidence indicates significant disturbances of serotonin metabolism in patients with AD and vascular dementia, particularly those with aggression (Chen et al., 1996; Gottfries et al., 1983; Procter, Francis et al., 1992). This provides a theoretical rationale for the use of selective serotonin reuptake inhibitors (SSRIs). As indicated in Table 8.6, the evidence for efficacy of SSRIs in treating agitation in dementia is variable. Mixed results were reported in older studies of alaproclate, with no more recent studies (see Tariot, 1996, for a review). In a retrospective review of nine prior double-blind, placebo-controlled studies of citalopram, some beneficial behavioral effects were noted (Nyth & Gottfries, 1990). This is supported by two more recent open trials (Pollock et al., 1997; Ragneskog, Eriksson, Karlsson, & Gottfries et al., 1996). One small placebo-controlled trial of fluoxetine and two placebo-controlled trials of fluvoxamine did not demonstrate benefit. There are only anecdotes available about other agents, all suggesting the possibility of benefit in at least some patients. Although generally well-tolerated, side effects of serotonergic agents can include gastrointestinal symptoms, anorexia, weight loss, sedation, insomnia, sexual dysfunction, and occasional increased anxiety or even agitation. Motor symptoms such as tremor can sometimes occur. The exact role of SSRIs in the therapeutic armamentarium is not well-established at this juncture; confirmatory clinical trials are needed.

ANTICONVULSANTS

Specific anticonvulsants have been used in psychiatry for the treatment of acute mania and have been assayed by clinicians for treatment of other neuropsychiatric disorders. Anticonvulsants have been considered for treatment of agitation in patients who also have manic-like features, depressive features, and/or possibly in those with prominent impulsivity, lability, or "nonspecific" outbursts of aggression.

Carbamazepine has psychotropic properties similar to lithium when used in mania, although carbamazepine is associated with less neurotoxicity. Case reports from a variety of patient populations suggest beneficial effects on agitation. With respect to dementia specifically, case reports and pilot studies subsequently suggested that carbamazepine may be effective in the treatment of some agitated behaviors (see Tariot & Schneider, 1998; Table 8.7). There have been three placebo-controlled studies. One small placebo-controlled crossover study in 19 women with a number of

TABLE 8.6 Selective Serotonin Reuptake Inhibitors

Study	Diagnosis	*N*	Design	Dose (mg/day) Duration	Response	Adverse Effects
CITALOPRAM						
Ragneskog et al., 1996	Dementia	93	Open, 2 centers	30, 4 weeks	Decreased CGI or Gottfries-Brane-Steen (GBS) for irritability, depression (60%)	Asthenia/tiredness (15); dizziness (14); drowsiness, sleep disturbances, restlessness (4), aggression (3), anxiety (2)
Pollock et al., 1997	AD	15	Open	20, 2 weeks	Decreased agitation, hostility, delusions, disinhibition	Drop-outs from nausea (1), myoclonus (1)
FLUOXETINE						
Geldmacher, Waldman, Doty, & Heilman, 1994	AD	5	Chart review	40, 4 weeks	No improvement on GBS	Agitation, dizziness, confusion
Auchus & Bissey-Black, 1997	AD	15	DB, PC parallel group vs. haloperidol	20, 6 weeks	Neither more effective than placebo for agitation	Anxiety, nervousness, confusion, tremor

Continued

TABLE 8.6 Continued

Study	Diagnosis	N	Design	Dose (mg/day) Duragion	Response	Adverse Effects
SERTRALINE						
Volicer, Rheaume, & Cyr, 1994	Severe AD	10	Open	Variable dose, duration	Improved affect (8), improved food intake (6)	None reported
Burke, Folks, Roccaforte, & Wengel, 1994	AD	3	Open	50, 1–4 weeks	Decreased psychosis (3), wandering, crying (1)	None reported
Burke et al., 1997	AD, NOS dementia	19	Chart review	50, Variable duration	Improved on CGIC (10/11 AD; 4/8 NOS)	None reported

Note: See Table 8.2 footnote for abbreviations.

TABLE 8.7 Anticonvulsants

Study	Diagnosis	*N*	Design	Dose (mg/day) Duration	Response	Adverse Effects
CARBAMAZEPINE						
Tariot et al., 1994	AD, vascular dementia	25	Crossover, PC (some other psychotropics permitted)	300 modal, 5 weeks	Decreased agitation (16 vs. 4 placebo)	Tics (1), sedation
Lemke, 1995	Severe AD	15	Open (some on haloperidol)	100–600, 4 weeks	Decreased agitation	Ataxia (3), leukopenia (2), nausea (1)
Cooney, Mortimer, Smith, & Newton, 1996	AD	6	Randomized, PC, crossover	Up to 600, 8 weeks	Decreased aggression (all 6)	Sedation over 300 mg
Tariot & Schneider, 1998	dementia	51	Randomized PC (no psychotropics except chloral hydrate as needed)	300 modal, 6 weeks	Improved on CGI (20/26 on drug; none on placebo); also improved on OAS, BPRS, BRSD	Ataxia (9 vs. 3 placebo), disorientation (4 vs. 0 placebo), tics (1), sedation

Note: See Table 8.2 footnote for abbreviations.

methodologic limitations was reported as negative (Chambers, Bain, Rosbottom, Ballinger, & McLaren, 1982). By contrast, positive different results were obtained from a preliminary crossover study in 25 nursing home patients with dementia, treated with an average dose of 300 mg per day (Tariot & Schneider, et al., 1994). A follow-up study in 51 patients found essentially similar results (Tariot et al., 1998). Interestingly, nursing home staff also reported spending less time providing care for behavioral problems in the drug group versus the placebo group in this latter study. In the two recent placebo-controlled studies, tolerability was generally good, although two patients developed tics, and there were mild side effects more commonly on drug than placebo (primarily sedation and ataxia) (Tariot, Schneider, & Katz, et al., 1995; Tariot & Schneider, 1998). Side effects not seen in the controlled studies might be more likely to occur with uncontrolled use, including rash, sedation, ataxia, hematologic abnormalities, hepatic dysfunction, and electrolyte disturbances (Tariot et al., 1995). Further, there are numerous known drug/drug interactions associated with the use of carbamazepine. While the carbamazepine data support the concept that anticonvulsants may be relevant for treatment of agitation in dementia, it is possible that alternative, potentially safer, agents would be as effective and better tolerated.

Valproic acid, along with its better-tolerated enteric-coated derivative, divalproex sodium, is an anticonvulsant structurally different from carbamazepine but with similar psychotropic effects in the treatment of mania. It has generally fewer side effects, and reduced potential for drug/drug interactions. In the US, divalproex is approved by the FDA for treatment of mania associated with bipolar disorder, as well as for the prophylactic treatment of migraine. In other clinical populations, it has a favorable side effect profile compared to alternative antimanic agents. In dementia, there are now numerous open series and case reports suggesting beneficial effect, occurring in roughly two-thirds of patients described (Table 8.8). This is supported by preliminary results from a placebo-controlled trial conducted by our group (unpublished data), in which 56 nursing home patients with dementia and agitation were randomized to clinically optimal doses of divalproex sodium or placebo. The average divalproex dose achieved was roughly 840 mg/day, with an average level of 46 mcg/ml. Trend level improvement was found in primary measures of agitation ($p<.10$) with generally good tolerability (significant adverse effects occurred with equal frequency in the drug and placebo groups, about 10%). Side effects seen commonly in other clinical populations include sedation, weight gain, hair loss, thrombocytopenia, and hepatic dysfunction. In our studies so far in patients with dementia, sedation and gastrointestinal disturbance appeared to be the most common side effects (Porsteinsson, Tariot, Erb, & Gaile, 1997; Tariot, 1999).

TABLE 8.8 Anticonvulsants

Study	Diagnosis	*N*	Design	Dose (mg/day) Duration	Response	Adverse Effects
VALPROATE						
Sival, Haffmans, Van Gent, & Van Nieuwkerk, 1994	AD, PD, vascular dementia	23	Retrospective review	240–1200 (mean=248), duration variable	Decreased aggression (12)	Drowsiness (2), ataxia (1)
Horne & Lindley, 1995	AD	1	Case report	NR, (level=62)	Decreased agitation	None reported
Lott, McElroy, & Keys, 1995	AD, PD, vascular dementia	10	Open	375-750 (mean =525), (mean level= 37 µmol/L), 4-34 weeks	Decreased agitation (9)	Worsening of tremor (1) , sedation (1)
Sandborn, Bendfeldt, & Hamdy, 1995	AD, vascular dementia	4	Open	1000–1500, (level=24-55), duration variable	Decreased agitation, aggression (2)	Sedation (2), ambulatory problems (2), incontinence (1)
Puryear, Kunik, & Workman, 1995	Severe organic mental disorder NOS, mixed (not all dementia)	13	Retrospective review (concurrent psychotropics in most patients)	500–1750, (mean level=61), 7 months	Improved on BPRS (9)	Dry mouth (5), low sexual interest (4), fatigue (4), tremor (3), nervousness (4), delirium (1), sedation

Continued

TABLE 8.8 Anticonvulsants (Continued)

Study	Diagnosis	*N*	Design	Dose (mg/day) Duration	Response	Adverse Effects
Haas, Vincent, Holt, & Lippmann, 1997	AD, vascular dementia, Wernicke-Korsakoff	12	Open	750–1500 (mean =938), (mean level=63), duration variable	Decreased aggression (all 12)	None reported
Kasckow, 1997	AD, alcohol, vascular dementia	10	Open (PRN chloral hydrate and lorazepam)	500–2250 (mean =1188), (mean level=63), 2–5 weeks	Improved on BEHAVE-AD, CGI (5)	Increased agitation (2), sedation (1), decreased platelets (1)
Porsteinsson et al., 1997	AD, vascular dementia, mental retardation	13	Open (PRN lorazepam and chloral hydrate)	250–1500 (mean =802), (mean level=54), 5–21 weeks	Improved on CGIC (10); increased weight (2)	Sedation (4), apraxia (3), anorexia(1)

TABLE 8.8 Continued

Study	Diagnosis	*N*	Design	Dose (mg/day) Duration	Response	Adverse Effects
Narayan & Nelson, 1997	AD, vascular dementia, PD dementia, other dementia	25	Retrospective review	250–4000 (mean =1650), (mean level=64), duration variable	11/16 with AD improved 3/9 with other dementia improved	Sedation (8), gait disturbance (1), confusion (1)
Herrmann et al., 1998	AD, LB, vascular dementia	16	Open	750–2500 (mean =1331), (mean level=459 µM/l), 5–34 weeks	Improved on CMAI, BEHAVE-AD (11)	Sedation, ataxia, diarrhea (1)
Kunik et al., 1998	Dementia	13	Retrospective review (concurrent BDZs, anti-psychotics)	500–1750 (mean =846), (mean level =48), duration variable	Decreased physical not verbal agitation and aggression on CMAI (10)	None reported; drug interaction with phenytoin noted (1)

The potential role of the more novel anticonvulsant agents, such as lamotrigene, gabapentin, and topiramate is not currently established, although there is at least once case report of benefit from treatment with gabapentin plus haloperidol (Regan & Gordon, 1997). Because anticonvulsants as a group have relatively benign side effects based on years of experience in other clinical populations, evidence of significant efficacy of one or more individual anticonvulsants will very likely influence clinical practice in the future.

Selegiline

Selegiline, also known as L-deprenyl, is a relatively selective inhibitor of monoamine oxidase (MAO) type B at lower doses (e.g., 10 mg/day), while it nonselectively inhibits MAO type A and B at higher doses. It has been used primarily in the treatment of patients with Parkinson's disease, but some reports also suggest beneficial effects in patients with dementia and agitation (see Table 8.9). In a meta-analysis of several controlled trials, Tolbert and Fuller (1996) found that all single blind and open-label studies that assessed behavioral improvement recorded a positive effect for selegiline, while two of five double-blind, placebo-controlled studies did so. The authors did not come to a definitive conclusion in favor of selegiline therapy for this purpose. A similar conclusion is drawn from a Cochrane meta-analysis of 11 randomized control double-blind trials, which 4 of 11 were reported to have beneficial behavioral effects (Birks & Flicker, 1998).

Our own interpretation of the literature is that, where beneficial behavioral effects were found, psychopathology had to have been present at baseline. Conversely, where psychopathology was absent, there was a ceiling effect, and no improvement could be discerned (e.g. Tariot & Schneider, 1998). Given the fact that there is some potential for drug/drug interactions, as well as some potential for side effects, selegiline is not typically considered a first rank choice for medication treatment for agitation. Its role for the treatment of cognitive dysfunction, or as a neuroprotective agent, has not fully been elucidated.

BETA BLOCKERS

Beta blockers have not been extensively studied in patients with diagnoses of dementia, although there are a number of older reports in patients with mixed organic brain syndromes (see Tariot et al., 1995). Shankle, Nielson, & Cotman (1995) recently reported that aspects of aggression improved in 8 of 12 patients with dementia receiving low dose propranolol (30–80 mg/day), with only one case of bradycardia. The entire literature regarding use of beta blockers for agitation associated with dementia is limited, concomitant psychoactive medications were typically permitted; all studies are small; and most are open trials. Adverse reactions, which appear more likely to occur with propranolol than pindolol, include bradycardia, hypotension, potential worsening of congestive heart failure or asthma, blockade of symptomatic consequences of hypoglycemia in diabetics, sedation, confusion, hallucinosis, depression, and increased AV block. Since there are no placebo-controlled, randomized, blinded parallel group studies of this strategy, and since the available literature is primarily anecdotal, it is unclear that this medication has a meaningful role in the treatment of agitation associated with dementia.

LITHIUM

Lithium therapy was originally advocated for use in dementia based on case reports and studies of anti-aggression efficacy in other patient populations (Risse & Barnes, 1986). There were a few case reports in the early 1980s, with no new reports since that time (Tariot & Schneider, 1998). This limited literature indicates that the majority of patients with dementia and agitation did not show behavioral improvement with lithium, with some exceptions.

CHOLINERGIC THERAPY

Several investigators have reported behavioral effects of cholinergic agents (see Table 8.10). Cummings, Gorman, and Shapiro (1993) reported that physostigmine ameliorated delusions in patients with AD. This was supported by work conducted by Harrell, Callaway, Morere, & Falgout (1990), and a case report by Molchan, Vitiello, Minichiello, & Sunderland (1991). Kaufer, Cummings, and Christina (1996) reviewed a series of patients treated only with tacrine, reporting some positive behavioral effects in a subgroup. A retrospective analysis of available behavioral data, which were limited in extent, from one of the pivotal tacrine trials reported improvement in delusions on tacrine therapy versus placebo (67% of patients versus 41%, respectively) and in pacing (70% versus 54%, respectively) and lack of deterioration in measures of cooperation in patients on tacrine versus placebo (Raskind et al., 1997). However, a Cochrane meta-analysis of controlled, randomized, double-blind trials of tacrine that conformed to the meta-analysis requirements found no difference from placebo in various behavioral measures (Qizilbash et al., 1999).

TABLE 8.9 Selegiline

Study	Diagnosis	*N*	Design	Dose (mg/day) Duration	Response	Adverse Effects
Tolbert & Fuller, 1996	AD	25 8 230	Meta-analysis of 2 open 1 single-blind 5 DB	NR 3 weeks–2 years	Improvement "behavior" 2/2 open trials 1/1 single-blind 2/5 double-blind	None reported
Lawlor, Aisen, Green, Fine, & Schmeidler, 1997	AD	25	Randomized, DB, PC	10, 6 weeks	Significant benefit measured by BPRS	None reported
Sano et al., 1997	Moderate AD	341	Randomized, MC, DB, PC comparison with vitamin E or combination	10, up to 2 years	Decreased behavioral (BRSD) symptoms with combined therapy, other comparisons were not significantly different from placebo	Syncope (9 selegiline vs. 3 placebo), falls (8 selegiline vs. 4 placebo), dental events (6 selegiline vs. 0 placebo)

TABLE 8.9 Continued

Study	Diagnosis	*N*	Design	Dose (mg/day) Duration	Response	Adverse Effects
Tariot & Schneider, 1998	Mild-moderate AD	50	Randomized, DB, crossover vs. placebo	10, 8 weeks	No significant effect on behavior, ability to function on a day-to-day basis or global ratings scale	None reported
Freedman et al., 1998	Probable AD	60	Randomized, DB, PC	10, 25 weeks	No significant short term affect on general behavior or neuropsychiatric symptoms	Dizziness (30%vs. 20% placebo), irritability (23% vs. 16% placebo), dry mouth (20% vs. 12% placebo), restlessness (19% vs. 12% placebo)
Birks & Flicher, 1998	AD		Meta-analysis of 11 randomized, PC, DB	Various	Benefit in treatment of behavior and mood in 4/11 trials	

TABLE 8.10 Cholinergics

Study	Diagnosis	*N*	Design	Dose (mg/day) Duration	Response	Adverse Effects
CHOLINESTERASE INHIBITORS TACRINE						
Hutchinson & Fazzini, 1996	PD dementia	7	Open	60 2 months	Decreased hallucinations (in all 7)	None reported
Kaufer et al., 1996	Mild-severe AD	28	Open	40–160 6 weeks	Significant decline NPI at >120 mg (9); more benefit in moderate AD (63% reduction) *vs* mild or severe	None reported
Raskind et al., 1997	Mild-mod AD	419	Retrospective analysis, MC Randomized, PC, DB, parallel group	160 30 wk	Decreased delusions (67% tacrine vs. 41% placebo), pacing (70% tacrine *vs.* 54% placebo), improved cooperation (94% tacrine vs. 47% placebo) using ADAS-noncog	As per original report
Qizilbash, 1998	AD	>2K	Meta-analysis randomized, PC, DB	20–160 2 weeks–9 months	No difference from placebo ADAS-noncog	Elevated serum liver enzymes, diarrhea, anorexia, dyspepsia, abdominal pain
DONEPEZIL						
Shea et al., 1998	Lewy body disease	9	Case report (1 also on risperidone)	5 8–16 weeks	Decreased hallucinations (8)	Worsening of parkinsonian features (3)
Pettenati & Donato, 1998	Mild to severe AD	21	Open	5 2 months	Improvement on NPI	None reported

TABLE 8.10 Continued

Study	Diagnosis	*N*	Design	Dose (mg/day) Duration	Response	Adverse Effects
METRIFONATE						
Morris et al., 1998	Mild-mod AD	408	Randomized, MC, PC, DB, parallel group	30–60 (lower loading dose) 26 wk	CIBIC+, ADAS-noncog improved by 12 weeks, NPI mean score showed significant decrease in hallucinations	Nausea (3%), diarrhea (2%), dyspesia (1%) [in metrifonate patients]
CHOLINERGIC AGONISTS XANOMELINE						
Bodick et al., 1997	AD	343	Randomized, MC, PC, DB, parallel group	75, 150, 225 6 months	Reduced vocal outbursts, suspiciousness, delusions, agitation, hallucinations; response dose-dependent	GI, syncope; 50% drop-out at high dose (nausea, vomiting, diaphoreis)
NICOTINE						
Wilson et al., 1995	AD	6	PC, DB, crossover	Patch 8 days	No change in "behavior"	Decrease in sleep

Note: See Table 8.2 footnote for abbreviations.

More recently, a prospective clinical trial of metrifonate versus placebo found reduction in some neuropsychiatric symptoms on drug versus placebo (Morris et al., 1998). Specifically, hallucinations occurred significantly less often, with a trend toward reduced apathy on drug versus placebo. These clinical trials data are supported by recent abstracts or open trials with donepezil in patients with AD, and dementia with Lewy bodies, suggesting improvement (Pettenati et al., 1998; Shea, McKnight, & Rockwood, 1998;). In all instances, the cholinesterase inhibitors are known to have fairly consistent cholinergic side effects including GI distress in roughly 10–25% of patients, with rare side effects including bradycardia and muscle cramps. The concept of possible benefit of cholinominetic therapy for behavioral symptoms was supported by recent work with the muscarinic agonist xaenomeline, which was reported to be associated with the reduction in agitation on drug versus placebo (Bodick et al., 1997). This may not be clinically relevant, as it appears that the medication is no longer in active development. By way of overview, cholinergic therapy in dementia is likely to have selective behavioral effects in some patients with dementia. Given the apparently selective behavioral effects observed, it does not appear likely that an important "antiagitation" effect will be reliably achieved, however, although more definitive studies are pending.

HORMONAL THERAPY

Antiandrogens have been reported to show beneficial effects on aggression and agitation in a variety of case reports (Table 8.11). Side effects include increased sleep, hair loss, disturbed appetite, and mood. Similarly, there are case reports of estrogen showing some beneficial effect on physical aggression in men. One study showed a higher likelihood of aggression in postmenopausal women who did not receive estrogen replacement therapy (Wiseman et al., 1997). Finally, Kyomen, Satlin, and Wei (1997) reported a randomized double-blind placebo-controlled clinical trial in 13 patients, 12 of whom were female. With a combination of estrogen and progesterone there was a significant reduction in physical but not other types of aggression. Again, the anecdotal evidence does not amount to an endorsement of this approach, only a suggestion that it may be helpful.

SUMMARY OF CLINICAL TRIALS

Where psychotropic medications are used for agitation in dementia, they should be selected carefully, applied in the lowest effective doses, and for the least period of time possible. Most of the available evidence suggests

TABLE 8.11 Hormones

Study	Diagnosis	*N*	Design	Dose (mg/day) Duration	Response	Adverse Effects
ESTROGENS						
Kay et al., 1995	Dementia and Kluver	5 men 12 women,	Open Randomized	Transdermal estradiol 1–3 days	Decreased aggression	Gynecomastia (1)
Kyomen et al., 1997	Dementia	12 women, 1 man	Randomized DB, PC	Estradiol 0.625 & progester-one 2.5 4 weeks	Decreased physical aggression, not other types of aggression	None reported
Wiseman et al., 1997	Dementia	18 women	Chart review	Not reported	With no history estrogen, aggression score higher	None reported
ANTIANDROGENS LEUPROLIDE						
Ott, 1995	Dementia with Kluver Bucy	1 man	Open	Intramuscular 7.5 mg/month	Decreased sexual aggression and inappropriate behavior	None reported
LEUPROLIDE or MEDROXY-PROGESTERONE						
Amadeo, 1996	AD	3 men	Open	Variable 4 weeks	Both decreased aggression, impulsiveness & hostility, pacing	Sleepiness, hair loss, diabetes, increased appetite, depression, reduced ejaculation

that antipsychotics show most benefit for agitation associated with psychotic features, with mounting evidence suggesting benefit for some patients for agitation not associated with psychotic features. The side effects of typical agents are legion: data are emerging regarding the possible superior side-effect profile of atypical agents.

The evidence to date regarding non-antipsychotic medications ranges from case reports to double-blind, placebo-controlled, parallel-group studies. Carbamazepine and divalproex sodium have demonstrated efficacy in uncontrolled studies; carbamazepine has produced negative results in one small controlled study and positive results in two controlled studies; and valproate showed trend effects in a preliminary placebo-controlled study. Buspirone has shown some benefit in open trials. There are encouraging early findings regarding trazodone and selective serotonin reuptake inhibitors. These data suggest the possibility that medications other than traditional antipsychotics may be effective and reasonably well-tolerated.

As we look ahead to the next generation of agents, it is possible that advances in understanding of the mechanisms of psychotropic action in general, and new understanding of pathophysiology of disturbed behavior in dementia, will lead to novel forms of therapy. We will attempt a provocative preview of this arena in the closing portion of the chapter.

NEUROBIOLOGICAL CORRELATES OF BEHAVIORAL SYMPTOMS IN DEMENTIA

While the neural substrates for agitation, aggression, and psychosis are likely to be diverse, several studies have correlated neuropathological and biochemical findings with the presence of behavioral symptoms in dementia. In general, the neuropathology of AD involves the long ascending tracts, resulting in the hallmark loss of the cholinergic input to the cortex and hippocampus, as well as in complex changes in noradrenergic, dopaminergic, and serotonergic function. Additionally, intrinsic neurons in many cortical and limbic areas are affected, as evidenced by changes in glutamate, GABA, and a variety of neuropeptides and their receptors. Many of these neurotransmitter systems have been implicated in the behavioral symptoms of AD (Table 8.12). For instance, psychosis and agitation/disinhibition factor scores on the Neurobehavioral Rating Scale correlate with hypometabolic and perfusion abnormalities in the frontal and temporal cortices (Mentis et al., 1995; Starkstein et al., 1994; Sultzer et al., 1995; Volkow et al., 1995), regions of significant loss of the cholinergic innervation to both neurons and vasculature. Agitation, hostility and psychosis can be exacerbated by muscarinic antagonists (Sunderland et al., 1985, 1987), and various cholinergic agonists (Bodick et al., 1997) and cholinesterase inhibitors (Cummings et al., 1993; Hutchinson & Fazzini, 1996; Morris et al., 1998; Raskind et al., 1997; Shea et al., 1998) show occasional efficacy in treating agitation, delusions, and hallucinations, although they can also sometimes aggravate pre-existing agitation. These findings suggest that neuronal targets within the frontal cortex or temporal regions may be involved in the modulation of behavioral symptomatology, and that these sites may be regulated at least in part by cholinergic systems.

There is also some evidence that agitation in dementia is associated with changes in catecholaminergic function. Agitation correlates with elevated cerebrospinal fluid (CSF) levels of the noradrenergic metabolite MHPG (Brane et al., 1989; Raskind et al., 1984), suggesting increased noradrenergic turnover or hyperactivity. The severity of agitation and aggression is also correlated with plasma concentrations of the dopamine metabolite homovanillic acid (Sweet et al., 1997), consistent with a separate report of pathologically identified differences in substantia nigra neuron numbers in patients with AD with and without aggression (Victoroff, Zarow, Mack, Hsu, & Chi, 1996). Many of the pharmacotherapies effective in treating agitation and aggression target catecholamines. β-adrenergic receptor blockers have been used successfully for over 10 years to reduce physical and verbal aggression and agitation in patients with dementia. The traditional, and to a lesser degree the atypical, antipsychotic agents act via blockade of dopamine D_2 receptors. These data suggest that dopamine blockade may be beneficial. To the extent, however, that this blockade is associated with the appearance of significant extrapyramidal side effects, modifying other neurotransmitter systems may be useful.

Serotonin is likely to be involved in agitation, as it is correlated with decreased levels of cortical serotonin and increased levels of the serotonin metabolite 5-HIAA in AD (Procter et al., 1992), suggesting altered turnover. The relationship is not simple, however, as agitation can be increased by serotonergic agonists, while it is sometimes effectively treated (and sometimes exacerbated) by SSRIs and atypical antipsychotics, which are antagonists at serotonin 5-HT_{2A} autoreceptors. AD patients with depression also show more loss of raphe neurons and decreases in 5-HT in many brain areas (Chen et al., 1996; Zweig et al., 1988). Another agent which can increase serotonergic activity, the anxiolytic buspirone, may have some benefit for agitation.

The major class of anxiolytics, the benzodiazepines, act through a mechanism involving GABA receptors. The benzodiazepine binding site coordinates with the GABA binding site to increase chloride permeability, inhibiting neuronal activity. Similarly, the anticonvulsant drugs which are effective in treating agitation—carbamazepine, valproate, and gabapentin—also promote GABAergic inhibition of neuronal function.

TABLE 8.12 Neurobiological Correlates of Behavioral Symptoms in Alzheimer's Disease

	Acetylcholine	Dopamine	Norepinephrine	Serotonin	Other
AGITATION AND AGGRESSION	↑ by muscarinic antagonists[1]; can be ↓ by muscarinic agonists[2]	severity of agitation correlates with plasma HVA[3]; ↑ presynaptic DA and CSF HVA[4] SN neuron counts normal in aggressive patients, but ↓ in patients with no aggression[5]; agitation generally ↓ by DA antagonists[6,7]	↑ CSF NE metabolite MHPG8,9, sugggesting possible NE hyperactivity; ↑ by elevated NE following yohimbine challenge[10]	↓ 5-HT and increased 5-HIAA levels and ↑ 5-HT turnover in some cortical areas[11]; ↓ platelet 3H-imipramine binding density[12]	high levels of cholesterol associated with agitation but not aggression[13]; hypometabolic and perfusion abnormalities in frontal and temporal cortex[14,15]
PSYCHOSIS	ameliorated by muscarinic agonists[2], cholinesterase inhibitors[16-20]; ↑ by cholinergic antagonists[21,22]	not associated with presynaptic DA function[23]	monoaminergic nuclei preserved[24]; NE levels in SN, other subcortical areas and cortex ↑ or preserved[25]	↓ 5-HT in prosubiculum and trend toward ↓ levels in other cortical and subcortical regions[25]	correlates with hypometabolic and perfusion abnormalities in frontal and temporal cortex[14,26,27]; density of cortical senile plaques and neurofibrillary tangles ↑[25]

TABLE 8.12 Continued

	Acetylcholine	Dopamine	Norepinephrine	Serotonin	Other
WANDERING		correlates with ↑ striatal D2 receptors[23]			correlates with ↓ glucose utilization in temporal and frontal cortices[28]
APATHY					correlates with hypometabolic and perfusion abnormalities in frontal and temporal cortex[29]
DEPRESSION	no change with muscarinic or nicotinic agonists or cholinesterase inhibitors; ↑ loss cholinergic neurons[30]	associated with normal or ↓ DA levels and variable SN pathology[31]; CSF HVA ↓ or unchanged[9]	more locus coeruleus neuron loss[24,30,32]; ↓ cortical NE levels but ↑ NE turnover[33]	loss of raphe neurons[24] and ↓ 5-HT in most brain areas[34]; ↓ 5-HT uptake sites in frontal and temporal cortex[34]	CRH ↑ in CSF[35]; ↓ cortisol suppression with dexamethasone[36]

1. Sunderland et al., 1987; 2. Bodick et al., 1997; 3. Sweet et al., 1997; 4. Eichelman, 1990; 5. Victoroff et al., 1996; 6. Devanand et al., 1998; 7. DeDeyn et al., 1999; 8. Raskind, Peskind, Halkr, & Jimerson, 1984; 9. Brane et al., 1989; 10. Raskind & Peskind, 1994; 11. Procter et al., 1992; 12. Schneider et al., 1988; 13. Orengo et al., 1996; 14. Sultzer et al., 1995; 15. Volkow et al., 1995; 16. Moris et al., 1998; 17. Shea et al., 1998; 18. Raskind et al., 1997; 19. Hutchinson & Fazzini, 1996; 20. Cummings et al., 1993; 21. Sunderland et al., 1985; 22. Sunderland et al., 1987; 23. Bierer et al., 1993; 24. Zweig et al., 1988; 25. Zubenko et al., 1991; 26. Mentis et al., 1995; 27. Starkstein et al., 1994; 28. Meguro et al., 1996 29. Craig et al., 1996; 30. Zubenko, 1992; 31. Chan-Palay & Asan, 1989; 32. Forstl Levy, Burns, Luthert, & Cairns, 1994; 33. Zubenko & Moosey, 1990; 34. Chen et al., 1996; 35. Banki, Karmacsi, Bissettz & Nemeroff, 36. O'Brien et al., 1996.

Note: See Table 8.2 footnote for abbreviations.

BRAIN REGIONS INVOLVED IN AGGRESSION AND AGITATION

From a variety of studies we know that aggression, like other motivated behaviors, is controlled by the medial hypothalamus, its inputs from the frontal cortex and extended amygdala, and outputs to autonomic and motor nuclei in the brainstem (Risold, Thompson, & Swanson, 1997). Damage to the hypothalamus in animals or in patients due to hypothalamic tumors (Reeves & Plum, 1969), can result in unprovoked aggression. By contrast, stereotactic damage of specific nuclei of the amygdala has been used successfully to treat patients with pathological aggressivity (Burzaco, 1985), although damage to other components can lead to aggression directed inappropriately. An important pathway from medial amygdala to medial hypothalamus and continuing on to the midbrain periaqueductal gray region controls predatory attack behavior in cats (Han, Shaikh, & Siegel, 1996). Thus, the extended amygdala has a complex role in integrating autonomic, endocrine and somatomotor aspects of emotional and motivational states (Heimer, Harlan, Alheid, Garcia, & de Olmos, 1997; Swayze et al., 1992; Trimble, Mendez, & Cummings, 1997). The frontal cortex provides another level of control over the hypothalamus, introducing flexibility, planning, and the ability to assess consequences of behaviors. Damage to the orbitofrontal cortex has been associated with disinhibition and violence, and dorsolateral lesions with social withdrawal and apathy (Krakowski, 1997).

There is neuropathology in all of these areas, including hypothalamus and brainstem autonomic and motor nuclei, at least at the later stages in AD (Swaab et al., 1993). Since the behavioral symptoms usually emerge within 2 years of the initial diagnosis, there may be secondary or parallel degenerative processes leading to behavioral and cognitive impairments. Initial damage to the hippocampus and entorhinal cortex may lead to deafferentation of the extended amygdala, which may in turn lead to sprouting of frontal cortical and intrinsic projections and increased responsiveness of meso-limbic dopamine systems. This sprouting and consequent neurochemical supersensitivity may underlie a variety of behavioral symptoms relating to psychosis and agitation, including the ability to inhibit unrewarded or inappropriate behaviors (Rolls, 1996), and may be responsible for the efficacy of some of the psychotropic agents in treating agitation. At present we can only conclude that the roles of the many neurochemical changes in dementia which may contribute to later-developing behavioral symptoms are likely to be complex and interdependent.

A PROPOSED COMMON MECHANISM FOR TREATMENTS OF AGITATION

In addition to the classical neurotransmitters known to be affected in patients with behavioral symptoms, there may be a role for several important neuropeptides and their receptors, which are also known to be altered in AD. Substance P is one of the earliest neurotransmitters to be affected in both AD and Huntington's disease, another neurodegenerative disorder with a high prevalence of aggressive symptoms. Early targets of the neurodegenerative process in AD are substance P-containing, deep cortical interneurons, while a substance P-containing subset of cholinergic neurons of the nucleus basalis of Meynert are affected at later stages (Ang & Shul, 1995; Kowall, Beal, Busciglio, Duffy, & Yankner, 1993). In AD, accompanying the loss of substance P neurons,there may also be sprouting in remaining neurons (Quigley & Kowall, 1991).

Converging evidence from clinical and experimental studies suggests that substance P may be involved in regulating affective behaviors, including aggression and agitation. For instance, preventing expression of the neurokinin-1 (NK-1) receptor gene in a mouse "knock-out" model eliminates both stress-induced analgesia and the aggressive response to territorial challenge (DeFelipe et al., 1998). Injection of synthetic substance P fragments can elicit isolation-induced fighting in normal mice (Hall & Stewart, 1984), while chronic capsaicin treatment leads to aggressive behavior in mice which correlates with the level of reduction in hypothalamic substance P (Bigi, De Acetis, De Simone, Aloe, & Alleva, 1993). In addition, the amygdalo-hypothalamic pathway regulating aggression in cats utilizes substance P (Han et al., 1996). Importantly, Kramer and colleagues recently showed that Merck's NK-869, a highly selective substance P antagonist which blocks NK-1 receptors, shows benefit in certain animal models of anxiety and depression and ameliorates symptoms of depression and anxiety in depressed patients with high levels of anxiety (Kramer et al., 1998). These preliminary preclinical and clinical data at least provide support for the notion that modulation of substance P can influence at least some aspects of behavior.

Given (1) the relationship of substance P to behavioral measures of aggression and agitation, and (2) the degenerative and plastic responses of substance P neurons in AD and HD, it is most interesting to find that the majority of treatments for agitation in these patients also have effects on or interact with substance P in animal models. Anecdotes suggest that estrogen can sometimes reduce aggressive behavior in both men and women with dementia, and estrogen regulates substance P levels in both hypothalamus and amygdala (Rance & Young, 1991; Ricciardi & Blaustein, 1994; Turcotte & Blaustein, 1997). The antipsychotic haloperidol decreases substance P in the hypothalamus (Lau & Tang, 1995), striatum, nucleus accumbens, and substantia nigra (Jolkkonen, Jenner, & Marsden, 1994; Waters, Konkoy, & Davis, 1995), while increasing NK-1 receptor sensitivity in substantia nigra (Liminga & Gunne, 1993). The anmestic effect of benzodiazepine treatment is blocked by coadministration of substance P (Costa and Tomaz, 1998). Both lithium and the anticonvulsant carbamazepine dose-dependently increase substance P in striatum and substantia nigra, but not in the raphe nuclei (Mitsushio, Takashima, Mataga, & Toru, 1988). The anticonvulsants carbamazepine and valproate (Bianchi, Rossoni, Maggi, Panerai, & Berti, 1998; W. S. Lee et al., 1995) block dural plasma extravasion and bronchoconstriction induced by substance P stimulation; valproate also inhibits substance P-stimulated cortisol and ACTH secretion (Coiro et al., 1992).

Loss of substance P-containing neurons has previously only been discussed in terms of its putative role in memory, since iontophoretic application of substance P into the nucleus basalis facilitates memory (Huston & Hasenohrl, 1993). However, it is likely that loss of substance P in AD may contribute not only to cognitive and behavioral pathology, but in fact to continued neuronal degeneration, since it can play a neuroprotective role in blocking the neurotoxic (Kowall et al., 1991) effects of beta-amyloid.

INTO THE FUTURE

The fleeting nature of behavioral symptomatology, often lasting only minutes to hours, suggests that the neurobiological changes of behavioral symptomatology in AD are dynamic and multidetermined. Relevant factors are likely to include personality, environment, social, medical and biological at the least. The dynamism suggests that structural causes alone are not apt to account for the biological basis of these behaviors, and that biochemical variables are important. The course of symptomatology in AD further supports this conclusion. Cognitive symptoms generally decline progressively with minor fluctuations, whereas the behavioral changes frequently are of later onset, intermittent, and often recurrent. In the present chapter, we have reviewed the more recent clinical studies evaluating pharmacological and non-pharmacological treatments for agitation in patients with dementia. The diversity of symptoms and the wide variety of agents which are effective at least to some degree suggest widespread biochemical alterations in many neurotransmitter systems. It is attractive to consider that some unifying hypothesis may emerge which will facilitate rational choices of therapy and drug design. We propose that agents which modify substance P or its NK-1 receptors and associated G-protein transducing system in the frontal cortex, amygdala or hypothalamus, should be effective in treating agitation.

CONCLUSION

Agitation is a common and morbid manifestation of dementia. A key management principle is to follow a logical sequence of evaluations and interventions to establish the etiology of the change in behavior, to treat specifically if there is an identifiable medical or psychiatric precipitant, and to establish whether simple and safe non-pharmacologic interventions will be beneficial prior to considering symptomatic pharmacotherapy. When psychotropics are used, they should be used judiciously, in the lowest effective doses, and for the shortest period of time necessary. Medications which are ineffective should be stopped after an appropriate empirical trial. Furthermore, even medications which are effective should probably be empirically tapered and, if possible discontinued, in most patients to establish whether ongoing treatment is still necessary. As an anecdote to this effect, our own naturalistic study of antipsychotic withdrawal in agitated nursing home patients suggested that roughly half of patients who had been treated long-term with traditional antipsychotics were able to have these stopped without recurrence of symptoms during the 6-month observation period (Horwitz, Tariot, Mead, & Cox, 1995). Additionally, in a recent randomized, double-blind baseline neuroleptic-controlled trial, Bridges-Parlet, Knopman, and Steffes (1997) found no significant difference between withdrawn and not-withdrawn subjects in the number of observed episodes of physically aggressive behavior or the number of subjects completing the 4-week trial.

With respect to selection of treatment, it is important to remember that no psychotropic has been approved for treatment of agitation in dementia, or indeed any other disorder, by the U.S. Food and Drug Administration. In the absence of regulatory approval, clinicians use their own experience, data from clinical trials, and consensus guidelines. Of the available consensus guidelines, one (American Psychiatric Association, 1997) focused on evidence from controlled clinical trials, and emphasized primarily the use of traditional antipsychotics. The more recent, nonevidence-based consensus process (Alexopoulos et al., 1998) relied on the opinion of "experts" rather than on data. Predictably, the range of therapies considered appropriate for treatment were much broader as a result of this process.

Current evidence suggests but does not prove that alternatives to traditional antipsychotics exist for treatment of this problem. As more studies become available, and are published, we will have a better idea about which classes are most effective and tolerable. Clinical trials data are pending and currently unpublished from studies with divalproex sodium, haloperidol versus trazodone versus placebo, risperidone from two multicenter trials, olanzapine from one multicenter trial, quetiapine studied in an open trial as well as a controlled trial versus haloperidol and placebo, donepezil alone, and donepezil plus sertraline, as well as others. These data will undoubtedly have a major impact on how we care for our patients, and lead to revisions of current practice guidelines.

ACKNOWLEDGEMENTS

We thank Sidra Tayrein for assistance in preparing the references.

REFERENCES

Alexopoulos, G. S., Silver, J. M., Kahn, D. A., Frances, A., & Carpenter, D. (1998). Treatment of agitation in older persons with dementia. *Postgraduate Medicine, April,* 1–88.

Allen, R. L., Walker, Z., D'Ath, P. J., & Katona, C. L. (1995). Risperidone for psychotic and behavioural symptoms in Lewy body dementia. *Lancet, 346* (8968), 185.

Amadeo, M. (1996). Antiandrogen treatment of aggressivity in men suffering from dementia. *Journal of Geriatric Psychiatry & Neurology, 9*(3), 142–145.

American Psychiatric Association Work Group on Alzheimer's Disease and Related Dementias, Rabins, P., Blacker, D., Bland, W., Bright-Long, L., Cohen, E., Katz, I., Rovner, B., & Schneider, L. (1997). Practice guideline for the treatment of patients with Alzheimer's disease and other dementias of late life. *American Journal of Psychiatry, 154*(5), 1–39.

Ang, L. C., & Shul, D. D. (1995). Peptidergic neurons of subcortical white matter in aging and Alzheimer's brain. *Brain Research, 674*(2), 329–335.

Auchus, A. P., & Bissey-Black, C. (1997). Pilot study of haloperidol, fluoxetine, and placebo for agitation in Alzheimer's disease. *Journal of Neuropsychiatry & Clinical Neurosciences, 9*(4), 591–593.

Ballard, C., Grace, J., McKeith, I., & Holmes, C. (1998). Neuroleptic sensitivity in dementia with Lewy bodies and Alzheimer's disease [letter]. *Lancet, 351*(9108), 1032–1033.

Banki, C. M., Karmacsi, L., Bissette, G., & Nemeroff, C. B. (1992). Cerebrospinal fluid neuropeptides in mood disorder and dementia. *Journal of Affective Disorders, 25*(1), 39–45.

Barnes, R., Veith, R., Okimoto, J., Raskind, M., & Gumbrecht, G. (1982). Efficacy of antipsychotic medications in behaviorally disturbed dementia patients. *American Journal of Psychiatry, 139*(9), 1170–1174.

Barton, R., & Hurst, L. (1966). Unnecessary use of tranquilizers in elderly patients. *British Journal of Psychiatry, 112*(491), 989–990.

Beber, C. R. (1965). Management of behavior in the institutionalized aged. *Diseases of the Nervous System, 26,* 591–595.

Bhandary, A. N., & Masand, P. S. (1997). Buspirone in the management of disruptive behaviors due to Huntington's disease and other neurological disorders. *Psychosomatics, 38*(4), 389–391.

Bianchi, M., Rossoni, G., Maggi, R., Panerai, A. E., & Berti, F. (1998). Effects of carbamazepine on plasma extravasation and bronchoconstriction induced by substance P, capsaicin, acetaldehyde and histamine in guinea-pig lower airways. *Fundamental & Clinical Pharmacology, 12* (1), 58–63.

Bierer, L. M., Knott, P. J., Schmeidler, J. M., Marin, D. B., Ryan, T.M., Haroutunian, V., Purohit, D. P., Perl, D. P., Mohs, R. C., & Davis, K. L. (1993). Post-mortem examination of dopaminergic parameters in Alzheimer's disease: relationship to noncognitive symptoms. *Psychiatry Research, 49*(3), 211–217.

Bigi, S., De Acetis, L., De Simone, R., Aloe, L., & Alleva, E. (1993). Neonatal capsaicin exposure affects isolation-induced aggressive behavior and hypothalamic substance P levels of adult male mice (Mus musculus). *Behavioral Neuroscience, 107*(2), 363–369.

Birks, J. and Flicker, L. The efficacy and safety of selegiline for the symptomatic treatment of Alzheimer's disease: a systematic review of the evidence (Cochrane Review). The Cochrane Library (2). 1998. (GENERIC)

Bodick, N. C., Offen, W. W., Levey, A. I., Cutler, N. R., Gauthier, S. G., Satlin, A., Shannon, H. E., Tollefson, G. D., Rasmussen, K., Bymaster, F. P., Hurley, D. J., Potter, W. Z., & Paul, S. M. (1997). Effects of xanomeline, a selective muscarinic receptor agonist, on cognitive function and behavioral symptoms in Alzheimer disease. *Archives of Neurology, 54*(4), 465–473.

Brane, G., Gottfries, C. G., Blennow, K., Karlsson, I., Lekman, A., Parnetti, L., Suennerholm, L., & Wallin, A. (1989). Monoamine metabolites in cerebrospinal fluid and behavioral ratings in patients with early and late onset of Alzheimer's disease. *Alzheimer Disease & Associated Disorders, 3,* 148–156.

Bridges-Parlet, S., Knopman, D., & Steffes, S. (1997). Withdrawal of neuroleptic medications from institutionalized dementia patients: results of a double-blind, baseline-treatment-controlled pilot study. *Journal of Geriatric Psychiatry & Neurology, 10*(3), 119–126.

Burke, W. J., Folks, D. G., Roccaforte, W. H., & Wengel, S. P. (1994). Serotonin reuptake inhibitors for the treatment of coexisting depression and psychosis in dementia of the Alzheimer type. *American Journal of Geriatric Psychiatry, 2*(4), 352–354.

Burke, W. J., Dewan, V., Wengel, S. P., Roccaforte, W. H., Nadolny, G. C., & Folks, D. G. (1997). The use of selective serotonin reuptake inhibitors for depression and psychosis complicating dementia. *International Journal of Geriatric Psychiatry, 12*(5), 519–525.

Burzaco, J. (1985). Stereotactic pallidotomy in extrapyramidal disorders. *Applied Neurophysiology, 48*(1-6), 283–287.

Caligiuri, M. P., Rockwell, E., & Jeste, D. V. (1998). Extrapyramidal side effects in patients with Alzheimer's disease treated with low-dose neuroleptic medication. *American Journal of Geriatric Psychiatry, 6*(1), 75–82.

Cantillon, M., Brunswick, R., Molina, D., & Bahro, M. (1996). Buspirone vs. haloperidol: a double-blind trial for agitation in a nursing home population with Alzheimer's disease. *American Journal of Geriatric Psychiatry, 4*(3), 263–267.

Chambers, C. A., Bain, J., Rosbottom, R., Ballinger, B. R., & McLaren, S. (1982). Carbamazepine in senile dementia and overactivity—a placebo controlled double blind trial. *IRCS Medical Science, 10;* 505–506.

Chan-Palay, V., & Asan, E. (1989). Alterations in catecholamine neurons of the locus coeruleus in senile dementia of the Alzheimer type and in Parkinson's disease with and without dementia and depression. *Journal of Comparative Neurology, 287*(3), 373–392.

Chen, C. P., Alder, J. T., Bowen, D. M., Esiri, M. M., McDonald, B., Hope, T., Jobst, K. A., & Francis, P. T. (1996). Presynaptic serotonergic markers in community-acquired cases of Alzheimer's disease: Correlations with depression and neuroleptic medication. *Journal of Neurochemistry, 66*(4), 1592–1598.

Chesrow, R. J., Kaplitz, S. E., Vetra, H. (1965). Blind study of oxazepam in the management of geriatric patients with behavioral problems. *Clinical Medicine, 13,* 1001–1005.

Christensen, D. B., & Benfield, W. R. (1998). Alprazolam as an alternative to low-dose haloperidol in older, cognitively impaired nursing facility patients. *Journal of the American Geriatrics Society, 46*(5), 620–625.

Coccaro, E. F., Kramer, E., Zemishlany, Z., Thorne, A., Rice, C. M., Giordani, B., Duvvi, K., Patel, B.M., Torres, J., & Nora, R. (1990). Pharmacologic treatment of noncognitive behavioral disturbances in elderly demented patients. *American Journal of Psychiatry, 147*(12), 1640–1645.

Coiro, V., Capretti, L., Volpi, R., Davoli, C., Marcato, A., Cavazzini, U., Caffarri, G., Rossi, G., & Chiodera, P. (1992). Stimulation of ACTH/cortisol by intravenously infused substance P in normal men: Inhibition by sodium valproate. *Neuroendocrinology, 56*(4), 459–463.

Cooney, C., Mortimer, A., Smith, A., & Newton, K. (1996). Carbamazepine use in aggressive behavior associated with senile dementia. *International Journal of Geriatric Psychiatry, 11*(10), 901–905.

Costa, J. C., & Tomaz, C. (1998). Posttraining administration of substance P and its N-terminal fragment block the amnestic effects of diazepam. *Neurobiology of Learning & Memory, 69*(1), 65–70.

Craig, A. H., Cummings, J. L., Fairbanks, L., Itti, L., Miller, B. L., Li, J., & Mena, I. (1996). Cerebral blood flow correlates of apathy in Alzheimer disease. *Archives of Neurology, 53*(11), 1116–1120.

Cummings, J. L., Gorman, D. G., & Shapira, J. (1993). Physostigmine ameliorates the delusions of Alzheimer's disease. *Biological Psychiatry, 33*(7), 536–541.

De Deyn, P. P., Rabheru, K., Rasmussen, A., Bocksberger, J. P., Dautzenberg, P. L. J., Eriksson, S., & Lawlor, B. A. (1999). A randomized trial of risperidone, placebo, and haloperidol for behavioral symptoms of demetia. *Neurology,* in press.

DeFelipe, C., Herrero, J. F., O'Brien, J. A., Doyle, C. A., Smith, A. J., Laird, J. M., Belmonte, C., Cervero, F., & Hunt, S. P. (1998). Altered nociception, analgesia and aggression in mice lacking the receptor for substance P. *Nature, 392,* 394–397.

DeLemos, G. P., Clement, W. R., & Nickels, E. (1965). Effect of diazepam suspension in geriatric patients hospitalized for psychiatric illnesses. *Journal of the American Geriatrics Society, 13,* 355–359.

Devanand, D. P., Marder, K., Michaels, K., Sackeim, H. A., Bell, K., Sullivan, M., Cooper, T., Pelton, G. H., & Mayeux, R. (1998). A randomized, placebo-controlled, dose-comparison trial of haloperidol for psychosis and disruptive behaviors in Alzheimer's disease. *American Journal of Psychiatry, 155,* 1512–1520.

Dysken, M. W., Johnson, S. B., Holden, L., Vatassery, G., Nygren, J., Jelinski, M., Kuskowski, M., Schut, L., McCarten, J.R., Knopman, D., Maletta, G. J., & Skare, S. (1994). Haloperidol concentrations in patinets with Alzheimer's dementia. *American Journal of Geriatric Psychiatry, 2*(2), 124–133.

Eichelman, B. S. (1990). Neurochemical and psychopharmacologic aspects of aggressive behavior. *Annual Review of Medicine, 41,* 149–158.

Factor, S. A., Brown, D., Molho, E. S., & Podskalny, G. D. (1994). Clozapine: A 2-year open trial in Parkinson's disease patients with psychosis. *Neurology, 44*(3), 544–546.

Findlay, D. J. (1989). Double-blind controlled withdrawal of thioridazine treatment in elderly female inpatients with senile dementia. *International Journal of Geriatric Psychiatry, 4*(2)

Finkel, S. I., Lyons, J. S., Anderson, R. L., Sherrell, K., Davis, J., Cohen-Mansfield, J., Schwartz, A., Gandy, J., & Scheide, L. (1995). A randomized, placebo-controlled trial of thiothixene in agitated, demented nursing home patients. *International Journal of Geriatric Psychiatry, 10*(2), 129–136.

Forstl, H., Levy, R., Burns, Luthert, P., & Cairns, N. (1994). Disproportionate loss of noradrenergic and cholinergic neurons as cause of depression in Alzheimer's disease: A hypothesis. *Pharmacopsychiatry, 27*(1), 11–15.

Frankenburg, F. R., & Kalunian, D. (1994). Clozapine in the elderly. *Journal of Geriatric Psychiatry & Neurology, 7*(2), 129–132.

Freedman, M., Rewilak, D., Xerri, T., Cohen, S., Gordon, A. S., Shandling, M., & Logan, A. G. (1998). L-deprenyl in Alzheimer's disease: Cognitive and behavioral effects. *Neurology, 50*(3), 660–668.

Freinhar, J. P., & Alvarez, W. A. (1986). Clonazepam treatment of organic brain syndromes in three elderly patients. *Journal of Clinical Psychiatry, 47*(10), 525–526.

Frenchman, I. B., & Prince, T. (1997). Clinical experience with risperidone, haloperidol, and thioridazine for dementia-associated behavioral disturbances. *International Psychogeriatrics, 9*(4), 431–435.

Geldmacher, D. S., Waldman, A. J., Doty, L., & Heilman, K. M. (1994). Fluoxetine in dementia of the Alzheimer's type: Prominent adverse effects and failure to improve cognition. *Journal of Clinical Psychiatry, 55*(4), 161

Ginsburg, M. L. (1991). Clonazepam for agitated patients with Alzheimer's disease. *Canadian Journal of Psychiatry, 36*(3), 237–238.

Goldberg, R. J., & Goldberg, J. (1997). Risperidone for dementia-related disturbed behavior in nursing home residents: A clinical experience. *International Psychogeriatrics, 9*(1), 65–68.

Gottfries, C. G., Adolfsson, R., Aquilonius, S. M., Eckernas, S. A., Svennerholm, L., Wiberg, A., & Winblad, B. (1983). Biochemical changes in dementia disorders of Alzheimer type (AD/SDAT). *Neurobiology of Aging, 4*, 261–271.

Gutzmann, H., Kuhl, K.P., Kanowski, S., & Khan-Boluki, J. (1997). Measuring the efficacy of psychopharmacological treatment of psychomotoric restlessness in dementia: Clinical evaluation of tiapride. *Pharmacopsychiatry, 30*(1), 6–11.

Haas, S., Vincent, K., Holt, J., & Lippmann, S. (1997). Divalproex: A possible treatment alternative for demented, elderly aggressive patients. *Annals of Clinical Psychiatry, 9*(3), 145–147.

Hall, M. E., & Stewart, J. M. (1984). Modulation of isolation-induced fighting by N- and C-terminal analogs of substance P: Evidence for multiple recognition sites. *Peptides, 5*(1), 85–89.

Hamner, M., Huber, M., & Gauthier, S. G. (1996). Patient with progressive dementia and choreaothetoid treated with buspirone. *Journal of Clinical Psychopharmacology, 16*(3), 261–262.

Han, Y., Shaikh, M. B., & Siegel, A. (1996). Medial amygdaloid suppression of predatory attack behavior in the cat: I Role of a substance P pathway from the medial amygdala to the medial hypothalamus. *Brain Research, 716*(1–2), 59–71.

Harrell, L. E., Callaway, R., Morere, D., & Falgout, J. (1990). The effect of long-term physostigmine administration in Alzheimer's disease. *Neurology, 40*(9), 1350–1354.

Hayashi, T., Yamawaki, S., Nishikawa, T., & Jeste, D. V. (1995). Usage and side effects of neuroleptics in elderly japanese patients. *American Journal of Geriatric Psychiatry, 3*(4), 308–316.

Heimer, L., Harlan, R. E., Alheid, G. F., Garcia, M. M., & de Olmos, J. (1997). Substantia innominata: A notion which impedes clinical-anatomical correlations in neuropsychiatric disorders. *Neuroscience, 76*(4), 957–1006.

Herrmann, N. (1998). Valproic acid treatment of agitation in dementia. *Canadian Journal of Psychiatry, 43*(1), 69–72.

Herrmann N., Rivard, M. F., Flynn, M., Ward, C., Rabheru, K., & Campbell, S. (1998). Risperidone for the treatment of behavioral disturbances in dementia: A case series. *Journal of Neuropsychiatry & Clinical Neurosciences, 10*(2), 220–223.

Holzer, J. C., Gitelman, D. R., & Price, B. H. (1995). Efficacy of buspirone in the treatment of dementia with aggression. *American Journal of Psychiatry, 152*(5), 812.

Horne, M., & Lindley, S. (1995). Divalproex dosium in the treatment of aggressive behaviour and dysphoria in patients with organic brain syndromes. *Journal of Clinical Psychiatry, 56*, 430–431.

Horwitz, G. J., Tariot, P. N., Mead, K., & Cox, C. (1995). Discontinuation of antipsychotics in nursing home patients with dementia. *American Journal of Geriatric Psychiatry, 3*(4), 290–299.

Houlihan, D. J., Mulsant, B. H., Sweet, R. A., Rifai, A. H., Pasternak, R., Rosen, J., & Zubenko, G. S. (1994). A naturalistic study of trazodone in the treatment of behavioral complications of dementia. *American Journal of Geriatric Psychiatry, 2*(1), 78–85.

Huston, J. P., & Hasenohrl, R. U. (1995). The role of neuropeptides in learning: Focus on the neurokinin substance P. *Behavioural Brain Research, 66*(1-2), 117–127.

Hutchinson, M., & Fazzini, E. (1996). Cholinesterase inhibition in Parkinson's disease. *Journal of Neurology, Neurosurgery & Psychiatry, 61,* 324–326.

Jackson, C. W., Pitner, J. K., & Mintzer, J. E. (1996). Zolpidem for the treatment of agitation in elderly demented patients. *Journal of Clinical Psychiatry, 57*(8), 372–373.

Jeanblanc, W., & Davis, Y. B. (1995). Risperidone for treating dementia-associated aggression. *American Journal of Psychiatry, 152*(8), 1239

Jolkkonen, J., Jenner, P., & Marsden, C. D. (1994). GABAergic modulation of striatal peptide expression in rats and the alterations induced by dopamine antagonist treatment. *Neuroscience Letters, 180*(2), 273–276.

Kasckow, J. W., McElroy, S. L., Cameron, R. L., Mahler, L. L., & Fudala, S. J. (1997). A pilot study on the use of divalproex sodium in the treatment of behavioral agitation in elderly patients with dementia: Assessment with the BEHAVE-AD and CGI rating scales. *Current Therapeutic Research, 58*(12)

Katz, I., Jeste, D.V., Mintzer, J. E., Clyde, C., Napolitano, J., & Brecher, M. (1999). Comparison of risperidone and placebo for pychosis and behavioral diturbances associated with dementia: A randomized, double-blind trial. *Journal of Clinical Psychiatry, 60,* 107–115.

Kaufer, D. I., Cummings, J. L., & Christine, D. (1996). Effect of tacrine on behavioral symptoms in Alzheimer's disease: An open-label study. *Journal of Geriatric Psychiatry & Neurology, 9*(1), 1–6.

Kay, P. A. J., Yurkow, J., Forman, L. J., Chopra, A. (1995). Transdermal estradiol in the management of aggressive behaviors in male patients with dementia. *Clinical Gerontologist, 15*(3), 54–58.

Kopala, L. C., & Honer, W. G. (1997). The use of risperidone in severely demented patients with persistent vocalizations. *International Journal of Geriatric Psychiatry, 12,* 73–77.

Kowall, N. W., Beal, M. F., Busciglio, J., Duffy, L. K., & Yankner, B. A. (1991). An in vivo model for the neurodegenerative effects of beta amyloid and protection by substance P. *Proceedings of the National Academy of Sciences of the United States of America, 88*(16), 7247–7251.

Kowall, N. W., Quigley, B. J. J., Krause, J. E., Lu, F., Kosofsky, B. E., & Ferrante, R. J. (1993). Substance P and substance P receptor histochemistry in human neurodegenerative diseases. *Regulatory Peptides, 46*(1-2), 174–185.

Krakowski, M. (1997). Neurologic and Neuropsychologic correlates to violence. *Psychiatric Annals 27,* 674–678.

Kramer, M. S., Cutler, N., Feighner, J., Shrivastava, R., Carman, J., Sramek, J. J., Reines, S. A., Liu, G., Snavely, D., Wyatt-Knowles, E., Hale, J. J., Mills, S. G., MacCoss, M., Swain, C. J., Harrison, T., Hill, R. G., Hefti, F., Scolnick, E. M., Cascieri, M. A., Chicchi, G. G., Sadowski,

S., Williams, A. R., Hewson, L., Smith, P., & Rupniak, N.M. (1998). Distinct mechanism for antidepressant activity by blockade of central substance P receptors. *Science, 281*(5383), 1640–1645.

Kunik, M. E., Puryear, L., Orengo, C. A., Molinari, V., Workman, R. H. (1998). The efficacy and tolerability of divalproex sodium in elderly demented patients with behavioral disturbances. *International Journal of Geriatric Psychiatry, 13*(1), 29–34.

Kyomen, H. H., Satlin, A., & Wei, J. Y. (1997, November). *Estrogen therapy decreases the frequency of physically aggressive behaviors in severely demented elderly patients.* Paper presented at 105th Annual Meeting, American Psychological Society, Chicago, IL.

Lanctot, K. L., Best, T. S., Mittmann, N., Liu, B. A., Oh, P. I., Einarson, T. R., & Naranjo, C. A. (1998). Efficacy and safety of neuroleptics in behavioral disorders associated with dementia. *Journal of Clinical Psychiatry, 59*(10), 550–561.

Lau, S. M., & Tang, F. (1995). The effect of haloperidol on met-enkephalin, beta-endorphin, cholecystokinin and substance P in the pituitary, the hypothalamus and the striatum of rats during aging. *Progress in Neuro-Psychopharmacology & Biological Psychiatry, 19*(7), 1163–1175.

Lavretsky, H., & Sultzer, D. (1998). A structured trial of risperidone for the treatment of agitation in dementia. *American Journal of Geriatric Psychiatry, 6*(2), 127–135.

Lawlor, B. A. (1994). A pilot placebo-controlled study of trazodone and buspirone in Alzheimer's disease. *International Journal of Geriatric Psychiatry, 9*(1), 55–59.

Lawlor, B. A., Aisen, P. S., Green, C., Fine, E., & Schmeidler, J. (1997). Selegiline in the treatment of behavioural disturbance in Alzheimer's disease. *International Journal of Geriatric Psychiatry, 12*(3), 319–322.

Lebert, F., Pasquier, F., & Petit, H. (1994). Behavioral effects of trazodone in Alzheimer's disease. *Journal of Clinical Psychiatry, 55*(12), 536–538.

Lee, H., Cooney, J. M., & Lawlor, B. A. (1994). The use of risperidone, an atypical neuroleptic, in Lewy body disease. *International Journal of Geriatric Psychiatry, 9*(5), 415–417.

Lee, W. S., Limmroth, V., Ayata, C., Cutrer, F. M., Waeber, C., Yu, X., & Moskowitz, M. A. (1995). Peripheral GABAA receptor-mediated effects of sodium valproate on dural plasma protein extravasation to substance P and trigeminal stimulation. *British Journal of Pharmacology, 116*(1), 1661–1667.

Lemke, M. R. (1995). Effect of carbamazepine on agitation in Alzheimer's inpatients refractory to neuroleptics. *Journal of Clinical Psychiatry, 56*(8), 354–357.

Levy, M. A., Burgio, L. D., Sweet, R., Bonino, P., Janosky, J., & Perel, J. (1994). A trial of buspirone for the control of disruptive behaviors in community-dwelling patients with dementia. *International Journal of Geriatric Psychiatry, 9*(10), 841–848.

Liminga, U., & Gunne, L. M. (1993). Intranigral stimulation of oral movements by [Pro9] substance P, a neurokinin-1 receptor agonist, is enhanced in chronically neuroleptic-treated rats. *Behavioural Brain Research, 57*(1), 93–99.

Lott, A. D., McElroy, S. L., & Keys, M. A. (1995). Valproate in the treatment of behavioral agitation in elderly patients with dementia. *Journal of Neuropsychiatry & Clinical Neurosciences, 7*(3), 314–319.

Madhusoodanan, S., Brenner, R., Araujo, L., & Abaza, A. (1995). Efficacy of risperidone treatment for psychoses associated with schizophrenia, schizoaffective disorder, bipolar disorder, or senile dementia in 11 geriatric patients: A case series. *Journal of Clinical Psychiatry, 56*(11), 514–518.

McKeith, I. G., Ballard, C. G., & Harrison, R. W. (1995). Neuroleptic sensitivity to risperidone in Lewy body dementia. *Lancet, 346*(8976), 699

McManus, D. Q., Arvanitis, L. A., Kowalcyk, B. B., & Seroquel Trial 48 Study Group. (1999). "Seroquel" (Quetiapine), a novel antipsychotic: experience in elderly patients with psychotic disorders. *Journal of Clinical Psychiatry,* in press.

Meguro, K., Yamaguchi, S., Yamazaki, H., Itoh, Yamaguchi, T., Matsui, H., & Sasaki, H. (1996). Cortical glucose metabolism in psychiatric wandering patients with vascular dementia. *Psychiatry Research, 67*(1), 71–80.

Mentis, M. J., Weinstein, E. A., Horwitz, B., McIntosh, A. R., Pietrini, P., Alexander, G. E., Furey, M., & Murphy, D. G. (1995). Abnormal brain glucose metabolism in the delusional misidentification syndromes: A positron emission tomography study in Alzheimer disease. *Biological Psychiatry, 38*(7), 438–449.

Mitsushio, H., Takashima, M., Mataga, N., & Toru, M. (1988). Effects of chronic treatment with trihexyphenidyl and carbamazepine alone or in combination with haloperidol on substance P content in rat brain: A possible implication of substance P in affective disorders. *Journal of Pharmacology & Experimental Therapeutics, 245*(3), 982–989.

Molchan, S. E., Vitiello, B., Minichiello, M., & Sunderland, T. (1991). Reciprocal changes in psychosis and mood after physostigmine in a patient with Alzheimer's disease. *Archives of General Psychiatry, 48*(12), 1113–1114.

Morris, J. C., Cyrus, P. A., Orazem, J., Mas, J., Bieber, F., Ruzicka, B. B., & Gulanski, B. (1998). Metrifonate benefits cognitive, behavioral, and global function in patients with Alzheimer's disease. *Neurology, 50*(5), 1222–1230.

Myronuk, L., Geizer, M., & Ancill, R. J. (1997). Zuclopenthixol acetate in a demented elderly patient with agitation. *Canadian Journal of Psychiatry, 42*(3), 325.

Narayan, M., & Nelson, J. C. (1997). Treatment of dementia with behavioral disturbance using divalproex or a combination of divalproex and a neuroleptic. *Journal of Clinical Psychiatry, 58*(8), 351–354.

Nygaard, H. A., Bakke, K., Brudvik, E., Elgen, K., & Lien, G. K. (1994). Dosing of neuroleptics in elderly demented patients with aggressive and agitated behaviour: A double-blind study with zuclopenthixol. *Current Medical Research & Opinion, 13*(4), 222–232.

Nyth, A. L., & Gottfries, C. G. (1990). The clinical efficacy of citalopram in treatment of emotional disturbances in dementia disorders: A Nordic multicentre study. *British Journal of Psychiatry, 157*, 894–901.

O'Brien, J. T., Ames, D., Schweitzer, I., Colman, P., Desmond, P., & Tress, B. (1996). Clinical and magnetic resonance imaging correlates of hypothalamic-pituitary-adrenal axis function in depression and Alzheimer's disease. *British Journal of Psychiatry, 168*(6), 679–687.

Orengo, C. A., Kunik, M. E., Molinari, V. A., Teasdale, T. A., Workman, R. H., & Yudofsky, S. C. (1996). Association of serum cholesterol and triglyceride levels with agitation and cognitive function in a geropsychiatry unit. *Journal of Geriatric Psychiatry & Neurology, 9*(2), 53–56.

Ott, B. R. (1995). Leuprolide treatment of sexual aggression in a patient with Dementia and the Kluver-Bucy syndrome. *Clinical Neuropharmacology, 18*(5), 443–447.

Patel, S., & Tariot, P. N. (1991). Pharmacologic models of Alzheimer's disease. *Psychiatric Clinics of North America, 14*(2), 287–308.

Petrie, W. M., Ban, T. A., Berney, S., Fujimori, M., Guy, W., Ragheb, M., Wilson, W. H., & Schaffer, J. D. (1982). Loxapine in psychogeriatrics: A placebo- and standard-controlled clinical investigation. *Journal of Clinical Psychopharmacology, 2*(2), 122–126.

Pettenati, C., & Donato, M. F. (1998, July). Behavioral symptoms of Alzheimer's disease: Improvement by donepezil. *Presented at the Sixth International Conference on Alzheimer's Disease, Amsterdam.*

Pitner, J. K., Mintzer, J. E., Pennypacker, L. C., & Jackson, C. W. (1995). Efficacy and adverse effects of clozapine in four elderly psychotic patients. *Journal of Clinical Psychiatry, 56*(5), 180–185.

Pollock, B. G., Mulsant, B. H., Sweet, R., Burgio, L. D., Kirshner, M. A., Shuster, K., & Rosen, J. (1997). An open pilot study of citalopram for behavioral disturbances of dementia: Plasma levels and real-time observations. *American Journal of Geriatric Psychiatry, 5*(1), 70–78.

Porsteinsson, A. P., Tariot, P. N., Erb, R., & Gaile, S. (1997). An open trial of valproate for agitation in geriatric neuropsychiatric disorders. *American Journal of Geriatric Psychiatry, 5*(4), 344–351.

Procter, A. W., Francis, P. T., Stratmann, G. C., & Bowen, D. M. (1992). Serotonergic pathology is not widespread in Alzheimer patients without prominent aggressive symptoms. *Neurochemical Research, 17*(9), 917–922.

Puryear, L. J., Kunik, M. E., & Workman, R., Jr. (1995). Tolerability of divalproex sodium in elderly psychiatric patients with mixed diagnoses. *Journal of Geriatric Psychiatry & Neurology, 8*(4), 234–237.

Qizilbash, N. (1998). Tacrine meta-analysis. *Journal of the American Medical Association, 280*, 1777–1782.

Qizilbash, N., Birks, J., Lopez, A. J., Lewington, S., Szeto, S. (1999). Tacrine for Alzheimer's disease. *Cochrane Review*, Issue 2.

Quigley, B. J. J., & Kowall, N. W. (1991). Substance P-like immunoreactive neurons are depleted in Alzheimer's disease cerebral cortex. *Neuroscience, 41*(1), 41–60.

Ragneskog, H., Eriksson, S., Karlsson, I., & Gottfries, C. G. (1996). Long-term treatment of elderly individuals with emotional disturbances: An open study with citalopram. *International Psychogeriatrics, 8*(4), 659–668.

Rance, N. E., & Young, W. S. (1991). Hypertrophy and increased gene expression of neurons containing neurokinin-B and substance-P messenger ribonucleic acids in the hypothalami of postmenopausal women. *Endocrinology, 128*(5), 2239–2247.

Raskind, M. A., & Peskind, E. R. (1994). Neurobiologic bases of noncognitive behavioral problems in Alzheimer disease. *Alzheimer Disease & Associated Disorders, 8 Suppl 3*, 54–60.

Raskind, M. A., Peskind, E. R., Halter, J. B., & Jimerson, D. C. (1984). Norepinephrine and MHPG levels in CSF and plasma in Alzheimer's disease. *Archives of General Psychiatry, 41*(4), 343–346.

Raskind, M. A., Sadowsky, C. H., Sigmund, W. R., Beitler, P. J., Auster, S. B. (1997). Effect of tacrine on language, praxis, and noncognitive behavioral problems in Alzheimer disease. *Archives of Neurology, 54*(7), 836–840.

Reeves, A. G., & Plum, F. (1969). Hyperphagia, rage, and dementia accompanying a ventromedial hypothalamic neoplasm. *Archives of Neurology, 20*(6), 616–624.

Regan, W. M., & Gordon, S. M. (1997). Gabapentin for behavioral agitation in Alzheimer's disease. *Journal of Clinical Psychopharmacology, 17*(1), 59–60.

Reisberg, B., Borenstein, J., Salob, S. P., Ferris, S. H., Franssen, E., & Georgotas, A. (1987). Behavioral symptoms in Alzheimer's disease: Phenomenology and treatment. *Journal of Clinical Psychiatry, 48 Suppl*, 9–15.

Ricciardi, K. H., & Blaustein, J. D. (1994). Projections from ventrolateral hypothalamic neurons containing progestin receptor- and substance P-immunoreactivity to specific forebrain and midbrain areas in female guinea pigs. *Journal of Neuroendocrinology, 6*(2), 135–144.

Risold, P. Y., Thompson, R. H., & Swanson, L. W. (1997). The structural organization of connections between hypothalamus and cerebral cortex. *Brain Research Reviews, 24*(2–3), 197–254.

Risse, S. C., & Barnes, R. (1986). Pharmacologic treatment of agitation associated with dementia. *Journal of the American Geriatrics Society, 34*(5), 368–376.

Rolls, E. T. (1996). The orbitofrontal cortex. *Philosophical Transactions of the Royal Society of London - Series B: Biological Sciences, 351*(1346), 1433–1443.

Salzman, C., Vaccaro, B., Lieff, J., & Weiner, A. (1995). Clozapine in older patients with psychosis and behavioral disruption. *American Journal of Geriatric Psychiatry, 3*(1), 26–33.

Sandborn, W. D., Bendfeldt, F., & Hamdy, R. (1995). Valproic acid for physically aggressive behaviour in geriatric patients. *American Journal of Geriatric Psychiatry, 3,* 239–242.

Sano, M., Ernesto, C., Thomas, R. G., Klauber, M. R., Schafer, K., Grundman, M., Woodbury, P., Growdon, J., Cotman, C. W., Pfeiffer, E., Schneider, L. S., & Thal, L. J. (1997). A controlled trial of selegiline, alpha-tocopherol, or both as treatment for Alzheimer's disease. *New England Journal of Medicine, 336*(17), 1216–1222.

Satterlee, W. G., Reams, S. G., Burns, P. R., Hamilton, S., Tran, P. V., & Tollefson, G. D. (1995). A clinical update in olanzapine treatment in schizophrenia and in elderly Alzheimer's disease patients. *Psychopharmacology Bulletin, 31* 227–237.

Schneider, L. S., Pollock, V. E., & Lyness, S. A. (1990). A metaanalysis of controlled trials of neuroleptic treatment in dementia. *Journal of the American Geriatrics Society, 38*(5), 553–563.

Schneider, L. S., Severson, J. A., Chui, H. C., Pollock, V. E., Sloane, R. B., & Fredrickson, E. R. (1988). Platelet tritiated imipramine binding and MAO activity in Alzheimer's disease patients with agitation and delusions. *Psychiatry Research, 25*(3), 311–322.

Shankle, W. R., Nielson, K. A., & Cotman, C. W. (1995). Low-dose propranolol reduces aggression and agitation resembling that associated with orbitofrontal dysfunction in elderly demented patients. *Alzheimer Disease & Associated Disorders, 9*(4), 233–237.

Shea, C., MacKnight, C., & Rockwood, K. (1998). Donepezil for treatment of dementia with lewy bodies: a case series of nine patients. *International Psychogeriatrics, 10*(3), 229–238.

Shelton, P. S., & Hocking, L. B. (1997). Zolpidem for dementia-related insomnia and nighttime wandering. *Annals of Pharmacotherapy, 31*(3), 319–322.

Sival, R. C., Haffmans, P. M. J., Van Gent, P. P., & van Nieuwkerk, J. F. (1994). The effects of sodium valproate on disturbed behaviour in dementia. *Journal of the American Geriatrics Society, 42,* 906–907.

Starkstein, S. E., Vazquez, S., Petracca, G., Sabe, L., Migliorelli, R., Teson, A., & Leiguarda, R. (1994). A SPECT study of delusions in Alzheimer's disease. *Neurology, 44*(11), 2055–2059.

Street, J., Mitan, S., Tamura, R., Clark, W. S., Kadam, D., Sanger, T., Gannon, K. S., & Tollefson, G. D. (1998). Olanzapine in the treatment of psychosis and behavioral disturbances associated with Alzheimer's disease. *European Journal of Neurology, 5*(3), S39.

Sugerman, A. A., Williams, B. H., & Adlerstein, A. M. (1964). Haloperidol in the psychiatric disorders of old age. *American Journal of Psychiatry, 120,* 1190–1192.

Sultzer, D. L., Gray, K. F., Gunay, I., Berisford, M. A., & Mahler, M. E. (1997). A double-blind comparison of trazodone and haloperidol for treatment of agitation in patients with dementia. *American Journal of Geriatric Psychiatry, 5*(1), 60–69.

Sultzer, D. L., Mahler, M. E., Mandelkern, M. A., Cummings, J. L., Van, Gorp, W. G., Hinkin, C. H., & Berisford, M. A. (1995). The relationship between psychiatric symptoms and regional cortical metabolism in Alzheimer's disease. *Journal of Neuropsychiatry & Clinical Neurosciences, 7*(4), 476–484.

Sunderland, T., Tariot, P. N., Cohen, R. M., Weingartner, H., Mueller, E. A., & Murphy, D. L. (1987). Anticholinergic sensitivity in patients with dementia of the Alzheimer type and age-matched controls: A dose-response study. *Archives of General Psychiatry, 44*(5), 418–426.

Sunderland, T., Tariot, P. N., Mueller, E. A., Murphy, D. L., Weingartner, H., & Cohen, R.M. (1985). Cognitive and behavioral sensitivity to scopolamine in Alzheimer patients and controls. *Psychopharmacology Bulletin, 21*(3), 676–679.

Sunderland, T., Weingartner, H., Cohen, R. M., Tariot, P. N., Newhouse, P. A., Thompson, K. E., Lawlor, B. A., & Mueller, E. A. (1989). Low-dose oral lorazepam administration in Alzheimer subjects and age-matched controls. *Psychopharmacology, 99*(1), 129–133.

Swaab, D. F., Hofman, M. A., Lucassen, P. J., Purba, J. S., Raadsheer, F. C., & Van de Nes, J. A. (1993). Functional neuroanatomy and neuropathology of the human hypothalamus. *Anatomy & Embryology, 187*(4), 317–330.

Swayze, V. W., Andreasen, N. C., Alliger, R. J., Yuh, W. T., Ehrhardt, J. C. (1992). Subcortical and temporal structures in affective disorder and schizophrenia: a magnetic resonance imaging study. *Biological Psychiatry, 31*(3), 221–240.

Sweet, R. A., Mulsant, B. H., Pollock, B. G., Rosen, J., & Altieri, L. P. (1996). Neuroleptic-induced parkinsonism in elderly patients diagnosed with psychotic major depression and dementia of the Alzheimer type. *American Journal of Geriatric Psychiatry, 4,* 311–319.

Sweet, R. A., Pollock, B. G., Mulsant, B. H., Rosen, J., Lo, K. H., Yao, J. K., Henteleff, R. A., & Mazumdar, S. (1997). Association of plasma homovanillic acid with behavioral symptoms in patients diagnosed with dementia: A preliminary report. *Biological Psychiatry, 42*(11), 1016–1023.

Tariot, P. N. (1999). Divalproex in the treatment of mania associated dementia (unpublished data).

Tariot, P. N. (1996). Treatment strategies for agitation and psychosis in demential. *Journal of Clinical Psychiatry, 57*(Suppl 14), 21–29.

Tariot, P. N., Erb, R., Leibovici, A., Podgorski, C. A., Cox, C., Asnis, J., Kolassa, J., & Irvine, C. (1994). Carbamazepine treatment of agitation in nursing home patients with dementia: A preliminary study. *Journal of the American Geriatrics Society, 42,* 1160–1166.

Tariot, P. N., Erb, R., Podgorski, C. A., Cox, C., Patel, S., Jakimovich, L., & Irvine, C. (1998). Efficacy and tolerability of carbamazepine for agitation and aggression in dementia. *American Journal of Psychiatry, 155*(1), 54–61.

Tariot, P. N., Goldstein, B., Podgorski, C. A., Cox, C., & Frambes, N. (1998). Short-term administration of selegiline for mild-to-moderate dementia of the Alzheimer's type. *American Journal of Geriatric Psychiatry, 6*(2), 145–154.

Tariot, P. N., & Schneider, L. S. (1998). Nonneuroleptic treatment of complications of dementia: applying clinical research to practice. In J. C. Nelson (Ed.), *Geriatric psychopharmacology* (pp. 427–453). New York: Marcel Dekker.

Tariot, P. N., Schneider, L. S., & Katz, I. R. (1995). Anticonvulsant and other non-neuroleptic treatment of agitation in dementia. *Journal of Geriatric Psychiatry & Neurology, 8 Suppl 1,* S28–S39

Tolbert, S. R., & Fuller, M. A. (1996). Selegiline in treatment of behavioral and cognitive symptoms of Alzheimer disease. *Annals of Pharmacotherapy, 30*(10), 1122–1129.

Trimble, M. R., Mendez, M. F., & Cummings, J. L. (1997). Neuropsychiatric symptoms from the temporolimbic lobes. *Journal of Neuropsychiatry & Clinical Neurosciences, 9*(3), 429–438.

Tune, L. E., Steele, C., & Cooper, T. (1991). Neuroleptic drugs in the management of behavioral symptoms of Alzheimer's disease. *Psychiatric Clinics of North America, 14*(2), 353–373.

Turcotte, J. C., & Blaustein, J. D. (1997). Convergence of substance P and estrogen receptor immunoreactivity in the midbrain central gray of female guinea pigs. *Neuroendocrinology, 66*(1), 28–37.

Victoroff, J., Zarow, C., Mack, W. J., Hsu, E., & Chui, H. C. (1996). Physical aggression is associated with preservation of substantia nigra pars compacta in Alzheimer disease. *Archives of Neurology, 53*(5), 428–434.

Volicer, L., Rheaume, Y., & Cyr, D. (1994). Treatment of depression in advanced Alzheimer's disease using sertraline. *Journal of Geriatric Psychiatry & Neurology, 7*(4), 227–229.

Volkow, N. D., Tancredi, L. R., Grant, C., Gillespie, H., Valentine, A., Mullani, N., Wang, G. J., & Hollister, L. (1995). Brain glucose metabolism in violent psychiatric patients: a preliminary study. *Psychiatry Research, 61*(4), 243–253.

Wagner, M. L., Defilippi, J. L., Menza, M. A., & Sage, J. I. (1996). Clozapine for the treatment of psychosis in Parkinson's disease: Chart review of 49 patients. *Journal of Neuropsychiatry & Clinical Neurosciences, 8*(3), 276–280.

Waters, S. M., Konkoy, C. S., & Davis, T. P. (1995). Neuropeptide metabolism on intact, regional brain slices: E0ffect of dopaminergic agents on substance P, cholecystokinin and Met-enkephalin degradation. *Journal of Pharmacology & Experimental Therapeutics, 274*(2), 783–789.

Wilson, A. L., Langley, L. K., Monley, J., Bauer, T., Rottunda, S., McFalls, E., Kovera, C., & McCarten, J. R. (1995). Nicotine patches in Alzheimer's disease: Pilot study of learning, memory and safety. *Pharmacology, Biochemistry & Behavior, 51* , 509–514.

Wiseman, E. J., Souder, E., & Liem, P. H. (1997). Estrogen use and psychiatric symptoms in women with dementia. *Clinical Gerontologist, 18*(2), 81–84.

Workman, R. H., Orengo, C. A., Bakey, A. A., Molinari, V., & Kunik, M. E. (1997). The use of risperidone for psychosis and agitation in demented patients with Parkinson's disease. *Journal of Neuropsychiatry & Clinical Neurosciences, 9*(4), 594–597.

Wragg, R. E., & Jeste, D. V. (1988). Neuroleptics and alternative treatments: Management of behavioral symptoms and psychosis in Alzheimer's disease and related conditions. *Psychiatric Clinics of North America, 11*(1), 195–213.

Zubenko, G. S., Moossy, J., & Kopp, U. (1990). Neurochemical correlates of major depression in primary dementia. *Archives of Neurology, 47,* 209–214.

Zubenko, G. S., Moossy, J., Martinez, A. J., Rao, Claassen, D., Rosen, J., & Kopp, U. (1991). Neuropathologic and neurochemical correlates of psychosis in primary dementia. *Archives of Neurology, 48*(6), 619–624.

Zubenko, G. S. (1992). Biological correlates of clinical heterogeneity in primary dementia. *Neuropsychopharmacology, 6*(2), 77–93.

Zweig, R. M., Ross, C. A., & Hedreen, J. C., Steele, C., Cardillo, J. E., Whitehouse, P. J., Folstein, M. F., & Price, P. L. (1988). The neuropathology of aminergic nuclei in Alzheimer's disease. *Annals of Neurology, 24,* 233–242.

CHAPTER 9

Psychopharmacologic Interventions in Late-life Major Depression

WILLIAM APFELDORF & GEORGE ALEXOPOULOS
DEPARTMENT OF PSYCHIATRY
JOAN AND SANFORD I. WEILL MEDICAL COLLEGE
OF CORNELL UNIVERSITY

INTRODUCTION

Definition of Geriatric Depression

Geriatric depressive disorders are health problems with important medical, social, and financial consequences. Geriatric depression causes suffering to patients and their families, exacerbates medical illnesses, and contributes to disability that requires expensive support systems. Although the prevalence of depression does not appear to increase with age, the highest rates of suicide have been found in men age 75 and older[1]. Psychological autopsy studies of suicides in late life have found that most older suicide victims suffered from a psychiatric illness, usually late-onset depression; that most methods of suicide were violent, and that physical illness was the most common precipitant[2]. The main goals of treatment for geriatric depression include remission of depression and reduction in the risk of relapse and recurrence. Since depression often contributes to disability and excess medical morbidity, clinicians should expect improvements in both these areas.

Current diagnostic criteria for psychiatric disorders are codified in *Diagnostic and Statistical Manual for Mental Disorders, Fourth Edition,*[3] based on epidemiologic and field trials across age groups. However, diagnosis of psychiatric disorders in the elderly is complicated by several factors. First, the experience and expression of psychiatric symptoms are functions of age. Second, the criteria for psychiatric diagnosis must be applied age-appropriately. Third, the presence of multiple comorbid conditions is the rule, rather than the exception, in geriatric patients. The signs and symptoms of psychiatric disorders may overlap with signs of symptoms of many medical illnesses and may complicate diagnostic assessment[4]. Medical and neurological disorders may result in persistent psychiatric syndromes that will remit only when the underlying medical disorders are addressed. Fourth, psychiatric disorders may have late onset, so the clinician cannot be guided by previous history. Fifth, elderly patients may underreport psychological symptoms, or ascribe symptoms to other somatic concerns. Finally, there are currently no biological gold standard assessments or markers generally accepted for geriatric psychiatric disorders. To overcome these factors, clinicians may use the reports of family informants or caregivers to supplement information provided by the patient. In addition, the adoption of an inclusive approach allows consideration and treatment of psychiatric disorders while a search for medical or neurologic disorders is conducted.

SUBTYPES OF LATE-LIFE DEPRESSION

Late-Onset Depression

Geriatric depression with onset of first episode in late life (late-onset) is a heterogeneous entity that includes a large subgroup of patients who develop depression as part of a medical or neurological disorder that may or may not be clinically evident when the depression first appears[5]. Compared to patients who first experienced depression in early or midlife (early-onset), those with late-onset depression have a higher frequency of neuropsychological[6] and neuroradiological abnormalities[6,7,8,9], higher level of disability[10], and lower familial prevalence of affective disorders[11].

Vascular Depression

Cerebrovascular disease is frequent in elderly depressives. Felix Post noted a high incidence of cerebrovascular disease in elderly depressed patients and suggested that the resultant brain damage predisposess to late-life depression[12]. Depression is highly prevalent in patients with hypertension[13], coronary artery disease[14], and vascular dementia[15]. Depression is a frequent complication of stroke[16,17,18,19,20]. "Silent" cerebral infarction was observed in 94% of patients with onset of first depressive episode after 65 years of age[21]. On imaging, late-onset depressives exhibit white matter hyperintensitites more frequently than non-depressed, age-matched subjects[22,23]. Patients with vascular depression appear to have greater difficulty with initiation and perseveration, less insight, and less agitation and guilt, than comparison depressed patients without vascular risk factors[24]. Pharmacologic management of vascular depression provides new avenues for investigation[24]: studies can determine if drugs used in the prevention and treatment of cerebrovascular disease can reduce the risk for depression in patients with vascular risk factors or reduce chronicity, recurrence, cognitive impairment, and disability. Moreover, the long-term efficacy of specific antidepressants can be investigated in depressed patients at risk for new vascular lesions, since animal studies suggests that some antidepressants but not others promote recovery after ischemic brain lesions .

Depression with Pseudodementia

Geriatric depression with reversible dementia, the syndrome usually called pseudodementia, as a rule is a severe depression accompanied by a mild reversible dementia syndrome. Depressed elderly patients with pseudodementia often have a retarded and psychotic depressive syndrome[6]. While the dementia syndrome initially subsides after effective antidepressant treatment, in the long run, a high percentage of these patients develop irreversible dementia. With the advent of new pharmacologic treatments for dementia syndromes, it remains to be studied whether the identification of pseudodementia provides an early opportunity to pharmacologically intervene and improve the course of the underlying dementing illness.

Mood Disorder Secondary to Other Medical Conditions

In elderly persons, medical and neurological illnesses may predispose to or even cause depression. Drugs, medical illnesses, and dementing disorders may lead to depression. Steroids, reserpine, methyldopa, anti-Parkinsonian drugs, and β-blockers can cause depression. Viral infections, endocrinopathies such as thyroid or parathyroid abnormalities, and malignancies, such as lymphoma or pancreatic cancer, often are complicated by depression. While it is essential to diagnose and treat the underlying disease, depression may not remit until an antidepressant agent is used. Depression is especially common in patients with neurological brain diseases. Approximately 30–60% of stroke patients experience depression within 24 months after the stroke[25]. In Alzheimer's patients, major depression occurs in approximately 15% of patients and less severe depressive syndromes in 40–50% of patients[26].

GENERAL CONSIDERATIONS FOR PHARMACOLOGIC MANAGEMENT

The main goals of treatment for geriatric depression include: 1) remission of depression; and 2) reduction in the risk of relapse and recurrence. Older patients can benefit from the same psychopharmacological agents as younger patients. However, the clinician must be aware that aging and medical conditions associated with aging can have an impact on pharmacokinetics and can increase the sensitivity to side effects even at low plasma concentrations of antidepressants. Aging-induced changes in hepatic metabolism prolong the clearance of many psychopharmacological agents in older people, thus, increasing the likelihood that drugs and their active metabolites will accumulate and cause toxicity.

There is currently a paucity of research studies guiding the selection of one type of antidepressant over another, and the choice is often made based on side effect profile and to minimize potential drug-drug interactions. The sensitivity of geriatric patients to interventions may lead to treatment complications or undertreatment. Changes in pharmacokinetics and pharmacodynamics with age necessitate thorough knowledge of the effects of psychotropic drugs in the elderly[27]. Aging-induced changes in hepatic metabolism prolong the clearance of most psychotropics in older people, thus, increasing the likelihood that drugs and their active metabolites will accumulate and cause toxicity. Potential drug-drug interactions influence both choice of agent and dosing. Side effects of the medications must be monitored, including ongoing assessments weighing the potential benefits of improved behavior and functional outcomes against the risks of complications. Compliance with a prescribed regimen is often problematic in geriatric patients struggling with comorbid conditions which both impair their ability to maintain adherence and require attention: it is estimated that 70% of elderly patients fail to take 25–50% of their medications as prescribed[28]. Minimizing polypharmacy aids in preventing drug-drug interactions, iatrogenic illness, and compliance difficulties.

An orderly approach to the design of successive treatment trials is essential. When failure to respond to a specific treatment occurs, information is provided to guide the selection of the next intervention. Patients and their families can benefit from education and participation in the treatment decision process. Sharing responsibility with patients and families for important treatment decisions may reduce the risk of undertreatment, improve compliance, provide relief to a family system stressed by the presence of a psychiatric disorder, and assist the patient and caregivers in monitoring the effects of treatments. Since geriatric psychiatric disorders often lead to permanent disability, undertreatment may have severe consequences.

STAGES OF TREATMENT

Acute Phase

Treatment with antidepressants is effective in reducing signs and symptoms of geriatric depression. Antidepressants, regardless of class lead to improvement of depressive symptomatology in approximately 60% of elderly patients while the placebo response rate is 30–40%[29]. Even among responders, a significant number of elderly patients continue to have significant residual symptomatology. It is crucial that antidepressant drugs are given at adequate plasma levels or dosages for a sufficient length of time. Older patients are more likely than younger patients to develop delirium, constipation, urinary retention, dry mouth, and orthostatic hypotension. For this reason, the initial dosage of antidepressants is lower than that used with younger patients, and should be increased at a slower pace. An adequate antidepressant trial in the elderly is longer than that of younger adults and should last at least 7 to 9 weeks.

Continuation and Maintenance Phase

Depression is a recurrent disorder. Following the acute phase of treatment (2–3 months), the antidepressant should be continued for at least 6 months following remission of symptoms (continuation phase). Continuation treatment is used to prevent relapse of the episode which the patient most recently suffered. After being well for 6 months, patients are at risk for a new episode of depression (recurrence). History of three or more episodes is the strongest predictor of recurrence[30]. Other predictors of high severity of the initial episode and persisting anxiety[31]. Patients at high risk for recurrence should have maintenance treatment for at least 1 to 2 years. Unlike continuation treatment, which is used to prevent relapse of the initial depressive episode, maintenance treatments seek to prevent new episodes of depression. The dose and plasma level used for continuation and maintenance treatment should be the same as those used for effective acute treatment of depression[32].

SPECIFIC ANTIDEPRESSANTS BY CATEGORY

Four classes of antidepressants are available for the treatment of geriatric depression. These are: tricyclics, serotonin reuptake inhibitors, monoamine oxidase inhibitors, and atypical antidepressants.

Antidepressants Introduced Since 1985

Serotonin Reuptake Inhibitors (SRIs)

Studies of elderly outpatients observed that citalopram, fluoxetine, sertraline, and paroxetine are effective in reducing depressive symptoms during the acute treatment of depression[30,31,32,33,34,35]. There are few research studies using fluvoxamine to treat elderly depressives. While research inpatient studies are sparse, clinical experience suggests that these agents are effective in outpatients with a broad spectrum of depressive disorders. The initial dosages of SRIs for the elderly are lower than for younger adults; recommended starting daily dosages are citalopram 10 mg, fluoxetine 5–10 mg, paroxetine 5–10 mg, sertraline 25 mg, and fluvoxamine 25 mg. For most patients, daily dosages citalopram 30 mg, fluoxetine 20 mg, paroxetine 20 mg, sertraline 75 mg, and fluvoxamine 100 mg are sufficient, although higher doses are required by some.

The SRIs have minimal cardiac side effects and often are used as first-line agents in elderly patients with depression or in patients with cardiac disease. With the exception of allergy, they have few, if any, dangerous side effects, and are less toxic if overdosed. Nausea, restlessness, insomnia, headache, anorexia, diarrhea, and sexual dysfunction are the most frequent side effects in the elderly. Inappropriate secretion of antidiuretic hormone may lead to hyponatremia, confusion, and falls in the elderly. SRIs interact with drugs frequently used in the depressed elderly. These include interactions from inhibition of the hepatic cytochrome P450 isoenzyme system and from protein displacement of other drugs. Fluoxetine, sertraline, and paroxetine inhibit cytochrome P450 2D6 isoenzyme. This pathway is essential for the hydroxylation of nortriptyline and desipramine and the metabolism of antipsychotics, Type 1_A antiarrhythmic drugs (encainide, flecanide), (β-blockers, and verapamil, effectively raising their plasma levels. Therefore, drugs metabolized by this pathway may require reduction of dosages and monitoring of plasma levels in patients treated with fluoxetine, sertraline, and paroxetine. Citalopram has a minimal effect on the P450 isoenzymes and may be chosen in patients who receive other medications metabolized by the P450 system. Fluvoxamine inhibits to cytochrome P450 3A4 and 1A2 isoenzymes without inhibiting the 2D6 isoenzyme. The 3A4 isoenzyme is responsible for the metabolism of alprazolam, triazolam, carbamazepine, quinidine, erythromycin, terfenazine, and astemizol, and may lead to an increase in plasma levels of these agents. The coadministration of these agents and fluvoxamine should be avoided. Similarly, theophylline should be used cautiously in fluvoxamine-treated patients, since fluvoxamine may produce a three-fold decrease in theophylline clearance by the 1A2 pathway. Administration of SRIs to patients on other tightly protein-bound drugs, such as warfarin and digitoxin, may displace these drugs and lead to increased side effects.

Buproprion

There is limited research information on the use of buproprion in the elderly population[36]. Studies with younger patients suggest that buproprion is of comparable efficacy to tricyclics and SRIs. Buproprion has limited effect on cognitive function and on heart rate and rhythm, but may exacerbate preexisting hypertension. Seizures have been reported in 0.4% of patients treated with buproprion. The risk of seizures may be minimized by slow introduction of buproprion (75 mg daily), restriction of the total daily dosage to less than 450 mg daily, and the use of a sustained release buproprion preparation.

Nefazodone

Nefazodone has not been extensively investigated in geriatric patients[37]. However it has properties that may be desirable for the treatment of some elderly depressives. Nefazodone promotes sleep and has anxiolytic effects. Nefazodone is well-tolerated and safe in overdose, does not influence sleep architecture, and does not cause sexual dysfunction. Cognitive function examination should be done in patients treated with nefazodone, because the drug may lead to dose-related cognitive side effects. Nefazodone inhibits the cytochrome P450 3A4 isoenzyme, responsible for the metabolism of alprazolam, triazolam, carbamazepine, and erythromycin. Sedation and the need for twice-daily dosing may be a problem for some elderly patients. A total daily dosage of 300–500 mg may be required.

Venlafaxine

Venlafaxine inhibits serotonin uptake and at high dosages inhibits norepinephrine uptake. Clinical trials of elderly depressed subjects found venlafaxine well-tolerated and efficacious[38,39]. Venlafaxine was found effective in hospitalized depressed patients as well as drug-refractory depressives and in depressed patients with chronic pain. Elderly patients appear to require dosages comparable to those of younger adults, with daily dosages 100–200 mg adequate for the majority of elderly patients. There are few drug-drug interactions, except with MAOIs. Frequent side effects include nausea, insomnia, sweating, and mild increases in blood pressure requiring monitoring.

Mirtazapine

Mirtazapine is chemically dissimilar to the previously mentioned antidepressants, and acts to enhance noradrenergic and specific serotonergic activities. It has prominant antihistaminergic and moderate antimuscarinic actions, and frequent side effects include sedation, dry mouth, dizziness, constipation, and increased appetite. In a study of elderly outpatients with depression, initial dosages began at 5–10 mg and reached mean dosages of approximately 30 mg daily[40].

Reboxitane

Reboxitane is a specific noradrenaline reuptake inhibitor, used in Europe and Latin America and under investigation in the United States, now being used for the treatment of depressive disorders. It appears to have little affinity for serotonin and dopamine uptake sites, and acts primarily as a noradrenergic reuptake inhibitor. Reboxitane was compared with imipramine in elderly depressed patients, and demonstrated similar efficacy[41]. Side effects reported include tachycardia, extrasystolic arrhythmia, supraventricular tachycardia, and severe atrial fibrillation associated with elevated plasma levels. The maximum recommended dosage of reboxitane for elderly depressed patients is 4–6 mg total daily, administered in a divided dosing regimen.

Current Use of Older Antidepressants

Tricyclic Antidepressants

The tricyclic antidepressants nortriptyline and desipramine have been the best investigated antidepressants in geriatric depression. They have lower anticholinergic and sedative effects than other tricyclics, such as imipramine, amitriptyline, and doxepin. Nortriptyline appears to have a lower potential for orthostatic hypotension than other tricyclic antidepressants. Elderly patients require plasma levels similar to those of younger adults in order to respond to treatment with tricyclic antidepressants: nortriptyline plasma levels of 60–150 ng/ml and desipramine levels > 115 ng/ml[42]. Elderly patients often develop therapeutic plasma levels while on low daily dosages: nortriptyline 1–1.2 mg/kg body weight and desipramine 1.5–2 mg/kg. Monitoring plasma levels allow the clinician to determine treatment compliance. Elderly patients may require a longer acute antidepressant treatment than younger adults, with a significant response noted after 6–12 weeks of treatment. Elderly patients with cognitive impairment who develop depressive symptoms may respond to nortriptyline or desipramine at plasma levels lower than that needed to treat late-life depression.

Higher intellectual functions, orthostatic blood pressure, the electrocardiogram, and the ability to urinate should be monitored frequently in depressed elderly patients receiving nortriptyline or desipramine. Tricyclic antidepressants have anticholinergic properties, and should be avoided in patients with prostatic hypertrophy or patients with narrow angle glaucoma. Nortriptyline and desipramine have properties similar to Type 1_A antiarrhythmic drugs (quinidine-like). When administered to patients with right or left bundle branch blocks, tricyclics may cause second degree block in approximately 10% of cases. The Type 1_A properties necessitate cautious use of these drugs in patients with ischemic heart disease. Elderly patients on nortriptyline often develop higher plasma levels of the nortriptyline metabolite 10-hydroxynortriptyline than do younger adults, which may contribute to cardiac conduction defects in elderly patients.

Monoamine Oxidase Inhibitors (MAOIs)

Phenelzine and tranylcypromine are effective agents in patients with major depression and other depressive disorders. Low dosages, phenelzine 30–45 mg daily or tranylcypromine 20–30 mg daily, should be used in the elderly. Orthostatic hypotension is the most frequent side effect of MAO inhibitors, and may lead to falls and fractures. Other side effects include weight gain, anergia, insomnia, and daytime somnolence with phenelzine, and include nervousness, insomnia, and excessive perspiration with tranylcypromine. Peripheral neuropathy occurs is a small percentage of patients on MAOIs and often responds to pyridoxine. Sympathomimetic amines, monoamine precursors, other antidepressants, demerol, and tyramine-rich food may cause a hypertensive crisis and should be avoided in patients on MAOIs. These drug interactions and diet restrictions often prevent the use of MAOIs in the elderly.

Meclobomide, a benzamide-derived reversible MAO-A inhibitor, was shown to be a safe, well-tolerated, and mildly effective antidepressant in elderly depressives[43] but other studies have failed to confirm significant benefit compared to placebo and nortriptyline[44]. Meclobomide shows little affinity for muscarinic receptors and carries less risk for hypertensive crisis.

Psychostimulants

Dextroamphetamine and methylphenidate are relatively ineffective in elderly patients with primary major depression. However, psychostimulants appear to improve apathy and anergy in medically ill patients or cognitively impaired patients. Dextroamphetamine or methylphenidate at dosages 5–10 mg in the morning and at noon are sufficient. Psychostimulants have rapid onset of action, minimal side effects, limited potential for tolerance, and low risk of addiction when used for these indications[45].

Combination Regimens

Combinations of antidepressant drugs have been used to improve the response of partially remitted geriatric depression. Lithium may augment tricyclic antidepressant response in elderly patients[46]. The dose of lithium required by depressed elderly patients receiving tricyclics may be one-third to one-half that of younger adults. In younger depressives, combinations of tricyclics with SRIs have led to an antidepressant response sooner than tricyclics alone. Other augmentation techniques, include combinations of tricyclics or SRIs with thyroid hormones, psychostimulants, bupropion, pindolol, and other agents. Clinical experience suggests that augmentation techniques can be effective in some depressed geriatric patients with incomplete response to a single antidepressant agent. However, systematic studies of such combinations are lacking in the elderly.

SPECIAL CONSIDERATIONS

Treatment of Psychotic Depression

Psychotic depression is rather frequent in the elderly population and occurs in 3.6% of elderly depressives living in the community[47] and in 20 to 45% of hospitalized elderly depressives[48]. Psychotic depression is a severe illness with profound depressive symptomatology accompanied by delusions and less frequently by hallucinations. Delusions occur in successive episodes of geriatric depression if the severity of episodes is high[49,50]. However, in geriatric patients, psychotic depression is not merely a consequence of high severity of depression since high percentages of severely depressed elderly patients do not develop delusions[49,50]. Psychotic depression is associated with a risk for suicide[51] usually with violent means[52]. For this reason, it is crucial to diagnose and treat psychotic depression.

There is evidence that elderly patients with psychotic depression respond poorly to acute treatment with tricyclic antidepressants alone[53]. Poor response to tricyclic antidepressants is not explained by the high severity of depression alone[54]. Combinations of tricyclic antidepressants and neuroleptics appear to be effective in psychotic depression both in controlled studies of younger patients[55,56] and in naturalistic treatment studies of elderly patients[49,52]. The most frequently prescribed antidepressants are nortriptyline or desipramine at plasma levels comparable to those of younger adults (60–150 ng/ml for nortriptyline or above 115 ng/ml for desipramine). Perphenazine is the neuroleptic that has been used in most studies of psychotic depression[55] and appears to be effective at daily dosages of approximately 32 mg. It is unclear if elderly patients can respond to lower dosages of neuroleptics or whether risperidone, olanzapine, and quetiapine can be effective and better tolerated than perphenazine. Risperidone, olanzapine, and quetiapine appear to carry a lower risk of tardive dyskinesia and other side effects associated with traditional antipsychotics, and are often chosen over the better-studied agents. While there is agreement that psychotic depression requires combination drug therapy, these drugs may not be tolerated by elderly patients. For this reason, ECT frequently is the treatment of choice in psychotic depression. Studies comparing ECT with simulated ECT have demonstrated benefit in psychotic depression[57]. There is some evidence that bilateral ECT is more effective that unilateral ECT is psychotic depression[56].

The need for special treatment makes it crucial to diagnose psychotic depression. It often is difficult to distinguish depressive delusions from overvalued ideas of worthlessness and hopelessness. Nondelusional depressed patients, as a rule, are able to recognize the exaggerated nature of their overvalued ideas, although they are unable to stop being preoccupied with them. Depressive delusions can be distinguished from delusions of demented patients in that the latter are less systematized and less congruent to the affective disturbance[58]. In contrast, depressive delusions usually are organized ideas of hypochondriasis, nihilism, guilt, persecution, or jealousy.

Maintenance Treatment

Depression is a relapsing and remitting illness; 50 to 80% of patients who have had one depressive episode can expect a recurrence. The recurrence rate increases with each successive episode. In mixed-age unipolar depressives, 34% of patients have a depressive episode during the year after recovery[59,60], with the relapse (within 6 months from recovery) rate higher during the months immediately after recovery. The figures for relapse/recurrence in major depression (15–19%) in geriatric patients[61] are comparable to those of mixed-age populations (21%)[59,60]. In mixed-age populations, history of three or more previous depressive episodes and late age of depression onset are the strongest predictors of relapse/recurrence[59,60]. In geriatric populations, most studies suggest that the likelihood of relapse is increased in patients with history of frequent episodes, intercurrent medical illnesses, and possibly high severity of depression[62]. Most recently, lifetime history of myocardial infarction was found to predict frequent relapses in depressed medical outpatients[63]. The course of depressive disorder changes over time. There is evidence that the interepisode intervals tend to become shorter in successive episodes[63]. However, specific studies in geriatric depressives are lacking.

Controlled treatment studies of mixed-age depressives have shown that imipramine continuation therapy (intended to prevent relapse during the first 4–6 months after recovery) and maintenance therapy (intended to prevent recurrence after 4–6 months from recovery) succeeded in the survival of 50–80% of the population over 1 to 3 years[64,65]. In contrast, only 20% of placebo-treated patients remained well[64]. These observations suggest that tricyclic antidepressants are effective in preventing relapse and recurrence of major depression. Three controlled-treatment studies of elderly depressives suggest that antidepressant drugs may offer protection from relapse[32,66,67]. In a study of continuation treatment of elderly outpatients with major depression, nortriptyline or phenelzine treatment led to a relapse rate of 16.7% and 20.0% respectively[66]. An even lower relapse rate was reported by the other study[67].

With respect to recurrence, however, conflicting findings are reported. In an open-label study, maintenance treatment with nortriptyline was associated with low recurrence rate 14.8%[68]. In contrast, a placebo-controlled study showed that 1 year maintenance on nortriptyline resulted in a 53.8% recurrence rate, a percentage similar to that of placebo[69]. Nonetheless, maintenance on phenelzine led to a 13.3% recurrence rate[69]. The subjects of these studies were mainly outpatients with a mean age in the mid-60s. In a placebo-controlled study of geriatric patients with recurrent depression recovered after acute and continuation treatment with nortriptyline or interpersonal psychotherapy, maintenance treatment with nortriptyline and interpersonal psychotherapy had a recurrence rate of 20% over 3 years, compared to 43% with nortriptyline alone, 64% for interpersonal psychotherapy alone, and 90% for placebo treatment[32].

Since depression may be a severely debilitating or potentially lethal illness, older unipolar patients who have had two or more depressive episodes should receive maintenance treatment with antidepressants. The dosage of heterocyclic antidepressant used for maintenance therapy should be the same as the dosage used during the acute treatment phase. Lithium carbonate may be prescribed for unipolar patients who develop side effects while on maintenance antidepressant treatment and become noncompliant to treatment. Regardless of which medication is used for maintenance treatment, careful monitoring of dosages and plasma levels and appropriate adjustment are necessary as the patient ages. If a relapse or a recurrence occurs, using a regimen similar to that employed in the original depressive episode may lead to remission in 80% of depressed geriatric patients[31].

Patients whose depression has responded only to ECT should be placed on maintenance dosages of an antidepressant after their depression has abated. Antidepressants that failed to produce remissions should not be selected for maintenance treatment after ECT. Older patients who have had relapses on antidepressants or lithium, or who cannot take these drugs because of medical contraindications, should be considered for maintenance ECT. For these patients, clinical experience suggests that a single ECT treatment given every 4 to 6 weeks may prevent recurrence of depression.

For patients with history of manic episodes in addition to depression (bipolar disorder), antidepressant drugs may induce a manic episode. In bipolar mood disorder, lithium, valproate or carbamazepine are preferred to antidepressants for maintenance treatment[70].

The course and long-term treatment of geriatric psychotic depression are under investigation. Younger patients with psychotic depression have a poor outcome at least during the first 2 years from recovery[17] but their outcome over 8 to 40 years is similar to the outcome of non-psychotic depressives[71,72]. The long-term outcome of geriatric psychotic depression is to some extent comparable to that of younger adults. A geriatric study showed that approximately 80% of psychotic depressives recovered and only 50% had a relapse within 3.5 to 8.5 years[49]. The recurrence rate of psychotic depression was similar to that of non-psychotic depression, although psychotic depression often required hospitalization during recurrences. Relapses and recurrences are particularly frequent in elderly patients who only achieve partial recovery after acute treatment of psychotic depression[53]. Therefore, it is particularly important to treat the initial episode aggressively and provide continuation and maintenance therapy. Studies are underway to examine whether combinations of tricyclics and neuroleptics are necessary or whether antidepressants alone are sufficient for this purpose. It should be emphasized, however, that patients who recover after ECT should not receive continuation treatment with drugs that failed prior to ECT, since these drugs as a rule are unable to prevent relapse[59].

CONCLUSIONS

The treatment of geriatric patients with depression presents the clinician with challenges and opportunities. Difficulties in recognizing psychiatric syndromes, medical and psychiatric comorbidity, altered pharmacokinetics, and sensitivity to side effects, may complicate the treatment of the elderly. Untreated geriatric psychiatric syndromes carry significant morbidity and mortality, and can also adversely impact on families and caregivers. Correction of underlying medical abnormalities may be a necessary but often not a sufficient intervention. With advances in our knowledge of the geriatric depression subtypes and the availability of studies investigating specific antidepressants in the elderly, antidepressant selection may be guided by the patient's specific clinical symptoms and comorbidity. The failure of any one specific treatment trial can inform the selection of the next. Difficulties with compliance must be addressed to assure adequate treatment is delivered and overdosing is prevented.

REFERENCES

1. American Psychiatric Association. (1994)*Diagnostic and Statistical Manual of Mental Disorders* (4th ed.) Washington, DC: American Psychiatric Press.
2. Conwell Y., Brent D.(1995) Suicide in aging, I: patterns of psychiatric diagnosis. *Int. Psyhcogeriatr,* 7, 149–164.

3. Conwell, Y. (1994) "Suicide in elderly patients". In:*Diagnosis and treatment of depression in late life.* (eds. Schneider LS, Reyolds CF, Lebowitz BD, Friedhoff A.) Washington DC, American Psychiatric Press, 397–418.
4. National Institute of Health. (1992) Consensus Conf, JAMA.
5. Alexopoulos G. S., (1990) "Clinical and biological findings in late-onset depression": In:Tasman, A., Goldfinger, S.M., Kaufman, D.A., eds. *Review of Psychiatry,* Vol 9, Washington DC: American Psychiatric Press, 1990; pp. 249–262.
6. Alexopoulos G. S., Young R. C., Meyers B. S., (1993). Geriatric depression: Age of onset and dementia. *Biol Phychiatry,* 34, 141N145.
7. Alexopoulos G. S., Young R. C., Shindledecker R. (1992). Brain computed tomography in geriatric depression and primary degenerative dementia. *Biol Psychiatry,* 31, 591–599.
8. Jacoby R. J., Levy R. (1980). Computed tomography in the elderly. Affective disorder. *British Journal Psychiatry,* 136, 270–275.
9. Coffee D.E., Figiel G.S., Djang W.T., Cress M., Saunders W.B., Weiner R.D. (1988) Leukoencephalopathy in elderly depressed patients referred for ETC. *Biol Psychiatry,* 24, 143–161.
10. Alexopoulos G.S., Vrontou C., Kakuma T., Meyers B.S., Young RC, Klausner E., Clarkin J. (1996). Disability in geriatric depression. *American Journal Psychiatry,* 153, 877–885.
11. Baron M., Mendlewicz J., Klotz J. (1981) Age of onset and genetic transmission in affective disorders. *Acta Psychiatr Scand,* 64, 373–380.
12. Post F., Shculman K. (1985). New views on old age affective disorder. In *Recent Advances in Psychogeriatrics,* (pp. 119–140. New York: Churchill Livingston.
13. Rabkin J.G., Charles E., Kass F. (1983). Hypertension and DSM III depression in psychiatric outpatients. *American Journal Psychiatry,* 140, 1072–1074.
14. Carney R.M., Rich W.M., Telvelde A., Saini J., Clark K., Jaffe A.S. (1987). Major depressive disorder in coronary artery disease. *American Journal Cardiol,* 60, 1273–1275.
15. Sulzer D.L., Levin HJ.S., Mahler M.E., High W.M., Cummings J.L. (1993). A comparison of psychiatric symptoms in vascular dementia and Alzheimer's disease. *American Journal Psychiarty,* 150, 1806–1812.
16. Robinson R.G., Kubos K.L., Starr L.B., Rao K., Price T.R. (1984). Mood disorders in stroke patients: importance of location of lesion. *Brain,* 107, 81–93.
17. Robinson D.G., Spiker D.G. (1985). Delusional depression: A one year followup. *J Affect Disorder* 9, 79–83.

18. Starkstein S.E., Robinson R.G., Berthier M.L., et al. (1988). Depressive disorders following posterior circulation as compared with middle cerebral artery infarcts. *Brain*, 111, 387.
19. Folstein M.F., Maiberger R., McHugh P.R. (1971). Mood disorders as a specific complication of stroke. *Journal Neurol Neurosurg Psychiarty*, 40, 1018–1020.
20. Ebrahim S., Barer K., Nouri F. (1987). Affective illness after stroke. *British Journal Psychiatry*, 7, 1, 154, 170–182.
21. Fujikawa T., Yamawake S., Touhouda Y. (1993). Incidence of silent cerebral infarction in patients with major depression. *Stroke*, 24, 1631–1634.
22. Krishnan K.R.R., Goli V., Ellinwood E.H., France R.D., Blazaer D.Z., Nmemeoff C.B. (1988). Leukoencephalopathy in patient diagnosed as major depressive. *Biol Psychiatry*, 23, 519–522.
23. Coffey D.E., Figiel G.S., Djang W.T., Saunders W.B., Weiner R.D. (1989). White matter hyperintensity on MRI clinical and neuroanatomic correlates in the depressed elderly. *Journal Neuropsychiatry Clin Neurosci*, 1, 135–144.
24. Aalexopoulos G.S., Vrontou C., Kakuma T., Meyers B.S., Young R.C., Klausner E., Clarkin J. (1998). Disability in geriatric depression. *Am J Psychiatry*, 877–885.
25. Astrom M., Adofspm R., Asplund K. (1993). Major depression in stroke patients. A three year longitudinal study. *Stroke*, 24, 976–982.
26. Wragg R.E., Jeste D.V. (1989). Overview of depression and psychosis in Alzheimer's disease. *Am J. Psychiatry*, 146, 577–589.
27. Catterson M.L., Perskorn S.H., and Martin R.L. (1997). Pharmacodynamic and pharmacokinetic considerations in geriatric psychopharmacology. *Psychiatric Clinics of North America*, 20 (1), 205–218.
28. Perel J.M. (1994). "Geropharmacokinetics of Therapeutics, Toxic Effects, and Compliance" in Schneider S., Reynolds D.F., Lebowitz B.D. (Eds.) *Diagnosis and Treatment of Depression in Late Life*, 245–255.
29. Murphy E. (1994) "The Course and Outcome of Depression in Late Life." In Schneider S., Reynolds C.F., Lebowitz B.D. (Eds.), *Diagnosis and Treatment of Depression in Late Life*, 81–97.
30. Meyers B.S., Gabriele M., Kakuma T., Ippolito, Alexopoulos G.S. (1996) Anxiety and depression as predictors of recurrence in geriatric depression. *American Journal of Geriatric Psychiatry*, 4, 252–257.
31. Reynolds C.F., Frank E., Perel J.M., Miller M.D., Cornes C., Rifai H., Pollock B.G., Mazumar S., George C.J., Houck P.R., Kupfer D.J. (1994). Treatment of consecutive episodes of major depression in the elderly. *American Journal Psychiatry*, 151, 1740–1743.

32. Reynolds C.F., Frank, E., Perel J.P., Imber S.D., Cornes C., et al. (1/61999). Nortriptyline and interpersonal psychotherapy as maintenance therapies for recurrent major depression a randomized controlled trial in patients older than 59 years. *J Amer Med Assoc* (281:1), 39–45.
33. McEntee W.J., Coffee D.J., Bondareff W., Alpert M., Faj A.V., Rappaport S.A., Weiner M. F. (1996). Double-blind comparison of sertraline and nortriptyline in the treatment of depressed geriatric outpatients. Presented at Annual Meeting of the American Psychiatric Association, Philadelphia, PA.
34. Linden R.D., Newhouse P.A., Krishnan K.R.R., Farmer M., Goldstein B.J., Lazarus L.W. (1996). Sertraline and fluoxetine in geriatric depression. Presented at Annual Meeting of the American Psychiatric Association, Philadelphia, PA.
35. Linden R.D., Newhouse P.A., Krishnan K.R.R., Farmer M., Goldstein B.J., lazarus L.W. (1995). SSRIs in the Depressed Elderly: A Double-Blind Comparison of Sertraline and Fluoxetine in Depressed Geriatric Outpatients. Annual Meeting American Psychiatric Association, Poster Presentataion.
36. Branconnier R.J., Cole J.O., Ghazvinian S., et al. (1983). Clinical pharmacology of bupropion and imipramine in elderly depressives. *J. Clin Psychiatry*, 44 (5 Sect 2), 130–3.
37. Tourigny-Rivard M.F. (6/1997). Pharmacothery of affective disorders in old age. *Can J Psychiatry*, 42 (Suppl), 1, 10S–18S
38. Dierick M. (9/1996). An open-label evaluation of the long-term safety of oral vanlafaxine in depressed elderly patients. *Ann Clin Psychiatry*, 8 (3), 169–78.
39. Mahapatra S.N., Hackett D. (6/1997). A randomised, double-blind, parallel-group comparison of venlafaxine and dothiepin in geriatric patients with major depression. *Int J Clin Pract*, 54 (4), 209–13.
40. Hoyberg O.J., Maragakis B., Mullin J., Norum D., Stordal 1 E., Ekdahl P., Ose E., Moksnes K.M., Sennef C. (1996). A double-blind multicenter comparison of mirtazapine and amitriptyline in elderly depressed patients. *Acta Psychiatr Scand* , 93, 184–190.
41. Ban T.A., Dubini A., Giorgetti C., Petroccione A., Bercoff E., Chiu E. (1/1996). Multicentre, multinational double-blind study of the activity and tolerability of reboxetine versus imipramine in elderly patients suffering from depressive disorders. *Pharmacia Internal Report 9550089.*
42. Plotkin D.A., Gerson S.G., Jarvik L.F. (1987). "Antidepressant drug treatment in the elderly". In Meltzer H.Y. (Ed) *Psychopharmacology: the third generation of progress.* New York, Raven Press, 1149–1158.
43. Roth M., Montjoy C.Q., Amrein R. et al. (1996). Moclobemide in elderly patients with cognitive decline and depression. *British Journal of Psychiatry* 168, 149–157.

44. Nair, M.P.V., Amin M., Holm P., Katona D., Klitgaard N., et al. (1995). Moclobemide and nortriptyline in elderly depressed patients, A randomized, multicentre trial against placebo. *Journal of Affective Disorders,* 33, 1–9.
45. Satel S.L., Nelson J.C. (1989). Stimulants in the treatment of depression: A critical overview. *Journal of clinical Psychiatry,* 50, 241–249.
46. Salzman C. (1994). "Pharmacological treatment of depression in elderly patients" in Schneider S., Reynolds C.F., Lebowitz B.D. (Eds.) *Diagnosis and Treatment of Depression in Late Life,* 181–244.
47. Kivela S.L., Pahkala K. (1989) Delusional depression in the elderly: A community study. *Gerontology,* 22: 236–241.
48. Meyers B.S. (1992). Geriatric delusional depression. *Clin Geruiatr Med,* 8, 299–308.
49. Baldwin R.C. (1988) Delusional and non-delusional depression in late life. Evidence for distinct subytpes. *British Journal Psychiatry,* 152, 39–44.
50. Sands J.R., Harrow M. (1994). Psychotic unipolar depression at followup: factors related to psychosis in the affective disorders. *American Journal of Psychiatry,* 151, 995–1000.
51. Roose S. P., Glassman A.H., Walsh T., et al. (1983). Depression, delusions, and suicide. *American Journal of Psychiatry,* 140, 1150–1162.
52. Isometsa E., Henriksson M., Aro H., Heikkinen M., Kuoppasalmi K., Lonnqvist J. (1994). Suicide in psychotic major depression. *Journal of Affective Disorders (Netherlands), 31, 187–191.*
53. *Alexopoulos G.S., Young R.C., Meyers B.S. (1991).* Outcome of geriatric delusional depression. Abstract. American Psychiatriac Association, Annual Meeting, New Orleans.
54. Glassman A. H., Roose S.P. (1981). Delusional depression: A distinct entity? *Archives Gen Psychiatry,* 38, 424–427.
55. Spiker D.G., Weiss J.C., Dealy R.S., Griffin S.J., Hanin I., Neil J.F., Perel J.M., Rossi A.J., Soloff P.H. (1985). The pharmacological treatment of delusional depression. *American Journal of Psychiatry.* 142, 430–436.
56. Finlay-Jones R., Parker G. (1993). A consensus conference on psychotic depression. *Aust NZ J Psychiatry,* 27, 581–589.
57. Clinical Research Centre (1984). The Norwick Park ECT Trial: Predictors of response to real and simulated ETC. *British J Psychiatry,* 114, 227–237.
58. Greenwald B.S., Kramer-Ginsber E., Marin D.B., et al. (1989). Dementia with coexistent major depression. *American Journal of Psychiatry,* 146, 1472–1478.
59. Keller M.B., Klerman G.L., Lavori P.W., et al. (1984). Long-term outcome of episodes of major depression, *JAMA,* 252, 788–792.
60. Keller M., Lavori P.W., Lewis C. E., et al. (1983). Predictors of relapse in major depressive disorder. *JAMA,* 250, 3299–3304.

61. Alexopoulos G.S., Young R.C., Abrams R.C., et al. (1989), Chronicity and relapse in geriatric depression. *Biol Psychiatry* 26, 551–564.
62. Wells K.B., Rogers W., Burman M.A. et al. (1993). Course of depression in patients with hypertension, myocardial infarction or insulin-dependent deabetes. *american Journal of Psychiatry,* 150, 632–638.
63. Frank E., Kupfer D.J., Perel J., et al. (1990). Three year outcomes for maintenance therapies in recurrent depression. *Archives Gen Psychiatry,* 47, 1093–1099.
64. Montgomery S.A., Dufour H., Brion S., et al. (1988). The prophylactic efficacy of fluoxetine in unipolar depression. *British Journal Psychiatry* 153 (suppl 3), 69–76.
65. Georgotas A., McCue R.E., Cooper T.B. et al. (1988). How effective and safe is continuation therapy in elderly depressed patients? *Arch Gen Psychiatry,* 45, 929–932.
66. Reynolds C.E., Frank E., Perel J.M. et al. (1992). Combined pharmacotherapy and psychotherapy in the acute and continuation treatment of elderly patients with recurrent major depression: A preliminary report. *American Journal Psychiatry,* 149, 1687–1692.
67. Reynolds C.F., Perel J.M., Frank E. et al. (1989). Open trial maintenance pharmacotherapy in late life depression: survival analysis. *Psychiatry Res,* 27, 225–231.
68. Georgotas A., McCue R.E., Cooper T.B. (1989) A placebo-controlled comparison of nortriptyline and phenelzine in maintenance therapy of elderly depressed patients. *Arch Gen Psychiatry,* 46, 783–785.
69. Reynolds C.F., Frank E., Perel J. M., Miller M.D., Cornes C., Rifai H., Pollock B. G., Mazumar S., George C.J., Houck P.R., Kupfer D.J. (1994). Treatment of consecutive episodes of major depression in the elderly. *American J Psychiatry,* 151, 1740–1743.
70. Dilsaver S.C., Swann A.C., Shoaib A.M., Bowers T.C. (1993). The manic syndrome: factors which may predict a patient's response to lithium, carbamazepine and valproate. *J Psychiatry Neurosci,* 18, 61–66.
71. Coryell W., Tsuang M.T. (10/1982). Primary unipolar depression and the prognostic importance of delusions. *Arch Gen Psychiatry,* 39 (10), 1181–1184.
72. Tsuang D., Coryell W., (8/1993). An 8-year follow-up of patients withDSM-III-R psychotic depression, schizoaffective disorder, and schizophrenia. *Am J Psychiatrya* 150 (8), 1182–1188.

CHAPTER 10

Substance Use Disorders in Late Life

David W. Oslin
Geriatric and Addiction Psychiatry
University of Pennsylvania

Fred C. Blow
Department of Psychiatry
University of Michigan

INTRODUCTION

As the number of older adults increases, so too will the magnitude of mental health disorders. The public health impact of alcohol dependence, as well as that of other substance use disorders, will likely follow this trend. In addition to increases that follow the growth of the elderly population, the prevalence of late-life addiction is predicted to increase because of cohort changes. The current cohort of 30- to 50-year-old people represents a group who were raised during the 1950s and 1960s and as such participated in the increased use of and addiction to heroin, cocaine, tobacco, and alcohol. Both continued substance dependence and a history of substance dependence will have physical and mental health consequences for this cohort as it ages. This may be particularly true of younger women, who are showing increased use of alcohol compared to previous generations (Douglas, 1984). A recent study in Sweden found that the M:F ratio among older alcoholics admitted for addiction treatment decreased from 7.8:1 to 3.4:1 in the span of a decade ending in the late 1980s (Osterling & Berglund, 1994). As the current cohort of adults ages, there will be an immense need for knowledge about the continued use of alcohol and the sequelae of past alcohol use.

Although research in late-life addictions has developed slowly, recent studies have underscored the prevalence and disability related to substance abuse in late-life. Perhaps more importantly, recent research has demonstrated the efficacy of both psychotherapeutic and pharmacology treatments for older adults with alcohol abuse or dependence. Moreover, there is emerging evidence that reduction in alcohol use among older adults with alcohol dependence can lead to improvement in health-related quality of life. An area of continued need is a better understanding of other substance-related problems such as nicotine and benzodiazepine dependence. This chapter will highlight the recent advances in understanding and treating late-life addictions. The emphasis of this chapter will be on alcohol-related disability, as this is the area of the greatest current importance in older adults. Recent findings related to other substances will be included when appropriate.

EXTENT OF SUBSTANCE ABUSE

Understanding the extent of addictive disorders in late-life has been hindered by the methods employed in epidemiological research. Most epidemiological studies in the past have either focused on use patterns, such as quantity or frequency of substance use, or ill-defined clinical impressions such as "alcoholism." The use of quantity and frequency measures is particularly problematic in older adults as the correlation between quantity consumed and a diagnosis of alcohol abuse or dependence is weaker than among younger adults (Grant & Hartford, 1989). Thus an older adult may meet diagnostic criteria for alcohol dependence when consuming 7–10 drinks per week, whereas a 30-year-old consuming the same amount is not likely to meet diagnostic criteria for abuse or dependence. Moreover, reliance upon current quantity and frequency of use also would not capture the effects of past abuse or dependence. Recent studies have appropriately moved toward the use of diagnostic criteria as defined by DSM-IIIR or DSM-IV or to the use of instruments that measure alcohol related problems such as the AUDIT, the Diagnostic Interview Schedule or the Addiction Severity Index (Frances, 1994; McLellan, Lubrosky, & O'Brien, 1980; Robins, Helzer, Croughan, & Ratcliff, 1981; Saunders, Aasland, Babor, Delafuente, & Grant, 1993; Spitzer, 1987).

The most recent studies examining the epidemiology of substance use disorders among the elderly have focused on care settings such as primary care physician practices, nursing homes, or hospitals. Barry and colleagues (1998) conducted an alcohol screening program in over 12,000 elderly primary care patients. Among those evaluated, 15% of the patients screened positive for alcohol problems based upon alcohol consumption, binge drinking, or the presence of alcohol-related problems. A similar project conducted by Callahan and Tierney (1995) found 10.6 % of 3954 primary care patients over age 60 had alcohol problems. Patients were considered to have an alcohol-related problem if they reported any drinking in the last year and scored ≥2 on the CAGE questionnaire. Among 140 patients enrolled in a geriatric mental health outpatient clinic, Holroyd and Duryee (1997) report a prevalence for alcohol dependence (DSM-IV diagnosis) of 8.6%. The authors also reported that 11.4 % of the patients were dependent upon benzodiazepines. Two recent studies have reported on the lifetime occurrence of alcohol dependence among veteran nursing home residents. Joseph, Ganzini, & Atkinson (1995) found that 49% of a sample of residents had a lifetime diagnosis of alcohol dependence with 18% reporting active symptoms of dependence within 1 year of admission to the nursing home. Similarly, Oslin and colleagues found 29% of the residents had a lifetime diagnosis of alcohol abuse or dependence, with 10% of the residents meeting criteria for abuse or dependence within 1 year of admission to the home (Oslin, Streim, Parmelee, Boyce, & Katz, 1997).

The prevalence of alcohol dependence among community-dwelling elderly has been estimated in two recent studies. Kandel and colleagues recently reported on symptoms of alcohol dependence using the National Household Surveys on Drug Abuse (Kandel, Chen, Warner, Kessler, & Grant, 1997). Study participants include noninstitutionalized adults over 12 years of age. The study was conducted between 1991 and 1993 and included 87,915 participants divided into several age groups, including those 50 and over. Among the oldest group, the prevalence of both alcohol use and cigarette use were common (54.9% reported alcohol use in the last year and 22.6% reported cigarette use). However, the prevalence of alcohol dependence was only 1.6% and that of nicotine dependence, 5.4%. The prevalence of marijuana and cocaine dependence was reported as 0.01% and 0.1% of those over age 50. Black and colleagues reported on a cohort of 865 elderly adults living in a public housing project in Baltimore (Black, Rabins, & McGuire, 1998). The prevalence of current alcohol related problems (currently drinking and ≥2 positive CAGE questions) was 4% with a lifetime prevalence of 22%.

These recent studies demonstrate that the prevalence of alcohol abuse or dependence is approximately 2–4% among elderly persons living in the community. Moreover, the prevalence of alcohol abuse or dependence is approximately 10% of those older adults seeking help in outpatient clinics. These prevalence rates are similar to those previously reported in a review article by Liberto and colleagues focused mostly on the literature from 1965 to 1993 (Liberto, Oslin, & Ruskin, 1992). Put into perspective the prevalence of alcohol dependence for elderly men exceeds the prevalence of major depression for elderly men (Robins & Regier, 1991).

Perhaps a unique problem with the elderly is the misuse of prescription and over-the-counter medications. This includes the misuse of substances such as sedative/hypnotics, narcotic and non-narcotic analgesics, diet aids, decongestants, and a wide variety of other over-the-counter medications. Indeed, benzodiazepines have historically been among the most commonly prescribed medications in the United States. The prevalence of benzodiazepine use increases with age and the elderly are more likely to take benzodiazepines chronically (Holroyd s & Duryee J., 1997; Simon, VonKorff, Barlow, Pabiniak, & Wagner, 1996). Studies mostly from the '70s and '80s suggested that 10–15% of the elderly were actively taking a benzodiazepine (Dunbar, Perera, & Jenner, 1989; Krska & MacLeod, 1995; Wright, Caplan, & Payne, 1994; Zisselman, Rovner, Kelly, & Wood, 1994). Previous research has also shown that benzodiazepines are often inappropriately prescribed for illnesses such as depression, psychosis, and chronic insomnia (Isacson, Bingefors, Wennberg, & Dahlstrom, 1993; Rickels, Case, Schweizer, Garcia-Espana, & Fridman, 1991; Simon et al., 1996; Straand & Rokstad, 1997; Zisselman et al., 1994). However, in the last decade, serotonin-specific re-uptake inhibitors (SSRIs) such as sertraline, paroxetine, and fluoxetine have consistently been among the most frequently prescribed medications in the U.S., and it is reasonable to speculate that significant components of the use of chronic benzodiazepines may have been supplanted by the use of SSRIs. Although efforts at physician and public education over the last decade regarding proper benzodiazepine use and the management of depression may have led to decreases in the inappropriate use of benzodiazepines, there has been little research into the extent to which benzodiazepine use in the elderly remains a significant medical and public health problem.

CONSEQUENCES OF SUBSTANCE ABUSE AMONG OLDER ADULTS

The health-related consequences of alcohol use and other drugs of abuse have been articulated in many articles and reviews. Alcohol dependence is associated with increased morbidity and mortality from disease-specific disorders, such as alcohol-induced cirrhosis or alcohol-related cardiomyopathy, as well as increasing the risks for such diseases as hypertension or trauma related to falls or motor vehicle accidents. Until recently, there have been few studies demonstrating the reversibility of this morbidity after the initiation of abstinence. Joseph and colleagues demonstrated that among veteran residents of a nursing home, those with a recent history of alcohol-related problems were more likely to be discharged (Joseph, Atkinson, & Ganzini, 1995). A similar study by Oslin and colleagues (1997) demonstrated that there was a relationship between initiation of abstinence and improvement in activities of daily living. Residents were characterized as having a recent history of abuse within 1 year of admission to the nursing home, a past history of alcohol abuse, or no history of alcohol abuse.

Assessments of functioning were made at admission to the home and on average 1.4 years after admission. At the time of follow-up, the residents who had been abusing alcohol just prior to admission had significantly improved in their ability to perform basic activities of daily living (ADLs) compared to the other residents. Moreover, those with a past history of alcohol abuse also demonstrated an improvement in ADLs that was intermediate in degree to the recently abusing group. Similar benefits have been reported after discontinuation of benzodiazepines. In a study by Habraken and associates (1997), 50 nursing home residents were randomly assigned to continue for 1 year on benzodiazepines or be withdrawn and continued on a placebo. At both 6 and 12 months, the placebo-treated group demonstrated improvement in ADLs compared to the residents who remained on benzodiazepines.

These reports of the reversibility of morbidity associated with alcohol use and benzodiazepine use provide perhaps the greatest argument for initiating addiction treatment in older adults. A study by Adams demonstrated that diseases related to alcohol dependence a number of hospitalizations for Medicare recipients equal to that for myocardial infarction (Adams, Yuan, Barboriak, & Rimm, 1993). Despite this, hospitalized elderly are seldom identified as having an alcohol disorder or referred for treatment (Curtis, Millman, Joseph, & Charles, 1986). However, treating alcohol dependence could potentially prove cost-effective in the elderly through reduced hospitalizations for medical complications, or reduced use of nursing homes, or of other costly health services. This would represent a departure from traditional addiction treatment outcomes such as years of potential life lost, work-related disability, and crime, all of which have less relevance for the elderly than middle-aged adults.

TREATMENT

Many factors have lead to a reduction in use of long-term residential or inpatient treatments for addictive disorders. However, one result of the loss of these facilities has been a renewed interest in outpatient treatment, both specialty-based and in primary care settings. A recent multisite study sponsored by NIAAA highlights the efficacy of three psychosocial treatments for younger and middle-aged outpatients with an alcohol use disorder (Cooney et al., 1997). The three treatments included a motivational enhancement model of brief therapy, a cognitive behavioral treatment, and a 12-step facilitation treatment. Each of these treatments are manualized and can be easily transferred to use in nonresearch community programs. All three treatments were efficacious in reducing alcohol consumption after 1 year. Unfortunately, this study included only a few elderly adults. However, the Center for Substance Abuse Treatment published a Treatment Improvement Protocol (TIP) focused upon the treatment of late-life substance abuse disorders (Blow, 1998). The TIP includes recent and past literature review as well as consensus opinion from experts in the field of geriatric addictions on the identification and treatment of late-life addictions.

Oslin and colleagues have reported that older adults are more compliant with addiction treatment than younger adults as measured by treatment attendance (older adults attended 94% of their scheduled appointments) (Oslin, Pettinati, Volpicelli, & Katz, 1997). Previous literature has suggested that compliance with addiction treatment is directly related to a better outcome (Volpicelli et al., 1997). If this relationship holds for older adults, the expectation would be that treatment outcome would be better in the elderly. Perhaps one of the reasons for the excellent compliance in this study was the type of psychotherapy used. This study used compliance enhancement therapy as the model treatment, delivered by a nurse practitioner in 30-minute sessions. This approach is much more aligned to a primary care model than to traditional addiction therapy involving group therapy. Indeed, when the effects of compliance enhancement therapy were compared to results from previous clinical trials that used age-specific alcohol counseling, there was greater compliance with treatment visits using compliance enhancement (Oslin et al., 1997). This suggests that older adults may respond better to a primary care or health-oriented treatment approach rather than traditional models of addiction treatment.

In support of these latter findings, two recent studies have underscored the effectiveness of primary care based treatment of younger and older adults with alcohol-related problems. Fleming and colleagues randomly assigned patients age 18 to 65 who screened positive for alcohol-related problems to receive either usual care in a primary care practice or an intervention consisting of two 15-minute counseling sessions given by the primary care physician (Fleming, Barry, Manwell, Johnson, & London, 1997). At the end of 12 months, there were significantly greater reductions in alcohol use in the intervention group compared to the usual care group. In a similarly designed study of elderly primary care patients, Barry and colleagues (1998) have shown that older problem drinkers also respond favorably to physician advice with a marked reduction in alcohol consumption.

Further studies will need to clarify the predictors of lack of response to primary care treatment and the need for referral to specialty care. To highlight this point, it is noted that the two primary care studies enrolled mostly patients with moderate alcohol consumption, many of whom did not meet criteria for alcohol dependence, while clinical trials of addiction treatment typically enroll patients with alcohol dependence and usually with more severe cases of alcohol dependence. Thus in terms of a public health perspective, this is not an either/or treatment option; rather, it is likely that patients with less severe disease can and should be treated in primary care settings, and that patients with more severe disease should be treated by the primary care physician in conjunction with specialty care.

PHARMACOTHERAPY OF ADDICTION

Pharmacologic treatments have not traditionally played a major role in the long-term treatment of older alcohol-dependent adults. Until recently, disulfiram was the only medication approved for the treatment of alcoholism, but was seldom used in older patients because of concerns related to adverse effects. In 1995, the opioid antagonist naltrexone was approved by the FDA for the treatment of alcoholism. The FDA approval of naltrexone was based upon studies by Volpicelli and colleagues and O'Malley and colleagues demonstrating the efficacy of naltrexone for the treatment of middle-aged patients with alcohol dependence (O'Malley et al., 1992; Volpicelli, Alterman, Hayashida, & O'Brien, 1992). In both studies, naltrexone was found to be safe and effective in preventing relapse and reducing the craving for alcohol. The use of naltrexone was based on studies demonstrating an interaction between endogenous endorphin activity and alcohol intake. Similar results have been reported by using nalmafene, also an opioid antagonist (Mason et al., 1994).

Oslin and colleagues have extended this line of research by studying a group of older veterans age 50 to 70, in a double-blind placebo-controlled randomized trial of naltrexone 50 mg per day (Oslin, Liberto, O'Brien, Krois, & Norbeck, 1997). The results were similar to the other clinical trials, with half as many naltrexone-treated subjects relapsing to significant drinking compared to those treated with placebo. It is important to note that there was no improvement in total abstinence, but improvement in relapse to heavy drinking. Thus, failure to achieve abstinence should not be seen as a failure of treatment. Although this study did not include subjects over 70 years of age, it does raise the hope that opioid antagonists may have clinical efficacy among older alcoholics.

Recently, acamprosate has been studied as a promising agent in the treatment of alcoholism. Although the exact action of acamprosate is still unknown, it is thought to reduce glutamate response through actions distinct from those of typical NMDA blockers (Spanagel, Zieglgansberger, & Hundt, 1996; Zeise, Madamba, Siggins, Putzke, & Zieglgansberger, 1994). The clinical evidence favoring acamprosate is impressive. Mann and colleagues have studied 272 alcohol-dependent subjects in Europe for up to 48 weeks using a randomized placebo-controlled study of acamprosate. Forty-three percent of the acamprosate treated group was abstinent at the conclusion of the study compared to 21% in the placebo group (Sass, Soyka, Mann, & Zieglgansberger, 1996). There have been no studies indicating the efficacy of acamprosate among elderly patients, and confirmation of the safety and efficacy in this population is an important area for research.

Treatment studies for other substance disorders are lacking among the elderly. Although smoking is clearly linked to increased disability and mortality in late-life, there have been relatively few studies of smoking cessation focused upon the elderly. Orleans and colleagues found that use of transdermal nicotine replacement resulted in a 29% self-reported quit rate and greater success in patients who received professional encouragement to stop (physician or pharmacist) (Orleans et al., 1994). This study was an open-label descriptive study of lower-income smokers. The antidepressants buproprion and nortriptyline have both been shown to be effective in improving quit rates among middle-aged smokers (Hall et al., 1998; Hurt et al., 1997). Future studies should include more elderly subjects, as there are clearly defined benefits from smoking cessation among the elderly (Maxwell & Hirdes, 1993; Paganinihill & Hsu, 1994). Finally, although Rickels and colleagues demonstrated that the elderly could successfully be withdrawn from chronic benzodiazepine use, they also demonstrated that the elderly are more likely to return to benzodiazepine use within 3 years of discontinuation (Rickels et al., 1991; Schwizer, Case, & Rickels, 1989).

SUMMARY

Over the last several years there has been a growing awareness that addictive disorders among the elderly are a common public health problem. Epidemiological studies suggest that alcoholism is present in up to 4% of the elderly and there is at least one report suggesting that the prevalence of alcoholism among older adults is on the rise (Liberto et al., 1992; Osterling & Berglund, 1994). Moreover, problem or hazardous drinking is estimated to be even more common among the elderly than alcoholism (Barry et al., 1998; Liberto et al., 1992). However, there continues to be a gap in the number of older adults who are referred for treatment or who receive treatment for addictive disorders. Although there are many reasons for patients not to be engaged in treatment, recommending treatment is partially based upon the availability of effective treatment. Towards this end, there needs to be better dissemination of information regarding currently available and efficacious treatments for alcoholism and other addictive disorders, as well as continued development of more effective treatments.

REFERENCES

Adams, W. L., Yuan, Z., Barboriak, J. J., & Rimm, A. A. (1993). Alcohol-related hospitalizations in elderly people: Prevalence and geographic variation in the United States. *Journal of the American Medical Associaiotn, 270,* 1222–1225.

American Psychiatric Association (1994). *Diagnostic and statistical manual of mental disorders* (4th ed.). Washington, DC: Author.

American Psychiatric Association (1987). *Diagnostic and statistical Manual of Mental Disorders* (3rd e-revised.) Washington, DC: Author.

Barry, K. L., Blow, F. C., Walton, M. A., Chernack, S. T., Mudd, S. A., Coyne, J. C., & Gombery, E. S. L. (1998). Elder-specific brief alcohol intervention: 3-month outcomes. *Alcoholism: Clinical and Experimental Research, 22,* 32A.

Black B. S., Rabins, P. V. & McGuire, M. H. (1998). Alcohol use disorder is a risk factor for mortality among older public housing residents. *International Psychogeriatrics, 10,* 309–327.

Blow, F. C. (19989). *Substance abuse among older Americans.* Washington, DC: US Government Printing Office.

Callahan, C. M., & Tierney, W. M. (1995). Health services use and mortality among older primary care patients with alcoholism. *Journal of the American Geriatrics Society, 43,* 1378–1383.

Cooney, N. L., DiClemente, C. C., Carbonari, J., Zweben, A., Longabaugh, R. H., Stout, R. L., Donovan, D., Babor, T. F., Delboca, F. K., Rounsaville, B. J., Carroll, K. M., Wirtz, P. W., Bailey, S., Brady, K., Cisler, R., Hester, R. K., Kivlahan, D. R., Nierenberg, T. K., Pate, L. A., Sturgis, E., Muenz, L., Cushman, P., Finney, J., Hingson, R., Klett, J., & Townsend, M. (1997). Matching alcoholism treatments to client heterogeneity: Project Match posttreatment drinking outcomes. *Journal of Studies on Alcohol, 58,* 7–29.

Curtis, J., Millman, E., Joseph, M. & Charles, J. (1986). Prevalence rates for alcoholism, associated depression and dementia on the Harlem Hospital medicine and surgery services. *Advances in Alcohol and Substance Abuse, 6,* 45–65.

Douglas, R. L. (1984). Aging and alcohol problems: Opportunities for socioepidemiological research. In M. Galanter (Ed.) *Recent development in alcoholism* (Vol. 2, pp. 251–266). New York: Plenum.

Dunbar, G. C., Perera, M. H., & Jenner, F. A. (1989). Patterns of benzodiazepine use in Great Britain as measured by a general population survey. *British Journal of Psychiatry, 155,* 836–841.

Fleming, M. F., Barry, K. L., Manwell, L. B., Johnson, K., & London, R. (1997). Brief physician advice for problem alcohol drinkers. *JAMA, 277,* 1039–1045.

Grant, B. F., & Hartford, T. C. (1989). The relationship between ethanol intake and DSM-III alcohol use disorders: A cross-perspective analysis. *Journal of Substance Abuse, 1,* 231–252.

Habraken, H., Soenen, K., Blondeel, L., Van Elsen, J. Bourda, J. Coppens, E., & Willeput, M. (1997). Gradual withdrawal form benzodiazepines in residents of homes for the elderly: Experience and suggestions for future research. *European Journal of Clinical Pharmacology, 51*(5), 355–8.

Hall, S. M. Reus, V. I., Munoz, R. F., Sees, K. L., Humfleet, G., Hartz, D. T., Frederick, S., & Triffleman, E. (1998). Nortriptyline and cognitive-behavioral therapy in the treatment of cigarette smoking. *Archives of General Psychiatry, 55,* 683–690.

Holroyd, S., & Duryee, J. (1997). Substance use disorders in a geriatric psychiatry outpatient clinic: Prevalence and epidemiologic characteristics. *Journal of Nervous & Mental Disease, 185*(10), 627–32.

Hurt, R. D., Sachs, D. P., Glover, E. D., Offord, K. P., Johnsonton, J. A., Dale, L. C., Khayrallah, M., Schroeder, D. R., Glover P. N., Sullivan C. R., Croghan, I. T., & Sullivan, P. M. (1997). A comparison of sustained-release buproprion and placebo for smoking cessation. *New England Journal of Medicine, 337,* 1195–1202.

Isacson, D., Bingefors, K., Wennberg, M., & Dahlstrom, M. (1993). Factors associated with high-quantity prescriptions of benzodiazepines in Sweden. *Social Science & Medicine, 36*(3), 343–51.

Joseph, C. L., Atkinson, R. M., & Ganzini, L. (1995). Problem drinking among residents of a VA nursing home. *International Journal of Geriatric Psychiatry, 10,* 243–248.

Joseph, C. L., Ganzini, L., & Atkinson, R. (1995). Screening for alcohol use disorders i the nursing home. *Journal of the American Geriatrics Society, 43,* 368–373.

Kandel, D., Chen, K., Warner, L. A. Kessler, R. C., & Grant, B. (1997). Prevalence and demographic correlates of symptoms of last year dependence on alcohol, nicotine, marijuana and cocaine in the U.S. population. *Drug & Alcohol Dependence, 44*(1), 11 29.

Krska, J., & MacLeod, T. N. (1995). Sleep quality and the use of benzodiazepine hypnotics in general practice. *Journal of Clinical Pharmacy & Therapeutics, 20*(2), 91–6.

Liberto, J. G., Oslin, D. W., & Ruskin, P. E. (1992). Alcoholism in older persons: A review of the literature. *Hospital & Community Psychiatry, 43*(10), 975–84.

Mason, B. J., Ritvo, E. C., Morgan, R. O., Salvato, F. R., Goldberg, G., Welch, B., & Mantero-Atienza, E. (1994). A double-blind, placebo-controlled pilot study to evaluate the efficacy and safety of oral nalmefene HCL for alcohol dependence. *Alcoholism: Clinical and Experimental Research, 18,* 1162–1167.

Maxwell, C. J., & Hirdes, J. P. (1993). The prevalence of smoking and implications for quality-of-life among the community-based elderly. *American Journal of Preventive Medicine, 9,* 338–345.

McLellan, A. T., Lubrosky, L., & O'Brien, C. P. (1980). An improved evaluation instrument for substance abuse patients: The Addiction Severity Index. *Journal of Nervous and Mental Diseases, 168,* 26–33.

O'Malley, S. S., Jaffe, Al. J., Chang, G., Schottenfeld, R. S., Meyer, R. E., & Rounsaville, B. (1992). Naltrexone and coping skills therapy for alcohol dependence: A controlled study. *Archives of General Psychiatry, 49,* 881–887.

Orleans, C., Resch, N., Noll, E., Keintz, M., Rimer, B., Brown, T., & Snedden, T. (1994). Use of transdermal nicotine in a state-level prescription plan for the elderly. *JAMA, 271,* 601–607.

Oslin, D., Liberto, J., O'Brien, J., Krois, S., & Borneck, J. (1997). Naltrexone as an adjunctive treatment for older patients with alcohol dependence. *American Journal of Geriatric Psychiatry, 5,* 324–332.

Oslin, D. W., Pettinati, H., Volpicelli, J. R., & Katz, I. R. (1997). Enhanced treatment compliance among elderly alcoholics using BRENDA: A model psychosocial intervention. *Gerontologist, 37,* 326.

Oslin, D. W., Streim, J. E., Parmelee, P., Boyce, A. A., & Katz, I. R. (1997). Alcohol abuse: A source of reversible functional disability among residents. *International Journal of Geriatric Psychiatry, 12*(8), 825–32.

Osterling, A., & Berglund, M. (1994). Elderly first-time admitted alcoholics: A descriptive study on gender differences in a clinical population. *Alcoholism: Clinical and Experimental Research, 18,* 1317–1321.

Paganini-hill, A., & Hsu, G. (1994). Smoking and mortality among residents of a California retirement community. *American Journal of Public Health, 84,* 992–995.

Rickels, K., Case, W. G., Schweizedr, E., Garcia-Espana, F., & Fridman, R. (1991). Long-term benzodiazepine users 3 years after participation in a discontinuation program. *American Journal of Psychiatry, 148*(6), 757–61.

Robins, L. N., Helzer, J. E., Croughan, J., & Ratcliff, K. S. (1981). National Institute of Mental Heath Diagnostic Interview Schedule: Its history, characteristics, and validity. *Archives of General Psychiatry, 38,* 381–389.

Robins, L. N., &Regier, D. A. (Eds.). (1991). *Psychiatric disorders in American, the Epidemiologic Catchment Area study.* New York: The Free Press.

Sass, H., Soyka, M., Mann, K., & Zieglgansberger, W. (1996). Relapse prevention by acamprosate: Results form a placebo-controlled study in alcohol dependence. *Archives of General Psychiatry, 53,* 673–680.

Saunders, J. B., Aasland, O. G., Babor, T. F., De la fuente, J. R., & Grant, M. (1993). Development of the alcohol-use disorders identification test

(AUDIT): WHO collaborative project on early detection of persons with harmful alcohol-consumption. *Addiction, 88,* 791–804.

Schweizer, E., Case, W. G., & Rickels, K. (1989). Benzodiazepine dependence and withdrawal in elderly patients. *American Journal of Psychiatry, 146*(4), 529–31.

Simon, G. E., VonKorff, M., Barlow, W., Pabiniak, C., & Wagner, E. (1996). Predictors of chronic benzodiazepine use in a health maintenance organization sample. *Journal of Clinical Epidemiology, 49*(9), 1067–73.

Spanagel, R., Zieglgansberger, W., & Hundt, W. (1996). Acamprosate and alcohol: III. Effects on alcohol discrimination int he rate. *European Journal of Pharmacology, 305,* 51–56.

Straand, J., & Rokstad, K. (1997). General practitioners' prescribing patterns of benzodiazepine hypnotics: are elderly patients at particular risk for overprescribing? A report from the More & Romsdal Prescription Study. *Scandinavian Journal of Primary Health Care, 15*(1), 16–21.

Volpicelli, J. R., Alterman, A. I., Hayashida, M., & O'Brien, C. P. (1992). Naltrexone in the treatment of alcohol dependence. *Archives of General Psychiatry, 49,* 876–880.

Volpicelli, J. R., Rhines, K. C., Rhines, J. S., Volpicelli, L. A., Alterman, A. I., & O'Brien, C. P. (1997). Naltrexone and alcohol dependence: Role of subject compliance. *Archives of General Psychiatry, 54,* 737–742.

Wright, N., Caplan, R., & Payne, S. (1994). Community survey of long term daytime use of benzodiazepines. *MBJ, 309*(6946), 27–8.

Zeise, M. L., Madamba, S. G., Siggins, G. R., Putzke, J., & Zieglgansberger, W. (1994). The anti-craving substance *Acmprosate* reduces glutamatergic synaptic transmission and high-threshold calcium current in neo-cortical and hippocampal pyramidal neurons. *Alcoholism: Clinical and Experimental Research, 18,* 36A.

Zisselman, M. H., Rovner, B. W., Kelly, K. G., & Woods, C. (1994). Benzodiazepine utilization in a university hospital. *American Journal of Medical Quality, 9*(3), 138–41.

CHAPTER 11

Late-Life Psychosis: Advances in Understanding and Treatment

ROBERT A. SWEET & BRUCE G. POLLOCK
WESTERN PSYCHIATRIC INSTITUTE AND CLINIC
UNIVERSITY OF PITTSBURGH MEDICAL CENTER

OVERVIEW

The most common late-life psychoses are those associated with dementia, major depression with psychotic features, and schizophrenia (and related schizoaffective disorders). The relative frequency with which these disorders are encountered is dependent on the clinical setting. Dementia and mood-related psychoses are most common in acute care and skilled nursing facilities. Schizophrenia is most common in psychiatric long-term care settings. The intent of this chapter is to provide an overview of recent advances pertinent to each of these major categories of late-life psychoses. The most significant progress to occur in late-life psychoses during the past 3 years, cutting across diagnostic categories, has been the advent of the new atypical neuroleptics. These agents, risperidone, olanzapine, and quetiapine have rapidly replaced the prototype atypical agent, clozapine for use in most elderly populations. Moreover, because of their generally favorable safety profile, they have made substantial inroads into the use of the typical neuroleptics in geriatric practice. We will review these agents, identifying both specific knowledge and important areas where knowledge is lacking, with regard to geriatric practice.

ADVANCES IN CLINICAL UNDERSTANDING AND PHENOMENOLOGY

Psychosis in Dementia

Most studies have found that the psychotic symptoms, delusions and hallucinations, occur in 30–40% of patients with dementia at some time during their illness (Wreagg & Jeste, 1989). With current estimates of dementia prevalence in the United States at 4 million affected individuals, that would yield a prevalence of dementia-related psychosis of approximately 1.4 million individuals, more than 0.5% of the current population. The best-studied of the dementias is Alzheimer's disease (AD). Psychotic symptoms in AD usually appear in the middle stages of disease progression, and are moderately persistent during follow-up (Devanand et al., 1997). It remains unclear whether it is more appropriate to consider delusions and hallucinations as linked or separate phenomena in AD. Some reports have identified significant associations between hallucinations and delusions in AD (Gilley, Whalon, Wilson, & Bennett, 1991; Zubenko, Rosen, Sweet, Mulsant, & Fifai, 1992.) Others, however, have not found delusions and hallucinations to load in the same factors on behavioral rating scales nor to occur together more often than by chance (Devanand et al., 1997; Mulsant et al., 1996; Tariot et al., 1995). Similarly, a recent report found that delusions, but not hallucinations, were independent predictors of the occurrence and frequency of physical aggression in AD (Gilley et al, 1997).

Another important recent advance in the understanding of the phenomenology of psychosis in dementia has been the development of consensus clinical and neuropathologic criteria for the diagnosis of dementia with Lewy bodies (DLB) (McKeith, et a., 1996). After AD, DLB appears to be the most frequent dementia in autopsy series, accounting for 20%–30% of cases previously diagnosed as AD (Ellis, Caligirui, Galaska, & Thal, 1996). Formed visual hallucinations are common in DLB, though the specificity of these symptoms for DLB remains uncertain and awaits prospective clinical-pathological validation.

Major Depression with Psychotic Features in Late Life

In acute psychiatric settings, estimates of the frequency of psychotic symptoms in elderly patients experiencing a depressive episode (major depression with psychotic features, MD+P) range from 28%-45% (Brodaty et al, 1997; Meyers & Greenberg, 1986; & Zubenko et al., 1994). There is evidence that MD+P rates are higher in the elderly than in midlife patients with depression (Brodaty et al, 1997). Despite the frequency of late life MD+P, relatively few studies have specifically examined this syndrome in the elderly (Meyers, 1995). Several differences between elderly MD+P patients and similarly aged nonpsychotic depressives have been described. Elderly MD+P patients have been observed to have higher degrees of cognitive impairment than their nonpsychotic peers (Martinez, Mulsant, Meyers, & Labowitz, 1996; Sewell, Jeste, Paulsen, Kramer, & Gillin, 1994). MD+P in late life may also confer a higher risk for suicide (Martinex et al., 1996). Finally, there is evidence that elderly MD+P patients have poorer outcomes than elderly patients with nonpsychotic depression (Flint & Rifat, 1998b). In this regard, elderly MD+P patients may resemble midlife MD+P groups (Meyers, 1995).

Late-Life Schizophrenia

Elderly patients diagnosed with schizophrenia have classically been split into two groups: early-onset schizophrenia (EOS, usually defined as age of onset before age 45) and late-onset schizophrenia (LOS, defined as age of onset after age 45) (Lacro & Jeste, 1997). However, it is unclear if this grouping identifies biologically and clinically relevant subtypes. Both groups demonstrate similar degrees of positive symptoms, chronicity of course, cognitive impairment, and nonspecific changes on brain imaging. In comparison to EOS, however, LOS patients are more often female, have fewer negative symptoms, typically require lower doses of antipsychotics, and have been found to have larger thalami on magnetic resonance imaging (Corey-Bloom, Jernigan, Archibald, Harris, & Jeste, 1995). Regardless of age of onset, perhaps the most striking aspect of late-life schizophrenia is its relative rarity. While a rate of 1% is the generally accepted estimate for the prevalence of schizophrenia in mixed-age samples, epidemiologic studies of schizophrenia in elderly populations, using current diagnostic criteria, find prevalence rates ranging from only 0.1% to 0.6% (Copeland et al., 1998). Thus, among the most important questions in late life schizophrenia is why there are fewer cases. Premature mortality and/or age-related degeneration of neurotransmitter systems which lead to amelioration of symptoms have both been postulated.

Consistent with the latter postulate are studies indicating that the symptom profile of schizophrenia changes with aging. With increasing age, schizophrenia patients demonstrate less severe positive symptoms (Davidson et al., 1995; Schultz et al, 1997). In contrast, negative symptoms either remain unchanged or become more severe (Davidson et al.,, 1995; Schultz et al., 1997). Recently, cognitive impairment has been recognized as a fundamental feature of schizophrenia, independent of negative symptoms, with impact on functional status and prognosis (Harvey et al, 1996). There is some disagreement on whether cognitive impairment emerges early in schizophrenia and remains static or progresses over time (Davidson et al., 1995; Mockler, Riordan, & Sharma, 1997). Even those studies suggesting an age effect on cognition in schizophrenia find age-related declines which are modest, approximating 10% of the age-related declines seen in patients with neurodegenerative dementia (Davidson et al., 1995). Regardless of the course of cognitive dysfunction in schizophrenia, certain populations of elderly schizophrenic patients evaluated cross-sectionally demonstrate moderate to severe cognitive impairment at an alarmingly high rate (Davidson et al., 1996; Harvey, Leff, Trieman,

Anderson, & Davidson, 1997). The severity of deficits in late-life schizophrenia are comparable to those seen in AD, though the pattern of affected cognitive domains differs between schizophrenia and AD (Davidson et al., 1996).

ADVANCES IN NEUROBIOLOGY

Psychosis in Dementia

Relatively few studies have examined the psychobiology of psychosis in AD or DLB. No firm conclusions can be drawn as yet with regard to the localization of neuropathologic changes in AD patients with psychosis (Bondareff, 1996). A number of investigations have examined the concentrations of neurotransmitters and their metabolites in postmortem brain of AD patients with and without psychosis. Brain concentrations of serotonin and its metabolite, 5-hydroxyindoleacetic acid have been reported to be reduced in some, but not all, studies in psychotic AD patients (Lawlor et al., 1995; Zubenko et al., 1991). One study identified increased norepinephrine concentration in the substantia nigra of psychotic AD patients (Zubenko et al., 1991). Several studies have found no association of the concentrations of dopamine and its metabolites with the presence or severity of psychosis in AD and DLB (Bierer et al., 1993; Perry et al., 1990; Zubenko et al., 1991). Similarly, we found no association of psychosis severity with in vivo measurement of the plasma concentration of the dopamine metabolite homovanillic acid (Sweet et al., 1997).

Recently, we reported that genetic variation in the dopamine$_1$ (D_1) and D_3 receptors was associated with psychosis in AD . Even though AD+P and AD-P patients may not differ in brain DA concentration, differences between these groups in DA receptor density or affinity could still yield between-group differences in DA signaling. We found that psychosis occurred more frequently in patients who were homozygous for D_1 receptor allele B2 or who were homozygous for either D_3 receptor allele 1 or allele 2. AD with psychosis was not associated with the examined polymorphisms in the D_2 and D_4 receptor genes. While the finding for D_1 was novel, the association of excess homozygosity for either D_3 allele with AD+P was identical to that reported in studies of the association of D_3 genotype with schizophrenia (for a review of 30 association studies reported in schizophrenia and a meta-analysis, see Williams et al, 1998). The convergence of the D_3 findings in AD with reports in schizophrenia suggests that D_3 genotype may be a common mechanism conferring an increased likelihood of expressing psychotic symptoms in individuals with a superimposed disease process (e.g. neurodegenerative in AD or neurodevelopmental in schizophrenia). While in schizophrenia the magnitude of the effect of D_3 receptor genotype is modest (meta-analytic odds ratio (O.R., 95% C.I.) of 1.2 (1.1, 1.4), we observed a more robust increase in risk in AD+P, with an O.R. of 2.8 (1.2, 6.9). A firm estimate, however, of the magnitude of the effect of D_3 genotype in AD+P awaits further replication.

Whether these genetic variations in the D_1 and D_3 receptors lead to phenotypic differences in their corresponding receptor expression or function in human brain is not currently known. We recently conducted a pilot study directly examining the associations of D_1 and D_3 receptor density and affinity with the presence of psychosis in AD (Sweet, Hamilton, Pollock, Heinteleff, & KeKosky, in press.) Selective saturation binding assays for these two receptors were performed in rostral striatum obtained post-mortem from AD patients. We found D_1 receptor density to be reduced by 20% in psychotic AD patients, without any change in D_1 receptor affinity. In contrast, D_3 receptor density was unchanged in psychotic patients, but D_3 receptor affinity increased by 41%. Though clearly still preliminary, findings from this and similar studies may ultimately provide a guide to the development of a more rational, and selective, pharmacotherapy for psychosis in dementia.

Major Depression with Psychotic Features in Late Life

In midlife patients there is evidence that the psychobiology of MD+P differs from nonpsychotic depression, with more severe disruption of serotonergic, dopaminergic, and hypothalamic-pituitary-adrenal axis function (Aberg-Wistedt, 1985; Schatzberg, Wistedt & Bertisson, 1995). There are few similar studies, comparing elderly MD+P with elderly non-psychotic depressives. No differences in dexamethasone suppression test results or in growth hormone release after growth hormone releasing factor challenge were seen in elderly MD+P versus nonpsychotic depressed patients (Contreras et al., 1996; Obrien et al., 1997). Several neurobiologic studies, however, are consistent with the clinical observation of increased cognitive impairment in elderly MD+P patients. Elderly MD+P patients have been found to demonstrate higher rates of vascular risk factors, and to demonstrate a trend towards more frequent deep white matter lesions on magnetic resonance imaging, than nonpsychotic depressives (Obrien et al., 1997). In a small study, late-life MD+P was associated with an increased APOE4 allele frequency, while no association of APOE4 and nonpsychotic depression was seen (Zubenko et al, 1996). Though in a preliminary report we identified differences between elderly patients with MD+P and AD patients with psychotic symptoms in their prolactin response after perphenazine challenge (Sweet et al., 1995), no difference between these diagnostic groups was found in a larger series of patients (Sweet, 1999, unpublished observations). These findings, in concert with the clinical observations, raise the question of whether MD+P in late life is better seen as a marker for other brain pathology (e.g. AD or cerebrovascular disease) than as a variant of major depression. Answering this question awaits longitudinal studies with post-mortem examination, though it is likely that elderly patients with MD+P are comprised of subgroups with and without underlying degenerative etiologies.

Late-Life Schizophrenia

With the exception of postmortem studies, which frequently utilize elderly, chronically institutionalized schizophrenia subjects, studies of the neurobiology of late-life schizophrenia are lacking. Recently, a series of neuropathologic examinations of elderly schizophrenics have examined whether the prominent cognitive impairments of elderly schizophrenics are due to underlying neurodegenerative disease. Consistent with the clinical findings described above, these studies have found no evidence of the histopathologic changes which define AD, or for that matter any other identified neurodegenerative dementia (Arnold & Trojanowski, 1996; Arnold et al., 1998; Purohit et al., 1998). Thus, despite the clinical imperative to identify efficacious treatments for cognitive impairments in late-life schizophrenia, few leads exist. One area of hope, however, has been the recognition that several of the new atypical antipsychotic drugs may improve cognition in schizophrenia patients (see below).

ADVANCES IN TREATMENT

Psychosis in Dementia

Treatment studies of psychosis in dementia have historically utilized conventional neuroleptics. Conventional neuroleptics as a class are nonselective antagonists of D_2 and D_3 receptors, with varying degrees of antagonism of other neurotransmitter receptors depending on the agent selected. Across studies, conventional neuroleptics have been shown to have moderate efficacy in treating behavioral disturbances associated with dementia, but cause high rates of neuroleptic-induced parkinsonism and tardive dyskinesia (Sweet et al., 1998). Recent examinations of conventional neuroleptics have focused on whether dose- and concentration-response relationships can be determined that will allow for continued drug efficacy while reducing the frequency of treatment-limiting side effects. Devanand et al. (Devanand et al., 1998) examined moderate-dose haloperidol (2-3 mg/day) versus low-dose haloperidol (0.5–0.75 mg/day) and placebo in the treatment of psychotic and agitated symptoms in outpatients diagnosed with Alzheimer's disease. The 2–3 mg/day dose group demonstrated significantly greater improvement in measures of psychosis than either the low dose or placebo groups. Low-dose haloperidol, in contrast, was no more effective than placebo. Moderate to severe EPS developed in 25% of the patients treated with moderate dose haloperidol, while patients treated with low-dose haloperidol developed EPS no more often than placebo-treated patients. Of interest, haloperidol plasma concentrations correlated more strongly with both antipsychotic effects and EPS than haloperidol dose, suggesting a role for plasma concentration-controlled treatment in dementia patients. We have similarly found that perphenazine at doses of 1 mg/kg/day (i.e. 6 mg/day in a 60 kg patient, or approximately equivalent to 1.5 mg haloperidol/day) was efficacious in elderly patients with psychosis and agitation associated with dementia, and caused minimal EPS (Mulsant et al., 1996; Sweet et al., 1999). Unlike the finding reported for haloperidol, we found no correlation of perphenazine plasma concentration with EPS onset. These studies, and other recent reports demonstrating that conventional neuroleptics used at low doses and/or concentrations can yield antipsychotic benefit with limited acute parkinsonian side effects (Dysken et al., 1994; Finkel, Lyons, Anderson, & Sherrell, 1995), emphasize the need for direct comparisons of new agents with low dose, conventional neuroleptics.

An exciting recent development has been the examination of agents acting on serotonin systems in the treatment of psychosis in dementia. This includes both the combined serotonin$_{2A}$/D_2 antagonists (new atypical neuroleptics, reviewed below) and the selective serotonin reuptake inhibitors (SSRIs). Two recent reports described SSRI treatment of psychosis in dementia patients. A retrospective review described 20 patients with both depression and psychotic symptoms complicating dementia (12 diagnosed with AD) (Burke et al., 1997). After treatment with either sertraline or paroxetine, 15/20 (75%) of patients, and 11/12 (92%) AD patients, were rated as having moderately to markedly improved depressive and psychotic symptoms. We conducted a prospective, uncontrolled study of the highly selective SSRI, citalopram, in 16 dementia patients with agitated and psychotic symptoms (13 diagnosed with AD) (Pollack et al., 1997). Unlike the prior report, patients with a current major depressive episode were excluded from participation. Citalopram treatment was associated with significant improvement in symptoms of suspicion, with a trend towards a significant reduction in other delusions. Symptoms of agitation/aggression were also significantly improved. Preliminary results of an ongoing, randomized, double-blind, placebo- and perphenazine-controlled study of citalopram in the treatment of behavioral disturbance associated with a dementia confirm the efficacy of this SSRI in reducing both psychotic and agitation symptoms (B. G. Pollock, 1999 data). The benefit of SSRI treatment in reducing psychosis in AD patients raises the interesting question of whether SSRIs act by direct effects on serotonin neurotransmission, or because of serotonin-induced reduction of dopamine neurotransmission (Smith et al., 1997). Regardless of mechanism, with the generally favorable risk/benefit ratio associated with this class of medication, further evaluation of SSRIs in the treatment of dementia-related psychosis is warranted.

Major Depression with Psychotic Features in Late Life

The emerging pharmacologic treatment data in MD+P is consistent with the above evidence that the psychobiology of late life MD+P differs from that of midlife MD+P. In midlife MD+P treated pharmacologically, response rates approximate 80% when combination antidepressant plus neuroleptic are used (Anton & Burch, 1990; Rothschild, Samson, Bessette, & Carter-Campbell, 1993; SPiker et al., 1985). This response rate is significant better than that seen with neuroleptic treatment or antidepressant treatment alone (Spiker et al., 1985). In contrast, a recent report in elderly MD+P patients indicated that only 2 of 8 (25%) patients responded to a 6-week course of therapeutic plasma concentration nortriptyline plus perphenazine at a mean dose of 18 mg/day (Flint & Rifat, 1998a). In that study, a comparison group of MD+P patients treated with electroconvulsive therapy (ECT) had 15 of 17 (88%) respond to treatment. We recently completed a randomized, double-blind study of therapeutic plasma concentration nortriptyline plus perphenazine versus therapeutic plasma concentration nortriptyline plus placebo in 54 elderly MD+P patients. Though treatments in the two groups were relatively well tolerated, both groups had only moderate response. Defining response as resolution of both depression and psychosis, 50% of completers responded to the combination pharmacotherapy versus 44% treated with nortriptyline alone, a nonsignificant difference (B. H. Mulsant, personal communication, January 1999). These studies, as well as a retrospective review (Meyers & Greenberg, 1986), which found response rates to pharmacotherapy of only 29% in elderly MD+P patients with a contrasting response rate of 86% to ECT, would suggest that ECT and not pharmacotherapy should be the first line treatment for elderly MD+P patients. The further question of appropriate maintenance pharmacotherapy after successful ECT treatment of late life MD+P remains an important area of ongoing investigation. Eight of 15 (53%) of elderly MD+P patients maintained on nortriptyline monotherapy after successful ECT treatment experienced relapse or recurrence. Finally, one possible exception to the conclusion that ECT should be first-line treatment of late life MD+P is a report of the efficacy of sertraline monotherapy in MD+P (Zanardil, Franchini, Gasperini,

Perez, & Smeraldi, 1996). Though not yet studied formally in late-life MD+P, this report is consistent with the observed benefits of SSRI treatment for psychotic symptoms complicating a dementia (see above), and has a low risk of significant treatment-induced morbidity.

Late-Life Schizophrenia

One of the most surprising findings in a review of the treatment of late-life psychoses, is the near absolute lack of controlled clinical trials in late-life schizophrenia. The prominent clinical differences between schizophrenia occurring late in life versus schizophrenia occurring earlier in the life span suggest that treatment success in younger patients cannot be readily extrapolated to the elderly. Despite this concern, at present, studies in late-life schizophrenia are confined to open trials of agents found successful in younger patients. As recent studies of this kind have involved the new atypical antipsychotics, they are reviewed separately below.

NEW ATYPICAL ANTIPSYCHOTICS

Conventional neuroleptic treatment has shortcomings for elderly patients with psychosis. Across diagnostic groups, the elderly are subject to high rates of tardive dyskinesia, beginning rapidly after initiation of conventional neuroleptic treatment (Jeste et al., 1995; Sweet et al., 1995). Similarly, neuroleptic-induced parkinsonism is more frequent in elderly than young patients, and among elderly patients those with AD or DLB may be most sensitive (Ayd, 1960; McKeith, Fairbairn, Perry, Thompson, & Perry, 1992; Sweet, Mulsant, Pollock, Rosen, & Athieri, 1996). Finally, as reviewed above, the efficacy of conventional neuroleptics in elderly psychotic patients with AD or MD+P may be inadequate, and in late-life schizophrenia there is a need to identify treatments which are effective for negative symptoms and cognitive impairment.

In contrast to the conventional neuroleptics, the new atypical agents, risperidone, olanzapine, and quetiapine, have demonstrated equal to or greater efficacy for positive psychotic symptoms, a greater reduction in acute negative symptoms, and significantly lower rates of parkinsonian side effects and TD in midlife patients diagnosed predominantly with schizophrenia (Arvanitis & Miller, 1997; Marder & Meibach, 1994; Tollefson & Sanger, 1997; Tollefson, Beasley,Tamura et al., 1997; Tollefson, Beasley, Tran et al., 1997). Psychiatrists and primary care physicians were quick to extrapolate from the observed benefits in younger patients and have begun prescribing the new atypical neuroleptics to elderly patients, largely in advance of controlled studies in geriatric populations (Carter et al., 1995).

Extrapolation from results observed in midlife patients diagnosed with schizophrenia to the large proportion of elderly psychotic patients diagnosed with AD or with MD+P is not straightforward, however, given the substantial clinical and neurobiologic differences between these disorders. In the sections below, we will review the emerging body of data with regard to the use of the available new atypical agents in late life psychoses. Though placebo-controlled data are limited, we have attempted to identify studies which are otherwise informative, including pharmacokinetic studies which provide guidance for dosage adjustments in the elderly, and case series which document important leads to the efficacious use of these agents in the elderly or to notable side effects occurring in geriatric patients.

Risperidone

As an atypical neuroleptic without the risk of agranulocytosis or the need for frequent leukocyte monitoring, risperidone was rapidly utilized by geriatric clinicians (Carter et al., 1995). Risperidone's advent was followed by a series of retrospective reviews and uncontrolled prospective studies describing its use in elderly patients (Aronson, Lingam, & Hasanat, 1995; Borison, Davidson, & Berman, 1994; Goldberg, 1995; Jeanblanc & Davis, 1995; Jeste et al., 1996; Madhusoodanan, Brenner, Aranjo, & Abaza, 1995). These reports indicated benefits of risperidone treatment for both positive and negative symptoms in late-life schizophrenia, and for control of psychosis and agitation in dementia. Mean doses varied across studies, with dementia patients tending to receive lower doses (0.5–2.5 mg/day) than schizophrenic patients (4–6 mg/day). When doses were judiciously titrated, few if any patients discontinued risperidone secondary to apparent side effects, though episodes of orthostasis were common (Jeste et al., 1996; Madhusoodanan, et al., 1995). Recently two double-blind placebo controlled studies of risperidone in elderly patients with behavioral symptoms complicating a dementia have been reported (Brecher, 1998; Lemmens, DeDyne, & DeSmet, 1998). In the first study (Brecher, 1998), 625 nursing home patients were randomized to receive placebo, risperidone 0.5 mg/day, risperidone 1.0 mg/day, or risperidone 2.0 mg/day for 12 weeks. Both risperidone 1.0 mg/day and 2.0 mg/day groups demonstrated significantly greater reductions in psychosis and aggression measures than the placebo-treated group. Risperidone doses up to 1.0 mg/day were not associated with greater side effects than placebo. At the highest risperidone dose, however, neuroleptic-induced parkinsonism led to a modest increase in patient discontinuation. Significantly, over 200 of these patients have been followed for a mean of 6 months on risperidone with no incident cases of tardive dyskinesia, a striking reduction in comparison to reports of tardive dyskinesia incidence in elderly patients treated with typical neuroleptics (Brecher, 1998; Jeste et al., 1995). In the second study (Lemmens et al., 1998), 344 patients were randomized under double-blind conditions to receive placebo, risperidone 0.5–4.0 mg/day, or haloperidol 0.5–4.0 mg/day. A flexible dose design was used. Mean risperidone dose at study endpoint was 1.1 mg/day, for haloperidol the mean dose at study endpoint was 1.2 mg/day. Risperidone treatment was associated with a significant reduction in aggression measures and ratings of total behavioral disturbance (BEHAVE-AD) in comparison to placebo, without an increase in parkinsonian symptoms. Specific benefit for psychotic symptoms was not described.

Relatively less information is available to guide the use of risperidone in elderly patients with psychosis associated with DLB or Parkinson's disease. Open studies of risperidone at low doses (mean dose 0.7–1.5 mg/day) have reported conflicting results regarding tolerability in these disorders (Ford, Lynch, & Greene, 1994; Meco, Allesandri, Bonifati, & Giustini, 1994; McKeith, Ballard, & Harrison, 1995). At low doses risperidone may be a useful adjunct in the treatment of some patients with Parkinson's disease or dementia with Lewy bodies. Risperidone may not represent an adequate substitute for clozapine, however, in those patients most sensitive to exacerbation of rigidity by neuroleptics (Rich, Friedman, & Ott, 1995).

There is some preliminary, but exciting evidence that risperidone treatment may improve cognition in elderly schizophrenic patients (Borison et al., 1994; Jeste et al., 1996). Berman, Merson, Allan, Alexis, & Losonczy conducted a prospective, randomized, double-blind comparison of risperidone with haloperidol in 20 elderly schizophrenic subjects to examine the cognitive effects of these two treatments. Risperidone-treated patients showed significant improvement on the Boston Naming Test and the Mini Mental State exam, while haloperidol-treated patients did not. Neither drug was associated with improvement in other cognitive tests such as digit span, digit symbol substitution, verbal fluency, or trails (Berman et al., 1995).

Pharmacokinetic data to guide risperidone dosing in the elderly, has emerged since its release into the United States market. Risperidone is principally metabolized by CYP 2D6 (Huang et al., 1993). Importantly, it's major metabolite, 9-hydroxyrisperidone, is both active (with a receptor binding profile similar to the parent drug) (Ereshefsky & Lacombe, 1993), and present in plasma at concentrations 3–5 times higher than that of risperidone (Heykants et al., 1994). Elderly patients typically require one third the dose used in younger patients to achieve similar plasma concentrations of both 9-hydroxyrisperidone and risperidone (Hoffman, Winer, Bartels, & Oxman, 1995), possibly reflecting the renal excretion of 9-hydroxyrisperidone (Snoeck et al., 1995). Moreover, after single doses the half-lives of 9-hydroxyrisperidone and of the active moiety (risperidone +

9-hydroxyrisperidone) are 23 and 24 hours, respectively in elderly subjects, longer than in younger subjects (Snoeck et al., 1995). As a consequence, our usual starting dose of risperidone in an elderly patient is 0.25–0.5 mg/day, given as a single dose. Based on both the pharmacokinetic data and data from controlled studies in the elderly, target doses should be 1–1.5 mg/day. Unlike clozapine, risperidone is a potent dopamine$_2$ receptor antagonist, with nanomolar affinity for this receptor (Leysen, Janssen, Schotte, Lyten, & Megens, 1993). Thus, the risk of inadvertently overestimating the risperidone dose requirement in an elderly patient is the loss of "atypicality," with the onset of neuroleptic-induced parkinsonism. Because of its high dopamine$_2$ receptor affinity, risperidone can also be seen to cause elevations in plasma prolactin concentrations in both young and elderly patients, though the clinical implications of elevated prolactin in the elderly are not clear (Huang et al., 1993; Sweet et al., 1996). Risperidone also potently binds alpha$_1$ and alpha$_2$ receptors, which may account for the reports of hypotension in some elderly patients (Leysen et al., 1993). Risperidone lacks significant anticholinergic effects, which may contribute to its positive cognitive profile. Despite these concerns, most evidence suggests that risperidone can be used safely, with good tolerance in elderly patients after accounting for age-related decrements in risperidone and 9-hydroxyrisperidone clearance.

Olanzapine

Few reports have examined olanzapine use in the elderly, though these include one randomized, double-blind, placebo-controlled study. Satterlee, Tollefson, Reams, Burns, & Hamilton (1995) assigned 238 patients, over the age of 65, and diagnosed with psychotic and behavioral symptoms associated with Alzheimer's disease, to receive either olanzapine 1-8 mg/day or placebo. Olanzapine doses used were low, as only 69 subjects received olanzapine at a daily dose ≥5mg. Olanzapine and placebo did not differ significantly in efficacy for behavioral symptoms, and there were no significant differences in the rates of extrapyramidal symptoms, orthostasis, liver function tests, or white blood cell counts. Other possible adverse effects were not described. Because of the overall good drug tolerance, and the low olanzapine doses used relative to effective doses in schizophrenia (Beasley, 1997), it remains to be seen if higher doses will reveal greater efficacy. In DLB and psychosis associated with Parkinson's disease, reports have been mixed with regard to olanzapine tolerance (Friedman, 1998; Jimenez-Jimenez et al., 1998; Wolters, Jansen, Tynman-Qua, & Bergmans, 1996). In the largest of these reports, an open study of 15 nondemented patients with psychotic symptoms occurring in the context of Parkinson's disease, olanzapine, in doses ranging from 2 to 15 mg (mean 6.5 ± 3.9 mg), was well tolerated (Wolters et al., 1996). Patients demonstrated significant improvement in psychotic symptoms with olanzapine, without worsening of parkinsonism. They were also able to tolerate further increases in dopaminomimetic drugs, with subsequent improved motor function, without exacerbation of psychosis. As with risperidone, however, olanzapine may not be an adequate substitute for clozapine in the patients most sensitive to neuroleptic-induced parkinsonism (Jimenez-Jimenez et al., 1998).

Ereshefsky (Ereshefsky, 1996) reported that the elimination half-life of olanzapine is increased by 68% in elderly men, and by 42% in elderly women, and recommended dose reductions on this basis. Olanzapine is primarily metabolized by CYP 1A2 with CYP 2D6 also contributing to olanzapine's clearance. In vitro studies indicate a greater likelihood for olanzapine's clearance to be affected by other medications, such as SSRIs, as opposed to its causing significant inhibitory interactions (Ring, Binkley, Vandenbranden, & Wrighton, 1996). Olanzapine also undergoes nonoxidative clearance by glucuronidation, a mechanism that can be effected in the oldest-old or in patients with Alzheimer's disease (Fisman et al., 1988; Sonne, Loft, Dossing, Boesgaard, & Andreasen, 1991). Despite these potential concerns for reduced olanzapine clearance in the elderly, the tolerance of olanzapine by elderly patients in the above studies has been quite good. The tolerance of olanzapine by elderly patients is all the more surprising, given that olanzapine was developed to have activity at a broad range of neurotransmitter receptors (Bymaster, 1997). As a potent in vitro antagonist of $muscarinic_1$, $histamine_1$ and $alpha_1$ receptors, in addition to $dopamine_2$ and $serotonin_{2A}$ receptors, side effects such as delirium, urinary retention, sedation, or hypotension would have been expected more frequently in the elderly. As discussed above, higher dose studies of the efficacy of olanzapine in treating behavioral symptoms complicating Alzheimer's disease need to be conducted. It will be important to monitor whether autonomic side effects and sedation, or for that matter extrapyramidal symptoms, emerge more frequently at these higher doses.

Quetiapine

Results from an uncontrolled study of quetiapine in elderly patients with idiopathic psychosis, psychosis associated with a dementia, or psychosis associated with Parkinson's disease have been reported (Targum & Arvanitis, 1997). 152 elderly patients were treated for 12 weeks with quetiapine in doses ranging from 25 to 450 mg/day. Somewhat surprisingly, median final doses were somewhat higher in patients with organic than idiopathic psychoses (100 mg/day versus 87.5 mg/day). Both idiopathic and organic patient groups demonstrated a reduction in positive and negative symptoms with treatment, without a difference in response rate between diagnostic groups. The incidence of all extrapyramidal symptoms (6%) was lower than that seen with placebo treatment during trials conducted in younger patients. The most frequent adverse events were somnolence (30%), dizziness (13%), and postural hypotension (12%), though only 3% of patients developed clinically significant orthostatic blood pressure changes. Overall, tolerance was good with only 39 (26%) patients withdrawing from the study, 14 (9%) due to adverse events. Though the impact of quetiapine treatment on cognition in these elderly patients was not described, there is a single case report of a younger schizophrenic patient who had a robust cognitive improvement with quetiapine treatment (Stip, Lussier, Babai, & Fabian, 1996). It is possible that positive effects on cognition, similar to those described for risperidone, will emerge for quetiapine as well.

The pharmacokinetics of quetiapine have also been examined in elderly schizophrenic patients (Thyrum et al., 1997). Quetiapine demonstrated linear pharmacokinetics over the dose range of 100 mg to 250 mg three times daily, with an elimination half-life of 6.2 to 6.8 hours. Oral clearance in these nine elderly patients was reduced by 30% to 50% in comparison to younger subjects. Thus, thrice daily dosing, with total oral doses 30% to 50% lower than used in younger patients are indicated in the elderly. The primary metabolic pathway of quetiapine appears to be sulfoxidation by CYP 3A4, with minor dependence on CYP 2D6 (Crimm, Stams, & Bui, 1997). Consistent with these in vitro observations, phenytoin treatment increases quetiapine clearance 5-fold (Wong et al., 1997). Quetiapine showed little in vitro propensity, however, to inhibit these isozymes, or CYP 1A2, CYP 2C9, or CYP 2C19 (Grimm et al., 1997). Pending confirmatory studies, however, caution should be used when prescribing quetiapine with other agents which inhibit CYP 3A4 or depend on CYP 3A4 for their metabolism. Though there are numerous metabolites of quetiapine present in vivo, they do not appear to contribute to its therapeutic action (Ereshefsky, 1996).

The most distinct aspect of the receptor binding profile of quetiapine is the low affinity of this agent for $dopamine_2$ receptors (Schotte et al., 1996). In this regard, quetiapine is more like clozapine than risperidone or olanzapine. It may be this low affinity which accounts for the essentially complete lack of drug-induced parkinsonism at all studied doses of quetiapine (Arvanitis & Miller, 1997; Targum & Arvanatis, 1997), another feature that differentiates it from olanzapine and risperidone. The remaining receptor binding profile of quetiapine is consistent with the observed adverse events described in the open study above. Quetiapine's most potent action is as an inhibitor of $histamine_1$ receptors, likely contributing to the frequency of somnolence. More modest $alpha_1$ antagonism and relatively less frequent postural hypotension are also seen. Of note, quetiapine displays essentially no affinity for muscarinic receptors (Schottee et al., 1996), nor are significant anticholinergic symptoms reported (Schotte et al., 1996). This absence of muscarinic antagonism may ultimately contribute to a favorable cognitive profile for this agent, though controlled studies of quetiapine's effects on cognition in elderly schizophrenic subjects are not yet reported.

SUMMARY

Late-life psychoses are highly prevalent and, given the rapidly expanding geriatric population, relatively understudied. Whether due to normal age-related changes in neuropharmacology, or disease-specific changes in neuropharmacology with aging, it is clear that neither the clinical presentations nor the treatment of late-life psychoses can be anticipated by the study of the psychoses of midlife. This is just as true for late-life MD+P and late-life schizophrenia as it is for dementia-related psychosis, for which there is no clear midlife analogue. The identification of leads to novel treatments specific for the late-life psychoses will require both examination of the neurobiology of psychosis in elderly groups, and the development of animal models of psychosis in aging. In the meantime, the above review identifies several areas where there is inadequate knowledge about the treatment of elderly patients with psychosis using currently available agents. In the psychoses associated with dementia, the results of ongoing studies of the other atypical neuroleptics are anticipated soon. Further studies of the effects of SSRIs in these syndromes are clearly indicated, however, as are head-to-head studies comparing the efficacy of atypical agents with SSRI treatment and with optimal-dose conventional neuroleptics. Sadly, it is almost oxymoronic to refer to a current state of knowledge of the pharmacotherapy of late-life MD+P. The need for studies of acute treatment with an SSRI alone versus an SSRI plus an atypical neuroleptic is glaring. Similarly, studies defining appropriate continuation and maintenance therapy following acute ECT treatment are sorely needed. Finally, definitive studies of atypical neuroleptics or other novel agents (e.g. amantadine) on the negative symptoms and cognitive deficits of late life schizophrenia should be conducted.

REFERENCES

Aberg-Wistedt, A., Wistedt, B., & Bertilsson, L. (1985). Higher CSF levels of HVA and 5-HIAA in delusional compared to nondelusional depression. *Archives of General Psychiatry, 42*, 925–926.

Anton, R. F., & Burch, E. A. (1990). Amoxapine versus amitriptyline combined with perphenazine in the treatment of psychotic depression. *American Journal of Psychiatry, 147*, 1203–1208.

Arnold, S. E., & Trojanowski, J. Q. (1996). Recent advances in defining the neuropathology of schizophrenia. *Acta Neuropathol, 92,* 217–231.

Arnold, S. E., Trojanowski, J. Q., Gur, R. E., Blackwell, P., Han, L., & Choi, C. (1998). Absence of neurodegeneration and neural injury in the cerebral cortex in a sample of elderly patients with schizophrenia. *Archives of General Psychiatry, 55*(Mar), 225–232.

Aronson, S. M., Lingam, V., & Hasanat, K. A. (1995, May). *Risperidone in geropsychiatry: Review of early experience in two public hospitals* [Abstract]. Presented at the American Psychiatric Association (APA) 148th Annual Meeting, Miami, FL.

Arvanitis, L. A., & Miller, B. G. (1997). Multiple fixed doses of "seroquel" (quetiapine) in patients with acute exacerbation of schizophrenia: A comparison with haloperidol and placebo. *Biological Psychiatry, 42,* 233–246.

Ayd, F. J., Jr. (1960). Drug-induced extrapyramidal reactions: their clinical manifestations and treatment with akineton. *Psychosomatics, 1,* 143–150.

Beasley, C. M. (1997). Efficacy of olanzapine: an overview of pivotal clinical trials. *Journal of Clinical Psychiatry Monograph Series, 15*(2), 16–18.

Berman, I., Merson, A., Allan, E., Alexis, C., & Losonczy, M. (1995). Effect of risperidone on cognitive performance in elderly schizophrenic patients: a double-blind comparison study with haloperidol. *Psychopharmacology Bulletin, 31*(3), 552–552.

Bierer, L. M., Knott, P. J., Schmeidler, J. M., Marin, D. B., Ryan, T. M., Haroutunian, V., Purohit, D. P., Perl, D. P., Mohs, R. C., & Davis, K. L. (1993). Post-mortem examination of dopaminergic parameters in Alzheimer's disease: Relationship to noncognitive symptoms. *Psychiatry Research, 49,* 211–217.

Bondareff, W. (1996). Neuropathology of psychotic symptoms in alzheimer's disease. *International Psychogeriatrics, 8*(Suppl. 3), 233–237.

Borison, R. L., Davidson, M., & Berman, I. (1994, May). *Risperidone treatment in elderly patients with schizophrenia or dementia* [Abstract]. Poster session presented at the annual meeting of the American Psychiatric Association 146th Annual Meeting, Washington, DC.

Brecher, M. B. (1998, May). Follow-up study of risperidone in the treatment of patients with dementia: Interim results on tardive dyskinesia and dyskinesia severity. Presented at the American Psychiatric Association (APA) 151st Annual Meeting, New Research, 16, Toronto, Canada.

Brodaty, H., Luscombe, G., Parker, G., Wilhelm, K., Hickie, I., Austin, M. P., & Mitchell, P. (1997). Increased rate of psychosis and psychomotor change in depression with age. *Psychological Medicine, 27,* 1205–1213.

Burke, W. J., Dewan, V., Wengel, S. P., Roccaforte, W. H., Nadolny, G. C., & Folks, D. G. (1997). The use of selective serotonin reuptake inhibitors for depression and psychosis complicating dementia. *International Journal of Geriatric Psychiatry, 12,* 519–525.

Bymaster, F. P. (1997). In vitro and in vivo biochemistry of olanzapine. *Journal of Clinical Psychiatry Monograph, 15*(2), 10–12.

Carter, C. S., Mulsant, B. H., Sweet, R. A., Maxwell, R. A., Coley, K., Ganguli, R., & Branch, R. (1995). Pharmacoeconomics made simple. Risperidone use in a teaching hospital during its first year after market approval: economic and clinical implications. *Psychopharmacology Bulletin, 31*(4), 719–725.

Contreras, F., Navarro, M. A., Menchon, J. M., Rosel, P., Serrallonga, J., Perez-Arnau, F., Urretavizcaya, M., & Vallejo, J. (1996). Growth hormone response to growth hormone releasing hormone in non-delusional and delusional depression and healthy controls. *Psychological Medicine, 26,* 301–307.

Copeland, J. R. M., Dewey, M. E., Scott, A., Gilmore, C., Larkin, B. A., Cleave, N., McCracken, C. F. M., & McKibbin, P. E. (1998). Schizophrenia and delusional disorder in older age: Community prevalence, incidence, comorbidity, and outcome. *Schizophrenia Bulletin, 24*(1), 153–161.

Corey-Bloom, J., Jernigan, T., Archibald, S., Harris, M. J., & Jeste, D. V. (1995). Quantitative magnetic resonance imaging of the brain in late-life schizophrenia. *American Journal of Psychiatry, 152*(3), 447–449.

Davidson, M., Harvey, P. D., Powchik, P., Parrella, M., White, L., Knobler, H. Y., Losonczy, M. F., Keefe, R. S. E., Katz, S., & Frecska, E. (1995). Severity of symptoms in chronically institutionalized geriatric schizophrenic patients. *American Journal of Psychiatry, 152*(2), 197–207.

Davidson, M., Harvey, P. D., Welsh, K. A., Powchik, P., Putnam, K. M., & Mohs, R. C. (1996). Cognitive functioning in late-life schizophrenia: A comparison of elderly schizophrenic patients and patients with Alzheimer's disease. *American Journal of Psychiatry, 153*(10), 1274–1279.

Devanand, D. P., Jacobs, D. M., Tang, M. X., Castillo-Castaneda, C. D., Sano, M., Marder, K., Bell, K., Bylsma, F. W., Brandt, J., Albert, M., & Stern, Y. (1997). The course of psychopathologic features in mild to moderate Alzheimer disease. *Archives of General Psychiatry, 54,* 257–263.

Devanand, D.P., Marder, K., Michaels, K. S., Sackeim, H. A., Bell, K., Sullivan, M. A., Cooper, T. B., Pelton, G. H., & Mayeux, R. (1998). A randomized, placebo-controlled, dose-comparison trial of haloperidol treatment for psychosis and disruptive behaviors in Alzheimer's disease. *American Journal of Psychiatry, 155,* 1512–1520.

Dysken, M.W., Johnson, S. B., Holden, L., Vatassery, G., Nygren, J., Jelinski, M., Kuskowski, M., Schut, L., McCarten, J. R., Knopman, D., Maletta, G. J., & Skare, S. (1994). Haloperidol concentrations in patients with Alzheimer's dementia. *American Journal of Geriatric Psychiatry, 2,* 124–133.

Ellis, R. J., Caligiuri, M., Galasko, D., & Thal, L. J. (1996). Extrapyramidal motor signs in clinically diagnosed Alzheimer disease. *Alzheimer Disease and Associated Disorders, 10*(2), 103–114.

Ereshefsky, L. (1996). Pharmacokinetics and drug interactions: Update for new antipsychotics. *Journal of Clinical Psychiatry, 57*(Suppl 11), 12–25.

Ereshefsky, L., & Lacombe, S. (1993). Pharmacological profile of risperidone. *Canadian Journal of Psychiatry, 38*(7, suppl. 3), S80–S88.

Finkel, S. I., Lyons, J. S., Anderson, R. L., & Sherrell, K. (1995). A randomized, placebo-controlled trial of thiothixene in agitated, demented nursing home patients. *International Journal of Geriatric Psychiatry, 10,* 129–136.

Fisman, M., Inaba, T., Kalow, W., Fox, H., Merskey, H., & Wong, C. (1988). Oxazepam as a probe of hepatic metabolism in patients with Alzheimer's disease. *Progress in Neuro-Psychopharmacology and Biological Psychiatry, 12,* 255–261.

Flint, A. J., & Rifat, S. L. (1998a). The Treatment of Psychotic Depression in Later Life: A Comparison of Pharmacotherapy and ECT. *Internation Journal of Geriatric Psychiatry, 13,* 23–28.

Flint, A. J., & Rifat, S. L. (1998b). Two-year Outcome of Psychotic Depression in Late Life. *American Journal of Psychiatry, 155*(2), 178–183.

Ford, B., Lynch, T., & Greene, P. (1994). Risperidone in Parkinson's disease. *Lancet, 344*(8923), 681.

Friedman, J. (1998). Olanzapine in the treatment of dopaminomimetic psychosis in patients with Parkinson's disease. *Neurology, 50*(April), 1195–1196.

Gilley, D. W., Whalen, M. E., Wilson, R. S., & Bennett, D. A. (1991). Hallucinations and associated factors in Alzheimer's disease. *Journal of Neuropsychiatry, 3,* 371–376.

Gilley, D. W., Wilson, R. S., Beckett, L. A., & Evans, D. A. (1997). Psychotic symptoms and physically aggressive behavior in Alzheimer's disease. *Journal of the American Geriatrics Society, 45,* 1074–1079.

Goldberg, R. J. (1995). *Risperidone for dementia-related disturbed behavior in nursing home residents: A clinical experience* Presented at the American Psychiatric Association (APA) 148th Annual Meeting, Miami, Fl.

Grimm, S. W., Stams, K. R., & Bui, K. (1997). In vitro prediction of potential metabolic drug interactions for quetiapine [Abstract]. *Proceedings of the American Psychiatric Association (APA) 150th Annual Meeting,* 135.

Harvey, P. D., Leff, J., Trieman, N., Andersen, J., & Davidson, M. (1997). Cognitive impairment in geriatric chronic schizophrenic patients: a cross-national study in new york and london. *International Journal of Geriatric Psychiatry, 12,* 1001–1007.

Harvey, P. D., Lombardi, J., Leibman, M., White, L., Parrella, M., Powchik, P., & Davidson, M. (1996). Cognitive impairment and negative symptoms in geriatric chronic schizophrenic patients: A follow-up study. *Schizophrenia Research, 22,* 223–231.

Heykants, J., Huang, M. L., Mannens, G., Meuldermans, W., Snoeck, E., Van Beijsterveldt, L. V., Peer, A. V., & Woestenborghs, R. (1994). The pharmacokinetcis of risperidone in humans: a summary. *Journal of Clinical Psychiatry, 55*(5, suppl.), 13–17.

Hoffman, D. W., Winer, M. S. T., Bartels, S., & Oxman, T. E. (1995). Therapeutic dose: Serum level relationships of risperidone and active metabolite in a geriatric population. *Psychopharmacology Bulletin, 31*(3), 525

Huang, M. L., Peer, A. V., Woestenborghs, R., De Coster, R., Heykants, J., Jansen, A. A. I., Zylicz, Z., Visscher, H. W., & Jonkman, J. H. G. (1993). Pharmacokinetics and drug disposition: pharmacokinetics of the novel antipsychotic agent risperidone and the prolactin response in healthy subjects. *Clinical Pharmacology and Therapeutics, 54,* 257–268.

Jeanblanc, W., & Davis, Y. B. (1995). Risperidone for treating dementia-associated aggression. *American Journal of Psychiatry, 152*(8), 1239.

Jeste, D. V., Caligiuri, M. P., Paulsen, J. S., Heaton, R. K., Lacro, J. P., Harris, M. J., Bailey, A., Fell, R. L., & McAdams, L. A. (1995). Risk of tardive dyskinesia in older patients: a prospective longitudinal study of 266 outpatients. *Archives of General Psychiatry, 52,* 756–765.

Jeste, D. V., Eastham, J. H., Lacro, J. P., Gierz, M., Field, M. G., & Harris, M. J. (1996). Management of late-life psychosis. *Journal of Clinical Psychiatry, 57*(suppl. 3), 39–45.

Jimenez-Jimenez, F. J., Tallon-Barranco, A., Orti-Pareja, M., Zurdo, M., Porta, J., & Molina, J. A. (1998). Olanzapine can worsen parkinsonism. *Neurology, 50*(April), 1183–1184.

Lacro, J. P., & Jeste, D. V. (1997). Geriatric Psychosis. *Psychiatric Quarterly, 68*(3), 247–260.

Lawlor, B. A., Ryan, T. M., Bierer, L. M., Schmeidler, J. , Haroutunian, V., Mohs, R., & Davis, K. L. (1995). Lack of association between clinical symptoms and postmortem indices of brain serotonin function in Alzheimer's disease. *Biological Psychiatry, 37,* 895–897.

Lemmens, P., DeDyne, P., & DeSmedt, G. (1998). *Risperidone in the treatment of behavioral disturbances in dementia* [Abstract]. Presented at the American Psychiatric Association (APA) 151st Annual Meeting, New Research, 16.

Leysen, J. E., Janssen, P. M. F., Schotte, A., Luyten, W. H. M. L., & Megens, A. A. H. P. (1993). Interaction of antipsychotic drugs with neurotransmitter receptor sites in vitro and in vivo in relation to pharmacological and clinical effects: role of $5HT_2$ receptors. *Psychopharmacology, 112,* S40–S54

Madhusoodanan, S., Brenner, R., Araujo, L., & Abaza, A. (1995). Efficacy of risperidone treatment for psychoses associated with schizophrenia, schizoaffective disorder, bipolar disorder, or senile dementia in 11 geriatric patients: a case series. *Journal of Clinical Psychiatry, 56*(11), 514–518.

Marder, S. R., & Meibach, R. C. (1994). Risperidone in the treatment of schizophrenia. *American Journal of Psychiatry, 151*(6), 825–835.

Martinez, R. A., Mulsant, B. H., Meyers, B. S., & Lebowitz, B. D. (1996). Delusional and psychotic depression in late life. *American Journal of Geriatric Psychiatry, 4,* 77–84.

McKeith, I., Fairbairn, A., Perry, R., Thompson, P., & Perry, E. (1992). Neuroleptic sensitivity in patients with senile dementia of Lewy body type. *British Medical Journal, 305,* 673–678.

McKeith, I. G., Ballard, C. G., & Harrison, R. W. S. (1995). Neuroleptic sensitivity to risperidone in Lewy body dementia. *Lancet, 346,* 699.

McKeith, I. G., Galasko, D., Kosaka, K., Perry, E. K., Dickson, D. W., Hansen, L. A., Salmon, D. P., Lowe, J., Mirra, S. S., Byrne, E. J., Lennox, G. , Quinn, N. P., Edwardson, J. A., Ince, P. G., Bergeron, C., Burns, A., Miller, B. L., Lovestone, S. , Collerton, D. , Jansen, E. N. H., Ballard, C., de Vos, R. A. I., Wilcock, G. K., Jellinger, K. A., & Perry, R. H. (1996). Consensus guidelines for the clinical and pathologic diagnosis of dementia with Lewy bodies (DLB): report of the consortium on DLB international workshop. *Neurology, 47,* 1113–1124.

Meco, G., Alessandria, A., Bonifati, V., & Giustini, P. (1994). Risperidone for hallucinations in levodopa-treated Parkinson's disease patients. *Lancet, 343,* 1370–1371.

Meyers, B. S. (1995). Late-life delusional depression: acute and long-term treatment. *International Psychogeriatrics, 7*(suppl), 113–124.

Meyers, B. S., & Greenberg, R. (1986). Late-life delusional depression. *Journal of Affective Disorders, 11,* 133–137.

Mockler, D., Riordan, J., & Sharma, T. (1997). Memory and intellectual deficits do not decline with age in schizophrenia. *Schizophrenia Research, 26,* 1–7.

Mulsant, B. H., Mazumdar, S., Pollock, B. G., Sweet, R. A., Rosen, J., & Lo, K. (1996). Methodological issues in characterizing treatment response in demented patients with behavioral disturbances. *International Journal of Geriatric Psychiatry, 12,* 537–547.

Obrien, J. T., Ames, D., Schweitzer, I., Desmond, P., Coleman, P., & Tress, B. (1997). Clinical, magnetic resonance imaging and endocrinological differences between delusional and non-delusional depression in the elderly. *International Journal of Geriatric Psychiatry, 12,* 211–218.

Perry, E. K., Marshall, E., Perry, R. H., Irving, D., Smith, C. J., Blessed, G., & Fairbairn, A. F. (1990). Cholinergic and dopaminergic activities in senile dementia of Lewy body type. *Alzheimer Disease and Associated Disorders, 4*(2), 87–95.

Perry, E. K., McKeith, I., Thompson, P., Marshall, E., Kerwin, J., Jabeen, S., Edwardson, J. A., Ince, P., Blessed, G., Irving, D., & Perry, R. H. (1991). Topography, extent, and clinical relevance of neurochemical deficits in dementia of Lewy body type, Parkinson's disease, and Alzheimer's disease. *Annals of the New York Academy of Sciences, 640,* 197–202.

Pollock, B. G. (1999). SSRI use in elderly (unpublished data).

Pollock, B. G., Mulsant, B. H., Sweet, R. A., Burgio, L. D., Kirshner, M. A., Shuster, K., & Rosen, J. (1997). An open pilot study of citalopram for behavioral disturbances of dementia: Plasma levels and real-time observations. *American Journal of Geriatric Psychiatry, 5*(1), 70–78.

Purohit, D. P., Perl, D. P., Haroutunian, V., Powchik, P., Davidson, M., & Davis, K. L. (1998). Alzheimer disease and related neurodegenerative diseases in elderly patients with schizophrenia. *Archives of General Psychiatry, 55*(March), 205–211.

Rich, S. S., Friedman, J. H., & Ott, B. R. (1995). Risperidone versus clozapine in the treatment of psychosis in six patients with Parkinson's disease and other akinetic-rigid syndromes. *Journal of Clinical Psychiatry, 56*(12), 556–559.

Ring, B. J., Binkley, S.N., Vandenbranden, M., & Wrighton, S. A. (1996). In vitro interaction of the antipsychotic agent olanzapine with human cytochromes P450 CYP2C9, CYP2C19, CYP2D6 and CYP3A. *British Journal of Clinical Pharmacology, 41,* 181–186.

Rothschild, A. J., Samson, J. A., Bessette, M. P., & Carter-Campbell, J. T. (1993). Efficacy of the combination of fluoxetine and perphenazine in the treatment of psychotic depression. *Journal of Clinical Psychiatry, 54,* 338–342.

Satterlee, W., Tollefson, G., Reams, S., Burns, P., & Hamilton, S. (1995). A clinical update on olanzapine treatment in schizophrenia and in elderly Alzheimer's disease patients [Abstract]. *Psychopharmacology Bulletin, 31,* 534.

Schatzberg, A. F., Posener, J. A., & Rothschild, A. J. (1995). The role of dopamine in psychotic depression. *Clinical Neuropharmacology, 18*(Suppl. 1), S66–S73

Schotte, A., Luyten, W. H. M. L., Van Gompel, P., Lesage, A. S., De Loore, K., & Leysen, J. E. (1996). Risperidone compared with new and reference antipsychotic drugs: in vitro and in vivo receptor binding. *Psychopharmacology, 124,* 57–73.

Schultz, S. K., Miller, D. D., Oliver, S. E., Arndt, S., Flaum, M., & Andreasen, N. C. (1997). The life course of schizophrenia: Age and symptom dimensions. *Schizophrenia Research, 23,* 15–23.

Sewell, D. D., Jeste, D. V., Paulsen, J. S., Kramer, R. L., & Gillin, J. C. (1994). Family history and neuropsychological correlates of late life psychotic depression [Abstract]. *American Journal of Geriatric Psychiatry, 2,* 267.

Smith, G. S., Dewey, S. L., Brodie, J. D., Logan, J., Vitkun, S. A., Simkowitz, P., Schloesser, R., Alexoff, D. A., Hurley, A., Cooper, T., & Volkow, N. D. (1997). Serotonergic modulation of dopamine measured with [11c] raclopride and pet in normal human subjects. *American Journal of Psychiatry, 154*(4), 490–496.

Snoeck, E., Peer, A. V., Sack, M., Horton, M., Mannens, G., Woestenborghs, R., Meibach, R., & Heykants, J. (1995). Influence of age, renal and liver impairment on the pharmacokinetics of risperidone in man. *Psychopharmacology, 122,* 223–229.

Sonne, J., Loft, S., Dossing, M., Boesgaard, S., & Andreasen, F. (1991). Single dose pharmacokinetics and pharmacodynamics of oral oxazepam in very elderly institutionalized subjects. *British Journal of Clinical Pharmacology, 31,* 719–722.

Spiker, D. G., Weiss, J. C., Dealy, R. S., Griffin, S. J., Hanin, I., Neil, J. F., Perel, J. M., Rossi, A. J., & Soloff, P. H. (1985). The pharmacological treatment of delusional depression. *American Journal of Psychiatry, 142,* 430–436.

Stip, E., Lussier, I., Babai, M., & Fabian, J. L. (1996). Seroquel and cognitive improvement in patients with schizophrenia. *Biological Psychiatry, 40,* 430–437.

Sweet, R. A., Hamilton, R. L., Pollock, B. G., Henteleff, R. A., & DeKosky, S. T. (in press). Dopamine receptor correlates of psychosis in dementia. *Journal of the American Geriatrics Society.*

Sweet, R. A., Mulsant, B. H., Gupta, B. , Rifai, A. H., Pasternak, R. E., McEachran, A., & Zubenko, G. S. (1995). Duration of neuroleptic treatment and prevalence of tardive dyskinesia in late life. *Archives of General Psychiatry, 52,* 478–486.

Sweet, R. A., Mulsant, B. H., Pollock, B. G., Rosen, J., & Altieri, L. P. (1996). Neuroleptic-induced Parkinsonism in elderly patients diagnosed with psychotic major depression and dementia of the Alzheimer type. *American Journal of Geriatric Psychiatry, 4*(4), 311–319.

Sweet, R. A., Nimgaonkar, V. L., Kamboh, M. I., Lopez, O. L., Zhang, F., & DeKosky, S. T. (1998). Dopamine receptor genetic variation, psychosis, and aggression in Alzheimer's disease. *Archives of Neurology, 55,* 1335–1340.

Sweet, R. A., & Pollock, B. G. (1998). New atypical antipsychotics: Experience and utility in the elderly. *Drugs and Aging, 12*(2), 115–127.

Sweet, R. A., Pollock, B. G., Mulsant, B. H., Rosen, J., & Henteleff, R. (1996). Atypical neuroleptics: Pharmacologic considerations [Abstract]. *European Neuropsychopharmacology, 6,* 27–28.

Sweet, R. A., Pollock, B. G., Mulsant, B. H., Rosen, J., & Henteleff, R. A. (1995). Prolactin response to neuroleptic challenge in late-life psychosis. *Psychopharmacology Bulletin, 31,* 651–657.

Sweet, R. A., Pollock, B. G., Mulsant, B. H., Rosen, J. , Lo, K. H., Yao, J. K., Henteleff, R. A. , & Mazumdar, S. (1997). Association of plasma homovanillate with behavioral symptoms in patients diagnosed with dementia: a preliminary report. *Biological Psychiatry, 42,* 1016–1023.

Sweet, R. A., Pollock, B. G., Mulsant, B. H., Rosen, J., Sorisio, D., Kirshner, M., Henteleff, R., & DeMichele, M. A. (in press). The pharmacologic profile of perphenazine's metabolites. *Journal of Clinical Psychopharmacology.*

Targum, S. D., & Arvanitis, L. A. (1997). Quetiapine: efficacy, safety, and tolerability in elderly subjects with psychotic disorders [Abstract]. *Proceedings of the New Clinical Drug Evaluation Unit Program 37th Annual Meeting,* 3.

Tariot, P. N., Mack, J. L., Patterson, M. B., Edland, S. D., Weiner, M. F., Fillenbaum, G., Blazina, L., Teri, L., Rubin, E., Mortimer, J. A., Stern, Y. , & Behavioral Pathology Committee of the Consortium to Establish a Registry for Alzheimer's Disease. (1995). The behavior rating scale for dementia of the consortium to establish a registry for Alzheimer's disease. *American Journal of Psychiatry, 152*(9), 1349–1357.

Thyrum, P. T., Jaskiw, G., Fuller, M., Wong, Y. W. J., Ewing, B. J., & Yeh, C. (1997). Multiple-dose pharmacokinetics of ICI 204,636 in elderly patients with selected psychotic disorders. *Psychopharmacology Bulletin, 32*(3), 524.

Tollefson, G. D., Beasley, C. M., Jr. , Tamura, R. N., Tran, P. V., & Potvin, J. H. (1997). Blind, Controlled, Long-Term Study of the Comparative Incidence of Treatment-Emergent Tardive Dyskinesia with Olanzapine or Halperidol. *American Journal of Psychiatry, 154*(9), 1248–1254.

Tollefson, G. D., Beasley, C. M., Jr., Tran, P. V., Street, J. S., Krueger, J. A., Tamura, R. N., Graffeo, K. A., & Thieme, M. E. (1997a). Olanzapine Versus Haloperidol in the Treatment of Schizophrenia and Schizoaffective and Schizophreniform Disorders: Results of an International Collaborative Trial. *American Journal of Psychiatry, 154*(4), 457–465.

Tollefson, G. D., & Sanger, T. M. (1997b). Negative Symptoms: A Path Analytic Approach to a Double-Blind, Placebo- and Haloperidol-Controlled Clinical Trial with Olanzapine. *American Journal of Psychiatry, 154*(4), 466–474.

Williams, J., Spurlock, G., Holmans, P., Mant, R., Murphy, K., Jones, L., Cardno, A., Asherson, P., Blackwood, D., Muir, W., Meszaros, K., Aschauer, H., Mallet, J., Laurent, C., Pekkarinen, P., Seppala, J., Stefanis, C.N., Papadimitriou, G. N., Macciardi, F., Verga, M., Pato, C., Azevedo, H., Crocq, M.A., Gurling, H., Kalsi, G., Curtis, D., McGuffin, P., & Owen, M. J. (1998). A meta-analysis and transmission disequilibrium study of association between the dopamine D3 receptor gene and schizophrenia. *Molecular Psychiatry, 3*(2), 141–149.

Wolters, E. C., Jansen, E. N. H., Tuynman-Qua, H. G., & Bergmans, P. L. M. (1996). Olanzapine in the treatment of dopaminomimetic psychosis in patients with Parkinson's disease. *Neurology, 47,* 1082–1087.

Wong, J. Y. W., Ewing, B. J., Thyrum, P. T., & Yeh, C. (1997). The effect of phenytoin and cimetidine on the pharmacokinetics of quetiapine [Abstract]. *Proceedings of the American Psychiatric Association (APA) 150th Annual Meeting, New Research,* 135–135.

Wragg, R. E., & Jeste, D. V. (1989). Overview of depression and psychosis in Alzheimer's disease. *American Journal of Psychiatry, 146,* 577–587.

Zanardil, R., Franchini, L., Gasperini, M., Perez, J., & Smeraldi, E. (1996). Double-blind controlled trial of sertraline versus paroxetine in the treatment of delusional depression. *American Journal of Psychiatry, 153,* 1631–1633.

Zubenko, G. S., Henderson, R., Stiffler, J. S., Stabler, S., Rosen, J., & Kaplan, B. B. (1996). Association of the APOE e4 allele with clinical subtypes of late life depression. *Society of Biological Psychiatry, 40,* 1008–1016.

Zubenko, G. S., Moossy, J., Martinez, A. J., Rao, G., Claassen, D., Rosen, J., & Kopp, U. (1991). Neuropathologic and neurochemical correlates of psychosis in primary dementia. *Archives of Neurology, 48,* 619–624.

Zubenko, G. S., Mulsant, B. H., Rifai, A. H., Sweet, R. A., Pasternak, R. E., Marino, L. J., & Tu, X. M. (1994). Impact of acute psychiatric inpatient treatment on major depression in late life and prediction of response. *American Journal of Psychiatry, 151,* 987–994.

Zubenko, G. S., Rosen, J., Sweet, R. A., Mulsant, B. H., & Rifai, A. H. (1992). Impact of psychiatric hospitalization on behavioral complications of Alzheimer's disease. *American Journal of Psychiatry, 149*(11), 1484–1491.

CHAPTER 12

ECT for Geriatric Depression and Future Trends

CATHERINE J. DATTO
GERIATRIC PSYCHIATRY
UNIVERSITY OF PENNSYLVANIA

SARAH H. LISANBY
COLUMBIA UNIVERSITY
COLUMBIA PRESBYTERIAN MEDICAL CENTER

INTRODUCTION

Electroconvulsive therapy (ECT) has been proven effective for the treatment of depression (American Psychiatric Association, 1990) and recent studies have shown that its use among depressed elderly patients is increasing. There are many more pharmacotherapy alternatives available to treat psychiatric disorders today than there were when electroconvulsive therapy was first developed in 1938 (Endler, 1988). Despite these numerous developments, however, a population of patients remains treatment-resistant or intolerant to currently available medications. In addition, for those whose psychiatric disorder has led to the development of life-threatening conditions, namely serious suicidal risk, pervasive disorganization or severe catatonia, a safe, rapid, and effective treatment like ECT is required. In this chapter, the use of ECT for geriatric patients with depression will be addressed, reviewing some of the most recent data on this topic and speculating where future research will be directed.

EPIDEMIOLOGY: USE OF ECT IN THE ELDERLY

Hermann (Hermann, Dorwart, Hoover, & Brody, 1995) estimated that ECT utilization rates across the 50 states range from 0.4 to 81.2 patients per 10,000 population, with some areas reporting no use. He found that the strongest predictors of ECT use were the number of psychiatrists, number of private hospital beds per capita, the number of primary care physicians, and stringency of state regulation of ECT, with regulation affecting care primarily in California and Texas (Reid, Keller, Leatherman, & Mason, 1998).

Westphal, Horswell, Kumar, & Rush (1997), used Medicare data for ECT utilization in Louisiana, for beneficiaries age 65 years and older, for fiscal years 1993 and 1994, and found the utilization rate to be 2.38 per 10,000 person-years. Olfson, Marcus, Sackeim, Thompson, and Pincus (1998) used data from the 1993 Healthcare Cost and Utilization Project to analyze the rate of adult inpatient ECT use for those with a principal discharge diagnosis of recurrent major depression. Patients aged 65 years and older had an estimated 6.7 times greater likelihood of receiving ECT than younger adults, aged 18 to 34 years.

While the use of ECT in certain states shows decline after changes in state regulations, its overall use in the nation stopped declining in 1980 (Thompson, Weiner, & Myers et al., 1994). Rosenbach, Hermann, and Dorwart et al., (1997), used Medicare part B enrollment and claims data for 1987 through 1992, and found that the rate of ECT use per 10,000 Medicare beneficiaries increased from 4.2 to 5.1, and the component provided as outpatient rose from 7% to 16%. Outpatient ECT expenditures, as a percentage of total part B ECT spending, showed considerable regional variation: 18.2 % in the Northeast, 19.1% in the North Central region, 12.1% in the South, and 9.8% in the West.

ECT PRACTICE GUIDELINES

In 1990, the American Psychiatric Association (APA) issued a Task Force Report outlining suggestions for ECT practice. This report recommended that referrals for ECT be made prior to a trial of psychotropic medications when:

1. a rapid and definitive response is needed on medical or psychiatric grounds;
2. when the risks of other treatments outweigh the risks of ECT;
3. when a poor drug response is observed;
4. when a good ECT response exists for previous illness episodes; or
5. patient preference.

It stated that ECT is an effective treatment for all subtypes of depression, including major depression, single-episode, and recurrent. It is also an effective treatment for all subtypes of bipolar major depression, bipolar disorder mixed, all subtypes of mania, and some forms of functional psychoses. There are no longer any absolute contraindications to using

ECT, but there are situations with substantial risk, requiring careful treatment modifications. Some of the more common high-risk situations and effective treatment modifications will be discussed later in this chapter.

ECT treatments can be administered as index, continuation, or maintenance treatments (APA, 1990). A series of ECT treatments administered to induce a clinical remission in a defined episode of ECT is called a course of ECT or index ECT. When the therapeutic intent shifts to maintaining a clinical remission and/or minimizing the likelihood of relapse, it is referred to as continuation ECT (CECT). Maintenance ECT (MECT) is empirically defined as the prophylactic use of ECT longer than 6 months past induction of a remission in the index episode. There are no established guidelines directing the frequency with which CECT or MECT should be administered.

Recommendations regarding the use of ambulatory ECT were included in part of the APA report and in 1996, the Association for Convulsive Therapy issued a task force report on ambulatory ECT (McDonald et al., 1998). The latter supported the use of ambulatory ECT for some part of the index course, CECT, or MECT, and stated that it requires a facility properly equipped to deliver care in this manner. Some of the conditions that weigh against outpatient status for ECT include: 1) suicide risk, 2) adverse behaviors, 3) systemic disease, 4) inanition, and 5) absence of a caretaker for safe management before and after each treatment. Like the APA, this task force held that there were no established principles to define the schedule of treatment. It recommended that caretakers should be encouraged to identify early symptom relapse to the ECT psychiatrist so that arrangements for an earlier ECT treatment can be made.

EFFICACY OF ECT IN THE ELDERLY

Philibert, Richards, Lynch, & Winokur et al., (1995) studied geriatric patients with unipolar depression and found those who received ECT were more likely to be alive at follow-up and demonstrated greater clinical improvement than those patients treated only with pharmacotherapy.

Several attempts have been made to identify the predictive features of depressed patients that are most likely to respond to ECT. These features include the presence of melancholia, psychomotor retardation, delusional symptoms, a positive or nonsuppression response to the dexamethasone suppression test (Abrams, 1997a), and a blunted response of thyroid-stimulating hormone or thyrotropin-releasing hormone. Although these predictors have been identified in several research studies, the two latter are not for routine clinical use and some have even questioned the utility of using these to predict ECT response (Sobin, Prudic, Devanand, Nobler, & Sackeim, 1996).

Many medication-resistant patients respond to ECT; however, patients with primary, unipolar, nonpsychotic major depression who have not responded to an adequate antidepressant medication trial are less likely to respond to ECT than patients who are not medication resistant (Prudic et al., 1996).

Preliminary findings from Coffey (1996) suggest that many patients with subcortical hyperintensities on MRI, cortical atrophy, and ventricular enlargement will achieve a good therapeutic response to bilateral ECT. However, they suggest that those with the greatest levels of cerebral impairment, as indicated by neurological signs and symptoms, EEG, and brain MRI, show the lowest response rates to brief pulse right unilateral ECT, perhaps because their seizure threshold may be elevated.

Older age and older age of onset of depression are associated with sleep onset REM (rapid eye movement) (SOREM), or shortened REM latency, as recorded on polysomnographic studies. SOREM, identified pre-ECT, did not predict treatment response to ECT (Grunhaus et al., 1994; Grunhaus et al., 1997). However, some 70% of patients who continue to have SOREM post-ECT have been shown to exhibit the return of significant depressive symptoms by 6 months after treatment. Thus SOREM may be a useful predictor of the post-ECT course of depression.

There has been speculation that concomitant use of antidepressant medication may be another predictor of ECT response. In a retrospective chart review, Nelson and Benjamin (1989) found that patients receiving a combination of ECT and tricyclic antidepressant medication needed fewer treatments for recovery.

PRE-ECT EVALUATION FOR THE GERIATRIC PATIENT

In the elderly, the issue of competency to consent to ECT can be significant. The Competency Interview Schedule (Bean, Nishisato, Rector, & Glancy, 1996) is a useful tool when working with the patients and families to gain informed consent. The combination of a do-not-resuscitate (DNR) status and a request for ECT treatment is also expected to arise more frequently for geriatric patients (Sullivan, Ward, & Laxton, 1992). Levine, Blank, Schwartz, and Rait (1991) illustrate the importance of family involvement in treatment decisions involving the elderly and ECT. Westreich, Levine, Ginsburg, and Wilets (1995) showed that the use of an informational video in the informed consent process does not result in improved knowledge of ECT by the patient but does increase interest for the families in the consent process.

The APA Practice Guidelines (APA, 1990) state that the minimum components of the pre-ECT evaluation should include:

1. psychiatric history and examination;
2. medical evaluation to define risk factors, namely medical history, physical examination, vital signs, hematocrit, serum electrolytes, electrocardiogram, and dental history;
3. anesthetic evaluation addressing risk;
4. informed consent; and
5. evaluation by the ECT psychiatrist.

The assessment of a patient's orientation and memory functioning should be made prior to the first ECT treatment by bedside assessment or more formal measures. Follow-up assessment should be repeated at least 24 hours after an ECT treatment to avoid measuring postictal effects. There are no established guidelines for the frequency of testing cognitive function during a course of ECT.

Electroencephalography, brain computed tomography, or magnetic resonance imaging should only be considered if other information suggests that an abnormality may be present. The routine use of spine x-rays has become less critical as a result of the routine use of muscular relaxation, but should be ordered if preexisting disease affecting the spinal column is suspected or known to be present. Nevertheless, Milstein and Milstein (1995) found that 40% of the respondents to their survey still routinely acquire pre-ECT spine and skull radiographs.

COGNITIVE EFFECTS OF ECT AND EFFECTIVE TREATMENT MODIFICATIONS

ECT has been proven not to cause structural brain damage (Devanand, Dwork, Hutchinson, Bolwig, & Sackeim, 1994). Coffey and associates (Coffey et al., 1988; Coffey, 1996) found that elderly depressed patients referred for ECT exhibit a high frequency of baseline structural changes in both cortical and subcortical brain regions, namely subcortical hyperintensities (SH) on MRI, lateral ventricular enlargement, and cortical atrophy. Patients with the most severe abnormalities on MRI were at higher risk of increased cognitive side effects of treatment.

Post-ECT delirium (Fink, 1993), is an acute confusional state accompanied by restlessness that can occur as the patient begins to wake after a seizure and continues for the 10–20 minutes usually required for recovery.

Estimates of the incidence of post-ECT delirium vary from <1% to as high as 12% of treatments, similar to the incidence of delirium from anesthesia alone. Among the conditions that have been correlated with the appearance of postictal delirium are the first seizure(s) in a series, underlying brain pathology, concurrent drug therapy, and recent drug withdrawal. Figiel, Coffey, Djang, Hoffman, & Doraiswamy (1990; Coffey, 1996) identify the higher risk of post-ECT delirium for patients who have subcortical hyperintensities by MRI. The concomitant use of lithium and dopaminergic medications (Aarsland, Larsen, Waage, & Langeveld, 1997) are associated with post-ECT delirium. The preferred treatment for post-ECT delirium is reassurance, but additional doses of the anesthetic agent may also need to be administered (Fink, 1993).

Most of the studies of cognitive change in the elderly receiving ECT contain limited numbers of patients but the following studies evidence important trends in this area. Rubin, Kinseberf, Figiel, & Zorunski, (1993), found that depressed patients receiving index ECT had a maximum MMSE change after two thirds of the treatments were delivered, with a return to pretreatment scores after cessation of ECT.

Kellner and associates (1992) found that elderly patients who received ECT only once a week improved in their mood symptoms more slowly when compared to elderly patients receiving three times per week treatments, without any difference in cognitive changes noted between the groups.

Zervas and colleagues (1993) studied depressed inpatients (aged 20–65) receiving bilateral ECT and found that older age predicted greater memory loss 24–72 hours after an ECT course. This effect was less apparent one month later, and minimal differences between older and younger patients on the neuropsychological batteries were still present 6 months after the ECT course.

Steif, Sackeim, Portnoy, Decina, and Malitz (1986) reported that prior to ECT, depressed patients manifested marked deficits in immediate memory or acquisition abilities, but no deficit in delayed memory, or retention skills. When reassessed after the seventh ECT treatment, these patients displayed reductions in both immediate and delayed memory. Four days after the ECT course, immediate memory scales returned to baseline but delayed memory performance remained impaired.

Sackeim and associates (1993) have performed several definitive studies systematically evaluating the effects of electrode placement, bilateral versus unilateral, and electrical charge intensity, low-dose versus high-dose. Across virtually all objective cognitive measures performed the week after an ECT course, bilateral electrode placement resulted in greater deficits than did right unilateral therapy, but adverse effects of the higher stimulus dose were not evident. After 2 months, cognitive function was similar across all treatment modalities. The effects of stimulus intensity on short-term cognitive side effects were not associated with the absolute electrical dose but with the extent to which the dosage exceeded the seizure threshold.

Sobin and colleagues (1995) studied depressed patients (mean age 53) and found that the pre-ECT MMSE, and the duration of postictal disorientation, were strong predictors of the magnitude of retrograde amnesia, seen in the week after ECT and 2-month follow-up. These relationships were maintained regardless of ECT technique, not only bilateral versus unilateral electrode placement, but also low versus high-intensity electrical charge.

Swartz and Evans (1996; Manly & Swartz, 1994) have been studying the technique of asymmetric bilateral electrode placement, and Letemendia and colleagues (1993) have been examining the effects of bifrontal electrode placement, in attempts to maximize effectiveness and minimize side effects. Although showing some potential, this work requires replication and further controlled trials.

Sommer, Satlin, Friedman, and Cole (1989) concluded that there was no difference in cognitive impairment following ECT treatments premedicated by either atropine or glycopyrrolate. Prudic, Sackeim, Devanand, Krueger, and Setternbrino (1994) determined that the administration of subconvulsive electrical stimulation also has no adverse cognitive consequences.

A recent review about medications that may be used to minimize the cognitive effect of ECT (Prudic, Sackeim, & Spicknall, et al., 1998), suggests that this is a useful area for research. An animal model of post-ECS (electroconvulsive stimulation) shows promise.

CARDIAC EFFECTS OF ECT AND EFFECTIVE TREATMENT MODIFICATIONS

ECT is a low-risk procedure, even for the elderly patient with cardiac risk factors. In absolute terms, deaths related to ECT number about 4 per 100,000 treatments, placing the risk of ECT at the same level as for general anesthesia inductions alone. Although extensive medical screenings prior to ECT may eliminate some of the higher-risk patients, it is the higher-risk geriatric cardiac patient that is fast becoming the modal candidate for this treatment (Abrams, 1997b). There is evidence that geriatric patients who received ECT were more likely to be alive at follow-up than those who had not received ECT treatments (Philibert et al., 1995).

The cardiac effect pictured by echocardiography before and immediately after ECT treatment are similar to the typical changes seen in the heart with acute exercise, all of which subsequently return to normal (Messina et al., 1992).

A case control, chart review study by Rice, Sombroto, Markowitz, and Leon (1994) concluded that improvements in ECT safety reflect improvement in screening techniques to identify the high-risk patients. Zielinski and associates (1993) compared older depressed patients, with and without cardiac risk factors, receiving ECT. The cardiovascular complications that developed during treatment appeared to be strongly related to the nature of the preexisting cardiac disease.

Applegate and colleagues (1997) reported that medical therapy should be continued and maximized in all patients with CAD that are being considered for ECT, and that their regular cardiac medications be administered 60–90 minutes prior to ECT. The actual risk of asystole, for older patients with cardiovascular disease, may be lower than for younger, healthier patients according to a recent study by Burd and Kettl (1998).

In a study by McCall, Zvora, Brooker, and Arias (1997), 18 depressed patients (mean age 69), who received a pre-ECT infusion of esmolol, to blunt the rise in heart rate and blood pressure during ECT, experienced shortened seizure duration. In addition, Zvara and colleagues (1997) concluded there was no benefit from esmolol in the prevention of ECG defined ischemia for 2 hours post-ECT.

Particular attention should be paid to patients with atrial fibrillation, according to Petrides and Fink (1996). They document the risk of cardioversion to normal sinus rhythm as a result of ECT, indicating prophylaxis with anticoagulants.

OTHER RISK FACTORS AND EFFECTIVE TREATMENT MODIFICATIONS

Patients with osteoporosis, or recent fracture, are at higher risk of fracture or injury during the seizure. In these cases, curariform, nondepolarizing muscle relaxants, are a good adjunct to the administration of succinylcholine, a depolarizing muscle relaxant (Janis, Hess, Fabian, & Gillis, 1995).

There are reports of patients with aortic aneurysms successfully being treated with ECT, even one patient with a history of a dissection of the aneurysm (Dowling & Francis, 1993). Two case reports detail ECT treatments for elderly patients with moderate to severe aortic stenosis (Rasmussen, 1997), normal left ventricular cardiac function, and absence of cardiac symptoms. During the treatments careful attention was directed toward monitoring blood pressure and heart rate. The same can be said for several case reports of patients with cerebral aneurysms and aneurysm repairs. Monitoring of vital signs and use of antihypertensives to prevent extreme increases in blood pressure and heart rate are essential for these high risk-cases (Farah, McCall, & Amundson, 1996).

OTHER IMPORTANT TREATMENT MODIFICATIONS FOR THE GERIATRIC PATIENT

Of particular concern for the older patient referred for ECT is a progressive rise in seizure threshold with age. This has led some to use augmentation strategies as the patient's seizure threshold reaches the upper limits of charge that the ECT device can produce. Despite its frequent use, there is limited data available about the efficacy of the use of caffeine to augment seizure duration. Kelsey and Grossberg (1995) found that caffeine was safe when used in elderly patients, average age 75 years and that it did effectively prolong seizure length. Calev and associates (1993) found that their patients, with ages ranging from 18–75, when pretreated with caffeine, showed quicker response to ECT and required fewer electrical stimulations to complete their course. The patients treated with caffeine also had slightly better cognitive scores than the group without caffeine. Caffeine appears to lengthen seizure duration without lowering the convulsive threshold (McCall, Reid, Rosenquist, Foreman, & Kieso-Webb, 1993) but may also predispose patients to the risk of supraventricular tachycardia when combined with other medications that also have this risk (Beale, Pritchett, & Kellner, 1994).

The barbituate anesthetics methohexital and thiopental remain the anesthetic agents of choice during ECT. They are both short-acting but they also reduce seizure duration, an effect that increases with dose (Bergsholm & Swartz, 1996). Propofol, a nonbarbituate anesthetic, which has been shown to improve hemodynamic stability during ECT, may allow for an earlier return of cognitive function after ECT (Fredman, & Etienne, Smith, Husain, & White, 1994), and a smaller degree of nausea relative to the barbiturates. Propofol does, however, significantly shorten seizure duration. Etomidate is a nonbarbiturate and has been shown to enhance seizure activity, but the rate of cognitive recovery can be prolonged after ECT treatments using etomidate. Moreover, this agent is relatively ineffective in blunting the hyperdynamic cardiac response of ECT (Avramov, Husain, & White, 1995; Trzepacz, Weniger, & Greenhouse, 1993).

MAINTENANCE TREATMENT

Kramer (1987) surveyed active members of the International Psychiatric Association for the Advancement of Electrotherapy (IPAAE). Of the 85 questionnaires returned, 51 psychiatrists had used MECT during the previous 5 years. Treatment schedules varied between clinicians, but depression remained the most commonly treated disorder using this technique. A lack of facilities and administrative and legal barriers accounted for about half of those who indicated that they did not perform MECT.

Jaffe and colleagues (1990) followed 32 outpatients (mean age of 68) in a naturalistic study of outpatient ECT for recurrent mood disorder. Ten of the thirty-two patients continued in active outpatient treatment for a mean of 15 months without rehospitalization, and 12 were discharged from the ECT treatments after clinical remission. This study concluded that outpatient ECT was safe for these elderly patients and effective, with 69% of its patients successfully treated.

McDonald and associates (1998) studied 15 unipolar depressed patients, more than 60 years of age, who were treated with either continuation medication (C-MED), or continuation ECT (CECT). In the first 6 months of the study, the relapse rate of the CECT patients was lower (11% versus 67%) but they had similar health care costs. After 12 months of continuation treatment, CECT patients showed improvements in quality of life, lower health care costs, and significantly lower relapse rates as compared to C-MED patients.

Continuation ECT (Petrides, Dhossche, Fink, & Francis, 1994) was shown, for patients with an average age of 51 years, to reduce the relapse rates for depressive disorders from 50–95% to 33% within one year of discharge after successful index ECT. The relapse rate observed for patients with delusional depression was 42%, lower than the 95% reported for patients with this diagnosis maintained on continuation pharmacotherapy.

Thornton, Mulsant, Dealy, and Reynolds (1990) reviewed the records of 10 patients receiving MECT monthly for treatment of depression. During the 18 months prior to the initiation of MECT, all patients were treated with at least two different psychotropic medications, including at least one tricyclic, and only one patient remained free of psychotropic medications during MECT. The patients had fewer hospitalizations in the 18 months after initiating MECT than during the 18 months preceding MECT, namely 0.3 vs 3.1, respectively.

The tolerability of MECT is addressed in a study by Vanelle and associates (1994) of 22 patients suffering from intractable recurrent unipolar or bipolar mood disorders. Eight of these patients did not complain of side effects. Nine patients mentioned concentration difficulties, disorientation post-MECT, memory troubles, and loss of drive. Three patients complained of transiently experiencing headache, insomnia, and asthenia after the treatments. Fear of MECT was mentioned by 6 patients. The patients spent, on average, 7% of the year in the psychiatric hospital during MECT, compared to 44% prior to initiation of this treatment.

FUTURE DIRECTIONS

An exciting area of research is the use of Transcranial Magnetic Stimulation (TMS). rTMS (rapid-rate TMS) allows for the noninvasive study of the cerebral cortex, resulting from current passing through a wire coil held over the scalp. The use of rTMS permits the stimulation of specific areas near the surface of the brain, enabling researchers to identify brain functioning localization, without the production of seizures (Kirkcaldie, Pridmore, & Reid, 1997). When rTMS has been used to stimulate the left prefrontal cortex in 22 geriatric patients with treatment-resistant depression, 23% of the patients responded, with most of the nonresponders having late-onset depression (Figiel et al., 1998). Although the numbers of the patients treated with rTMS is still small, there is great hope that the technique will prove to be effective, but not have the side effects of ECT, including complications from the seizure, anesthesia, and cognitive impairment.

CONCLUSIONS

ECT is a safe and effective treatment for geriatric depression that is underutilized in many areas. It has been stigmatized in movies and the media, which continue to affect patients and their families, sometimes causing them to refuse to undergo treatment. It is therefore in the best interest of psychiatric clinicians and researchers to encourage and promote the advancement of research in the field of ECT, and the promising field of rTMS, so there is hope to offer a patient suffering from drug-resistant depression. It is also critical that the clinician takes a systematic approach to the treatment of depression and use adequate antidepressant treatment trials, adequate in both dosage and duration, to minimize the misidentification of treatment resistance. If ECT treatment is indicated for the geriatric patient, it should be clear from this chapter that an organized approach to identifying patient risk factors and optimizing available modifications will substantially increase the likelihood of safety and efficacy for the patient.

REFERENCES

Aarsland, D., Larsen J. P., Waage O., & Langeveld J. (1997). Maintenace Electroconvulsive Therapy for Parkinson's Disease. *Convulsive Therapy, 13*(4), 274–277.

Abrams R. (1997). *Electroconvulsive Therapy.* Oxford, England: Oxford University Press.

Abrams R. (1997b). The Mortality Rate with ECT. *Convulsive Therapy, 13*(3), 125–127.

Americanercian Psychiatric Association. (1990). *The practice of electroconvulsive therapy: recommendations for treatment, training, and privileging.* Washington, DC: APA Press.

Applegate, R. J. (1997). Diagnosis and Management of Ischemic Heart Disease in the Patient Scheduled to Undergo Electroconvulsive Therapy. *Convulsive Therapy, 13*(3), 128–144.

Avramov, M. N., Husain, M. M., & White, P. F. (1995). The Comparative Effects of Methohexital, Propofol, and Etomidate for Electroconvulsive Therapy. *Anesth Analg 81:* 596–602.

Beale, M. D., Pritchett, J. T., & Kellner, C. H. (1994). Supraventricular Tachycardia in a Patient Receiving ECT, Clozapine, and Caffeine. *Convulsive Therapy, 10*(3), 228–231.

Bean, G., Nishisato, S., Rector, N. A., & Glancy, G. (March 1996). The Assessment of Competence to Make a Treatment Decision: and Empirical Approach. *Canadian Journal of Psychiatry, 41*(2), 85–92.

Bergsholm, P., & Swartz, C. M. (1996). Anesthesia in Electroconvulsive Therapy and Alternatives to Barbiturates. *Psychiatric Annals, 26*(11), 709–712.

Burd, J., & Kettl, P. (1998). Incidence of Asystole in Electroconvulsive Therapy in Elderly Patients. *The Americanerican Journal of Geriatric Psychiatry, 6*(3), 203–211.

Calev, A., Phil, D., Fink, M., Petrides, G., Francis, A., Fochtmann, & L. Caffeine (1993). Pretreatment Enhances Clinical Efficacy and Reduces Cognitive Effects of Electroconvulsive Therapy. *Convulsive Therapy, 9*(2), 95–100.

Coffey, C. E. (1996). Brain Morphology in Primary Mood Disorders: Implications for Electroconvulsive Therapy. *Psychiatric Annals, 26*(11), 713–716.

Coffey, C. E., Figiel, G. S., Djang, W. T., Cress M., Saunders, W. B., & Weiner, R. D. (1988) Leukoencephalopathy in Elderly Depressed Patients Referred for ECT. *Biological Psychiatry 24, 143–161.*

Devanand D. P., Dwork A. J., Hutchinson, E. R., Bolwig, T. G., & Sackeim, H. A. (1994). *Does ECT Alter Brain Structure?* American Journal of Psychiatry, 151(7), 957–970.

Dowling, F. G., & Francis, A. (1993). Aortic Aneurysm and Electroconvulsive Therapy. *ConvulsiveTherapy 9*(2), 121–127.

Endler, N. S. (1988). The Origins of Electroconvulsive Therapy. *Convulsive Therapy, 4*(1), 5–23.

Farah A., McCall, W. V., & Americanundson R. H. (1996). ECT After Cerebral Aneurysm Repair. *Convulsive Therapy, 12*(3), 165–170.

Figiel, G. S., Coffey, C. E., Djang, W. T., Hoffman, G., & Doraiswamy, P. M. (1990). Brain magnetic resonance imaging findings in ECT-induced delirium. *Journal of Neurpsychiatry Clinical Neurosci 2, 53–58.*

Figiel, G. S., Epstein, C., McDonald, W. M., Americanazon-Leece, J., Figiel, L., Saldivia, A., & Glover, S. (1988). *The Use of Rapid-Rate Transcranial Magnetic Stimulation (rTMS) in Refractory Depressed Patients.* The Journal of Neuropsychiatry and Clinical Neurosciences 10: 20–25.

Fink, M. (1993). Post-ECT Delirium. *Convulsive Therapy 9(4):* 326–330.

Fink, M., Abrams, R., Bailine, S., & Jaffe, R. (1996). Americanbulatory Electroconvulsive Therapy: Report of a Task Force of the Association for Convulsive Therapy. *Convulsive Therapy, 12*(1), 42–55.

Fredman, B., d'Etienne, J., Smith, I., Husain, M. M., & White, P. F. (1994). Anesthesia for Electroconvulsive Therapy: Effects of Propofol and Methohexital on Seizure Activity and Recovery. *Anesth Analg, 79:* 75–79.

Grunhaus, L., Shipley, J. E., Eiser, A., Pande, A. C., Tandon, R., Remen, A., & Greden, J. F. (1994). Shortened REM Latency Post-ECT is Associated with Rapid Recurrence Of Depressive Symptomatology. *Biological Psychiatry, 36:* 214–222.

Grunhaus, L., Shipley, J. E., Eiser, A., Pande, A. C., Tandon, R., Remen, A., & Greden, J. F. (1997). Polysomnographic Studies in Patients Referred for ECT: Pre-ECT Studies. *Convulsive Therapy, 12*(4), 224–231.

Hermann, R. C., Dorwart, R. A., Hoover, C. W., & Brody, J. (1995). Variation in ECT Use in the United States. *American Journal of Psychiatry 152:6,* 869–875.

Jaffe, R., Dubin, W., Shoyer, B., Roemer, R., Sharon, D., & Lipschutz, L. (1990). OutpatientElectroconvulsive Therapy: Efficacy and Safety. *Convulsive Therapy, 6*(3), 231–238.

Janis, K., Hess, J., Fabian, J. A., & Gillis, M. (1995). Substitution of Mivacurium for Succinylcholine for ECT in Elderly Patients. *Canadian Journal of Anaesthiology, 42*(7), 612–613.

Kellner, C. H., Monroe, R. R., Pritchett, J., Jarrell, M. P., Bernstein, H. J., & Burns, C. M. (1992). Weekly ECT in Geriatric Depression. *Convulsive Therapy, 8*(4), 245–252.

Kelsey, M. C., & Grossberg, G. T. (1995). Safety and Efficacy of Caffeine-Augmented ECT in Elderly Depressives: A Retrospective Study. *Journal of Geriatric Psychiatry And Neurology, 8:* 168–172.

Kirkcaldie, M., Pridmore, S., & Reid, P. (1997). Bridging the Skull: Electroconvulsive Therapy (ECT) and Repetive Transcranial Magnetic Stimulation (rTMS) in Psychiatry. *Convulsive Therapy, 13*(2), 83–91.

Kramer, B. A. (1987). Maintenance ECT: A Survey of Practice (1986). *Convulsive Therapy, 3*(4), 260–268.

Kramer, B. A. (1993). Anticholinergics and ECT. *Convulsive Therapy 9*(4), 293–300.

Letemendia, F. J. J., Delva, N. J., Rodenburg, M., Lawson, J. S., Inglis, J., Waldron, J. J., & Lywood, D. W. (1993). Therapeutic advantage of bifrontal electrode placement in ECT. *Psychological Medicine, 23:*349–360.

Levine, S. B., Blank, K., Schwartz, H. I., & Rait, D. S. (1991). Informed Consent in the Electroconvulsive Treatment of Geriatric Patients. *Bulletin of the Americanerican Academy of Psychiatry and the Law:19*(4), 395–403.

Manly, D. T., & Swartz, C. M. (1994). Asymmetric Bilateral Right Frontotemporal Left Frontal Stimulus Electrode Placement: Comparisons with Bifrontotemporal and Unilateral Placements. *Convulsive Therapy, 10*(4), 267–270.

McCall, W. V., Reid, S., Rosenquist, P., Foreman, A., Kiesow-& Webb, N. (1993). A Reappraisal of the Role of Caffeine in ECT. *American Journal of Psychiatry, 150*(10), 1543–1545.

McCall, W. V., Zvara, D., Brooker, R., & Arias, L. (1997). Effect of Esmolol Pretreatment on EEG Seizure Morphology in RUL ECT. *Convulsive Therapy, 13*(3), 175–180.

McDonald, W. M., Phillips, V. L., Figiel, G. S., Marsteller, F. A., Simpson, C. D., & Bailey, M. C. Cost-Effective Maintenance Treatment of Resistant Geriatric Depression. *Psychiatric Annals, 28*(1), 47–52. (1998).

Messina, A. G., Paranicas, M., Katz, B., Markowitz, J., Yao, F -S., & Devereux, R. B. (1992). Effect of electroconvulsive therapy on the electrocardiogram and echcardiogram. *Anesth Analgesia 75, 511–514.*

Milstein, V., Milstein, M. J., & Small, I. (1995). *Radigraphic Screening for ECT: Use and Usefulness.* Convulsive Therapy, 11(1), 38–44.

Nelson, J. P., & Benjamin, L. (1989). Efficacy and Safety of Combined ECT and Tricyclic Antidepressant Drugs in the Treatment of Depressed Geriatric Patients. *Convulsive Therapy, 5*(4), 321–329.

Olfson, M., Marcus, S., Sackeim, H. A., Thompson, J., & Pincus, H. A. (1998). Use of ECT for the Inpatient Treatment of Recurrent Major Depression. *American Journal of Psychiatry 155:1,* 22–29.

Petrides, G., Dhossche, D., Fink, M., & Francis, A. (1994). Continuation ECT: Relapse Prevention In Affective Disorders. *Convulsive Therapy, 10*(3), 189–194.

Petrides, G., & Fink, M. (1996). Atrial fibrillation., anticoagulation, and electroconvulsive therapy. *Convulsive Therapy, 12*(2), 91–98.

Philibert, R. A., Richards, L., Lynch, C. F., & Winokur, G. (1995). Effect of ECT on Mortality and Clinical Outcome in Geriatric Unipolar Depression. *Journal of Clinical Psychiatry, 56*(9), 390–394.

Prudic, J., Haskett R. F., Mulsant, B., Malone, K. M., Pettinati, H. M., Stephens, S., Greenberg, R., Rifas, S. L., & Sackeim, H. A. (1996). Resistance to Antidepressant Medications And Short-Term Clinical Response to ECT. *American Journal of Psychiatry, 153*(8), 985–992.

Prudic, J., Sackeim, H. A., Devanand D. P., Krueger, R. B., & Settembrino, J. M. (1994). Acute Cognitive Effects of Subconvulsive Electrical Stimulation. *Convulsive Therapy 10*(1), 4–24.

Prudic, J., Sackeim H. A., & Spicknall, K. (1998). Potential Pharmacologic Agents for the Cognitive Effects of Electroconvulsive Treatment. *Psychiatric Annals, 28*(1), 40–46.

Rasmussen, K. G. (1997). Electroconvulsive Therapy in Patients with Aortic Stenosis. *Convulsive Therapy, 13*(3), 196–199.

Reid, W. H., Keller, S., Leatherman, M., & Mason, M. (1998). ECT in Texas: 19 Months of Mandatory Reporting. *Journal of Clinical Psychiatry, 59*(1), 8–13.

Rice, E. H., Sombrotto, L. B., Markowitz, J. C., & Leon, A. C. (1994). Cardiovascular Morbidity in High-Risk Patients During ECT. *American Journal of Psychiatry, 151Z*(11), 1637–1641.

Riesenman, J. P., & Scanlan, M. R. (1995). ECT 2 Weeks Post Coronary Artery Bypass Graft Surgery. *Convulsive Therapy, 11*(4), 262–265.

Rosenbach, M. L., Hermann, R. C., & Dorwart, R. A. (1997). Use of Electroconvulsive Therapy in the Medicare Poulation Between 1987 and 1992. *Psychiatric Services, 49,*(12), 1537–1542.

Rubin, E. H., Kinscherf, D. A., Figiel, G. S., & Zorumski, C. F. (1993). The Nature and Time Course of Cognitive Side Effects During Electroconvulsive Therapy in the Elderly. *Journal Of Geriatric Psychiatry and Neurology, 6:* 78–83.

Sackeim, H. A., Prudic, J., Devanand, D. P., Kiersky, J. E., Fitzsimmons, L., Moody, B. J., McElhiney, M. C., Coleman, E. A., & Settembrino, J. M. (1993). Effects of Stimulus Intensity And Electrode Placement on the Efficacy and Cognitive Effects of Electroconvulsive Therapy. *The New England Journal of Medicine, 328*(12), 839–846.

Sobin, C., Prudic, J., Devanand, D. P., Nobler, M. S., & Sackeim, H. A. (1996). Who Responds to Electroconvulsive Therapy? A Comparison of Effective and Ineffective Forms of Treatment. *British Journal of Psychiatry, 169:* 322–328.

Sobin, C., Sackeim, H. A., Prudicm J., Devanand, D. P., Moody, B. J., & McElhiney, M. C. (1995). Predictors of Retrograde Americannesia Following ECT. *American Journal of Psychiatry, 152*(7), 995–1001.

Sommer, B. R, Satlin, A., Friedman, L., & Cole, J. O. (1989). Glycopyrrolate Versus Atropine in Post-ECT Americannesia in the Elderly. *Journal of Geriatric Psychiatry and Neurology, 2,* 18–21.

Steif, B. L., Sackeim, H. A., Portnoy, S., Decina, P., & Malitz, S. (1986). Effects of Depression and ECT on Anterograde Memory. *Biological Psychiatry, 21:*921–930.

Sullivan, M. D., Ward, N. G., & Laxton, A. (1992). The Woman Who Wanted Electronconvulsive Therapy and Do-Not-Resuscitate Status. Questions of Competence on a Medical-Psychiatry Unit. *General Hospital Psychiatry, 14*(3), 204–209.

Swartz, C. M., & Evans, C. M. (1996). Beyond Bitemporal and Right Unilateral Electrode Placements. *Psychiatric Annals, 26*(11), 705–708.

Thompson, J. W., Weiner, R. D, & Myers, C. P. (1994). Use of ECT in the United States in 1975, 1980, and 1986. *American Journal of Psychiatry 151,*(11), 1657–1661.

Thornton, J. E., Mulsant, B. H., Dealy, R., & Reynolds, C. F. (1990). A Retrospective Study of Maintenance Electroconvulsive Therapy in a University-Based Psychiatric Practice. *Convulsive Therapy, 6*(2), 121–129.

Trzepacz, P. T., Weniger, F. C., & Greenhouse, J. (1993). Etomidate Anesthesia Increases Seizure Duration During ECT. *General Hospital Psychiatry, 15* 115–120.

Vanelle, J -M., Loo, H., Galinowski, A., de Carvalho, W., Bourdel, M -C., Brochier, P., Bouvet, O., Brochier, T., & Olie, J -P. (1994). Maintenance ECT in Intractable Manic- Depressive Disorders. *ConvulsiveTherapy, 10*(3), 195–205.

Westphal, J. R., Horswell, R., Kumar, S., & Rush, J. (1997). Quantifying Utilization and Practice Variation of Electroconvulsive Therapy. *Convulsive Therapy, 13*(4), 242–252.

Westreich, L, . Levine, S., Ginsberg, P., & Wilets, I. (1995). Patient Knowledge About Electroconvulsive Therapy: Effect of an Informational Video. *Convulsive Therapy, 11*(1), 32–37.

Zervas, I. M, Calev, A., Phil, D., Jandorf, L., Schwartz, J., Gaudino, E., Tubi, N., Lerer, B., & Shapira, B. (1993). Age-Dependent Effects of Electroconvulsive Therapy on Memory. *Convulsive Therapy, 9*(1), 39–42.

Zielinski, R. J., Roose, S. P., Devanand, D. P., Woodring, S., & Sackeim, H. A. (1993). Cardiovascular Complications of ECT in Depressed Patients With Cardiovascular Disease. *American Journal of Psychiatry, 150*(6), 904–909.

Zvara, D. A,, Brooker, R. F, McCall, W. V., Foreman, A. S., Hewitt, C., Murphy, B. A., & Royster, R. L. (1997). The Effect of Esmolol on ST-Segment Depression and Arrhythmias After Electroconvulsive Therapy. *Convulsive Therapy, 13*(3), 165–174.

Index

Springer Publishing Company

The Many Dimensions of Aging

Robert L. Rubinstein, PhD,**Miriam Moss,** PhD, and **Morton Kleban,** PhD, Editors

Dedicated to M.Powell Lawton and his continuing work in the field of gerontology, this book contains a selection of essays by persons who have worked with him or with his ideas over the last few decades. Each contributor addresses some aspect of Dr. Lawton's contribution to the field and develops it into an essay. Authored by the most prestigious researchers in the field, the chapters address the latest research findings and their implications in the elderly. Topics include: the environment and aging; health and quality of life issues; emotions and the aged; issues of caregiving; and practice and policy outcomes.

This volume provides a broad overview of advances in the field for graduate students, researchers, and professionals.

Contents: Preface• Introduction • I:Theory and Practice of Place• II: The Ecological Theory of Aging• III: Adjusting "Person-Environment Systems"• IV: Time and Function •V: Assessing Quality of Care Among Chronic Care Populations •VI: Family and Nursing Home Staff's Perceptions of Quality of Life Dementia •VII: Style Versus Substance •VIII: The Assessment and Integration of Preferences into Care Practices for Persons with Dementia Residing in Nursing Homes •IX: Opportunities for Defining Late Life Depression ab initio• X: A Stage Theory Model of Adult Cognitive Development Revisited • XI: Caregiving Research • XII: Appraisals of Dependence Versus Independence Among Care Receiving Elderly Women • XIII: If You Want to Understand Something, Try to Change It• XIV: Community Planning and the Elderly XV: Research as a Resource for Planning •XVI: Outcomes for Research in Mental Disorders of Late Life

1999 256pp. 0-8261-1247-1 ww.springerpub.com

536 Broadway, New York, NY 10012-3955 • (212) 431-4370 • Fax (212) 941-7842

Springer Publishing Company

Neurogerontology
Aging and the Nervous System
James F. Willott, PhD

Neurogerontology examines how the aging brain affects all aspects of cognition and physical performance. It comprehensively links the principles of neuroscience with gerontology and psychology. Written largely from a behavioral neuroscience perspective, *Neurogerontology* explores the functional relationships between the central nervous system and the psychological phenomenon of aging, including perception, arousal, learning, cognition, and motor behavior. Willott emphasizes healthy aging, but dementia and other pathological conditions are discussed.

The evidence-based approach to the neuroscience of aging makes this a valuable reference for professionals, as well as an informative textbook for students in gerontology courses.

Contents: Introduction • The research methods of neurogerontology • Some basics of neuroanatomy and neurobiology and their neurogerontological implications • Principles of neural communication and their neurogerontological implications • Information processing by the nervous system • Regulation of vital functions • Obtaining information with the sensory systems • The storage of information: learning and memory • Movement and the production of behavior • Modulation of the nervous systems: emotion, arousal, and circadian rhythms • Cognitive integration and disintegration (dementia) • Sex and reproduction • Modification of age-related changes in the brain, behavior, and cognition

1999 384pp. 0-8261-1259-5 www.springerpub.com

536 Broadway, New York, NY 10012-3955 • (212) 431-4370 • Fax (212) 941-7842